Lecture Notes of the Institute
for Computer Sciences, Social Informatics
and Telecommunications Engineering 192

More information about this series at http://www.springer.com/series/8197

Paolo Perego · Giuseppe Andreoni
Giovanna Rizzo (Eds.)

Wireless Mobile Communication and Healthcare

6th International Conference, MobiHealth 2016
Milan, Italy, November 14–16, 2016
Proceedings

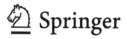 Springer

Editors
Paolo Perego
Politecnico di Milano
Design Department
Milan
Italy

Giovanna Rizzo
CNR - Istituto di Bioimmagini e Fisiologia
   Molecolare
Segrate, MI
Italy

Giuseppe Andreoni
Politecnico di Milano
Design Department
Milan
Italy

ISSN 1867-8211   ISSN 1867-822X   (electronic)
Lecture Notes of the Institute for Computer Sciences, Social Informatics
and Telecommunications Engineering
ISBN 978-3-319-58876-6   ISBN 978-3-319-58877-3   (eBook)
DOI 10.1007/978-3-319-58877-3

Library of Congress Control Number: 2017941501

Printed on acid-free paper

This Springer imprint is published by Springer Nature
The registered company is Springer International Publishing AG
The registered company address is: Gewerbestrasse 11, 6330 Cham, Switzerland

Preface

We are experiencing an era of profound transformation in which mobile ubiquitous connection makes it possible to have real innovation in health care and well-being services.

The market availability of wearable devices that are deeply integrated in everyday objects like watches and garments also enhances the possibility to have a continuous monitoring of parameters and functions. A huge amount of data are generated and new challenges emerge from their efficient management and processing.

This is the worldwide technological scenario of the so-called wearable decade, in which various tiny pieces of high technology become part of us, as computers and mobile phones did in the 2000s.

We operate in this infinitely mutable and extraordinarily fast scenario, with the aim to design innovations and new perspectives without forgetting the human dimension, which is the key and driving factor. For many years, technology has been the hub of innovation and development, forgetting that systems and devices are developed for humans, who should indeed be the center of the entire process. We believe that starting from the human dimension, taking a cue from disciplines such as ergonomics and design, can help researchers to develop and implement real tools fitting into everyday objects and life, which in the middle/long term means health.

In this edition of the 6th EAI International Conference on Wireless Mobile Communication and Health Care – MobiHealth 2016, held in Milan, Italy, November 14–16, 2016 – we tried to integrate this multidisciplinary approach and vision in order to bring together for the first time engineers with designers and other non-engineering professionals to create a heterogeneous community that can give life to a new way of innovation.

The conference was communicated through the standard Web channels in particular reaching out to the participants of previous editions with a call for papers, and sending a dedicated invitation to recognized experts in m-health and related topics.

We received 57 papers, about 70% from the first traditional channel and about 30% from selected invitations. Each paper was reviewed by at least two independent experts identified among the Organizing Committee and the EAI experts selected by keywords. Only papers that were positively assessed by both reviewers were accepted. Specific comments were made and sent to the authors to improve the final submission.

Moreover, in keeping with the scope of the conference, at MobiHealth 2016 three distinguished experts presented talks on mobile and pervasive health innovations:

- Giuseppe De Pietro – "Mobile Health Care and Electronic Health Records" – presented the frame of "smart" m-health applications for the personal citizen agenda (PCA) in Italy.
- Enrico Profumo – "How To Make It Happen: Which Are the Driving Forces Shaping Health Care" – analyzed the digitalization in health systems and the problem related to security.

– Maria Renata Guarneri – "Multidimensional ICT System for Motivating Behavioral Changes Toward Healthier Lifestyles for Overweight and Obesity Prevention" – presented the experience of the EU-funded PEGASO F4F project, which uses mobile apps, wearable devices, and videogames to encourage teenagers to adopt a healthy lifestyle.

The papers and related presentations were divided into ten sessions:

1. Technological development for m-health applications
2. Promotion of healthy lifestyle
3. Devices for m-health
4. Smart applications for clinical care
5. IOT for m-health
6. Mobile applications for health
7. Design approach for m-health solutions
8. Feel the fall
9. Machine learning in mH_applications
10. Systems and apps for movement analysis

The conference also included a special session on "Advances in Soft Wearable Technology for Mobile Health" and three workshops:

1. Advances in Personalized Health-Care Services, Wearable Mobile Monitoring, and Social Media Pervasive Technologies
2. Emerging Experiences into Receiving and Delivering Health Care Through Mobile and Embedded Solutions
3. e-Health: The 21st Century Games Revolution

The conference ended with a final round table bringing together the scientific representatives of high-level research projects (all EU-funded projects in the e-health field) to share experiences and lay out future directions.

We are grateful to Politecnico di Milano (especially to the design department) and to the European Alliance for Innovation for sponsoring and co-organizing this event. Furthermore, generous support for the conference was provided by Istituto di Bioimmagini e Fisiologia Molecolare - CNR.

Finally, we would like to thank all the participants for their hard work in preparing the manuscripts and the presentations. The papers included in these proceedings are the final result of a great amount of creative work and a highly selective review process. We hope that they will serve as a valuable source of information on the state of the art of mobile health and technology.

April 2017

Paolo Perego
Giuseppe Andreoni
Giovanna Rizzo

Organization

Steering Committee Chair

Imrich Chlamtac   University of Trento, Create-Net, Italy

Steering Committee Members

James C. Lin (Founding Chair)	University of Illinois at Chicago, USA
Dimitrios Koutsouris	National Technical University of Athens, Greece
Janet Lin	University of Illinois at Chicago, USA
Arye Nehorai	Washington University in St. Louis, USA
Konstantina S. Nikita	National Technical University of Athens, Greece
George Papadopoulos	University of Cyprus, Cyprus
Oscar Mayora	Create-Net, Italy

Founding Chairs

James C. Lin	University of Illinois at Chicago, USA
Konstantina S. Nikita	National Technical University of Athens, Greece

General Chairs and Co-chairs

Giuseppe Andreoni	Politecnico di Milano, Italy
Giovanna Rizzo	CNR, Italy
Roberto Sassi	UNIMI, Italy
Cees Lanting	CSEM, Switzerland

Technical Program Chairs

Paolo Perego	Politecnico di Milano, Italy
Renata Guarneri	Politecnico di Milano, Italy

Workshops Chair

Cristina de Capitani   CNR Istituto dei Polimeri, Compositi e Biomateriali Lombardy Cluster Technologies for Living Environments (TECHforLIFE), Italy

Publications Chairs

Giuseppe Andreoni	Politecnico di Milano, Italy
Paolo Perego	Politecnico di Milano, Italy

Publicity and Social Media Chairs

Alessandra Mazzola	Politecnico di Milano, Italy
Lia Tagliavini	Politecnico di Milano, Italy

Panels and Keynotes Committee Chair

Giuseppe Andreoni	Politecnico di Milano, Italy

Sponsorship and Exhibits Chairs

Cristina de Capitani	CNR Istituto dei Polimeri, Compositi e Biomateriali Lombardy Cluster Technologies for Living Environments (TECHforLIFE), Italy
Domenico Pannofino	Polihub, Italy

Demos Chair

Paolo Perego	Politecnico di Milano, Italy

Posters and PhD Track Chair

Carlo Emilio Standoli	Politecnico di Milano, Italy

Local Chairs

Alessandra Mazzola	Politecnico di Milano, Italy
Lia Tagliavini	Politecnico di Milano, Italy

Web Chairs

Carlo Emilio Standoli	Politecnico di Milano, Italy
Roberto Sironi	Politecnico di Milano, Italy

Technical Program Committee

Qammer H. Abbasi	Texas A&M University at Qatar
Yasir Alfadhl	Queen Mary University of London, UK
Akram Alomainy	Queen Mary University of London, UK
Ioannis Andreadis	National Technical University of Athens, Greece
Giuseppe Andreoni	Politecnico di Milano, Italy

Emmanouil Spanakis	Computational Medicine Laboratory (CML), Institute of Computer Science
Alessandro Tognetti	Research Center E. Piaggio, University of Pisa, Italy
Manolis Tsiknakis	Computational Medicine Laboratory (CML), Institute of Computer Science
Mark van Gils	VTT Technical Research Centre of Finland
Dimitrios Vergados	University of Piraeus, Greece
Lei Wang	SIAT, Chinese Academy of Sciences, China
Jianqing Wang	Nagoya Institute of Technology, Japan
Ouri Wolfson	University of Illinois, USA
Ken-ichi Yamakoshi	Kanazawa University, Japan
Geng Yang	Royal Institute of Technology (KTH), Sweden
Konstantia Zarkogianni	National Technical University of Athens, Greece
Maxim Zhadobov	Institute of Electronics and Telecommunications of Rennes (IETR), France
Lei Zhao	Jiangsu Normal University, China

Contents

Technological Development for m-Health Application

Self-Powered Implantable Electromagnetic Device for Cardiovascular
System Monitoring Through Arterial Wall Deformation 3
    Grigorios Marios Karageorgos, Christos Manopoulos,
    Sokrates Tsangaris, and Konstantina Nikita

A Custom Base Station for Collecting and Processing Data
of Research-Grade Motion Sensor Units 11
    Kamen Ivanov, Zhanyong Mei, Huihui Li, Wenjing Du, and Lei Wang

Energy-Efficient IoT-Enabled Fall Detection System
with Messenger-Based Notification 19
    Igor Tcarenko, Tuan Nguyen Gia, Amir M. Rahmani,
    Tomi Westerlund, Pasi Liljeberg, and Hannu Tenhunen

Promotion for Healthy Lifestyle

A Mobile Adviser of Healthy Eating by Reading Ingredient Labels 29
    Man Wai Wong, Qing Ye, Yuk Kai Chan Kylar, Wai-Man Pang,
    and Kin Chung Kwan

Investigating How to Measure Mobile User Engagement 38
    Stefano Carrino, Maurizio Caon, Omar Abou Khaled,
    and Elena Mugellini

Personalised Guidance Services for Optimising Lifestyle in Teen-Agers
Through Awareness, Motivation and Engagement – PEGASO:
A Pilot Study Protocol 45
    Fulvio Adorni, Federica Prinelli, Chiara Crespi, Elisa Puigdomènech,
    Santiago Felipe Gomez, Espallargues Carreras Mireia,
    Castell Abat Conxa, Brian McKinstry, Anne Martin,
    Lucy McCloughan, Alexandra Lang, Laura Condon,
    Sarah Atkinson, Rajeeb Rashid,
    and On Behalf of the PEGASO Consortium

PEGASO Companion: A Mobile App to Promote Healthy Lifestyles
Among Adolescents 53
    Maurizio Caon, Stefano Carrino, Laura Condon, Antonio Ascolese,
    Sara Facchinetti, Marco Mazzola, Paolo Perego, Filip Velickovski,
    Giuseppe Andreoni, and Elena Mugellini

Device for m-Health

SmartMATES for Medication Adherence Using Non-intrusive
Wearable Sensors   65
  A.H. Abdullah and T.H. Lim

Paradigm-Shifting Players for IoT: Smart-Watches for Intensive
Care Monitoring   71
  Francesca Stradolini, Eleonora Lavalle, Giovanni De Micheli,
  Paolo Motto Ros, Danilo Demarchi, and Sandro Carrara

Toward an Open-Source Flexible System for Mobile Health Monitoring   79
  Mathieu Bagot, Pascale Launay, and Frédéric Guidec

Smart Applications for Clinical Care

A System for Hypertension Management Assistance Based
on the Technologies of the Smart Spaces   85
  Alexander Borodin, Tatyana Kuznetsova, and Elena Andreeva

Enhancing the Early Warning Score System Using Data Confidence   91
  Maximilian Götzinger, Nima Taherinejad, Amir M. Rahmani,
  Pasi Liljeberg, Axel Jantsch, and Hannu Tenhunen

Application of Wearable Monitoring System in Tourette
Syndrome Assessment   100
  Sofia Scataglini, Marcello Fusca, Giuseppe Andreoni, and Mauro Porta

Assessment of Physiological Signals During Happiness, Sadness,
Pain or Anger   107
  Nima TaheriNejad and David Pollreisz

Customising the Cold Challenge: Pilot Study of an Altered Raynaud's
Phenomena Assessment Method for Data Generation   115
  Isobel Taylor

IOT - Internet of Things

A Context-Aware, Capability-Based, Role-Centric Access Control Model
for IoMT   125
  Flora Malamateniou, Marinos Themistocleous, Andriana Prentza,
  Despina Papakonstantinou, and George Vassilacopoulos

Modular IoT Platform for AAL and Home Care Using Bluetooth
Low Energy   132
  Johannes Kropf, Samat Kadyrov, and Lukas Roedl

Non-conventional Use of Smartphones: Remote Monitoring Powered
Wheelchairs in MARINER Project 138
    Paolo Meriggi, Ivana Olivieri, Cristina Fedeli, Diana Scurati,
    Giovanni Ludovico Montagnani, Elena Brazzoli, Marina Rodocanachi,
    and Lucia Angelini

Intelligent Automated EEG Artifacts Handling Using Wavelet Transform,
Independent Component Analysis and Hierarchal Clustering. 144
    Shaibal Barua, Shahina Begum, and Mobyen Uddin Ahmed

Mobile Application for Health

Crowdsourced Data Collection of Physical Activity and Health Status:
An App Solution. 151
    Daniel Kelly, Brian Caulfield, and Kevin Curran

Skinhealth, A Mobile Application for Supporting Teledermatology:
A Case Study in a Rural Area in Colombia 160
    Juan Pablo Sáenz, Mónica Paola Novoa, Darío Correal,
    and Bell Raj Eapen

Smartphone-Based Detection of Location Changes Using WiFi Data 164
    Anja Exler, Matthias Urschel, Andrea Schankin, and Michael Beigl

Adaptive Motif-Based Alerts for Mobile Health Monitoring 168
    Ekanath Rangan and Rahul Krishnan Pathinarupothi

A Portable Real Time ECG Device for Arrhythmia Detection
Using Raspberry Pi 177
    C.A. Valliappan, Advait Balaji, Sai Ruthvik Thandayam,
    Piyush Dhingra, and Veeky Baths

Design Approach for mHealth Solutions

A Didactic Experience in Designing Smart Systems for mHealth Services . . . 187
    Carlo Emilio Standoli, Maria Renata Guarneri, Marinella Ferrara,
    and Giuseppe Andreoni

DIABESITY: A Study for mHealth Integrated Solutions 195
    Italo Zoppis, Giancarlo Mauri, Ferancesco Sicurello, Eugenio Santoro,
    Giada Pietrabissa, and Gianluca Castelnuovo

A Reference Framework of mHealth Patents for Innovative Services 200
    Massimo Barbieri and Giuseppe Andreoni

Monitoring Patients in Ambulatory Palliative Care:
A Design for an Observational Study   207
    Vanessa C. Klaas, Alberto Calatroni, Michael Hardegger,
    Matthias Guckenberger, Gudrun Theile, and Gerhard Tröster

System for Fall Detection and Prediction

Fall Detection Using a Head-Worn Barometer   217
    Guglielmo Cola, Marco Avvenuti, Pierpaolo Piazza,
    and Alessio Vecchio

Investigation of Sensor Placement for Accurate Fall Detection   225
    Periklis Ntanasis, Evangelia Pippa, Ahmet Turan Özdemir,
    Billur Barshan, and Vasileios Megalooikonomou

Fall Detection with Orientation Calibration Using a Single Motion Sensor . . .   233
    Shuo Yu and Hsinchun Chen

A Neural Network Model Based on Co-occurrence Matrix
for Fall Prediction   241
    Masoud Hemmatpour, Renato Ferrero, Bartolomeo Montrucchio,
    and Maurizio Rebaudengo

Machine Learning in mHealth Applications

Using Smartwatch Sensors to Support the Acquisition of Sleep Quality
Data for Supervised Machine Learning   251
    Cinzia Bernardeschi, Mario G.C.A. Cimino, Andrea Domenici,
    and Gigliola Vaglini

Multilayer Radial Basis Function Kernel Machine   260
    Mashail Alsalamah and Saad Amin

Improving the Probability of Clinical Diagnosis of Coronary-Artery
Disease Using Extended Kalman Filters with Radial Basis
Function Network   269
    Mashail Alsalamah and Saad Amin

A Hypothetical Reasoning System for Mobile Health
and Wellness Applications   278
    Aniello Minutolo, Massimo Esposito, and Giuseppe De Pietro

Systems and Apps for Movement Analysis and Detection

Accuracy of the Microsoft Kinect System in the Identification
of the Body Posture 289
    Paolo Abbondanza, Silvio Giancola, Remo Sala, and Marco Tarabini

A Web Based Version of the Cervical Joint Position Error Test:
Reliability of Measurements from Face Tracking Software 297
    Angelo Basteris, Luke Hickey, Ebony Burgess-Gallop, Ashley Pedler,
    and Michele Sterling

Motion Capture: An Evaluation of Kinect V2 Body Tracking
for Upper Limb Motion Analysis 302
    Silvio Giancola, Andrea Corti, Franco Molteni, and Remo Sala

Use of Wearable Inertial Sensor in the Assessment of Timed-Up-and-Go
Test: Influence of Device Placement on Temporal Variable Estimation 310
    Stefano Negrini, Mauro Serpelloni, Cinzia Amici, Massimiliano Gobbo,
    Clara Silvestro, Riccardo Buraschi, Alberto Borboni, Diego Crovato,
    and Nicola Francesco Lopomo

Advances in Soft Wearable Technology for Mobile-Health

Development of a Sustainable and Ergonomic Interface for the EMG
Control of Prosthetic Hands 321
    Emanuele Lindo Secco, Cedric Moutschen, Andualem Tadesse Maereg,
    Mark Barrett-Baxendale, David Reid, and Atulya Kumar Nagar

Synergy-Driven Performance Enhancement of Vision-Based 3D Hand
Pose Reconstruction 328
    Simone Ciotti, Edoardo Battaglia, Iason Oikonomidis, Alexandros
    Makris, Aggeliki Tsoli, Antonio Bicchi, Antonis A. Argyros,
    and Matteo Bianchi

A Quantitative Evaluation of Drive Patterns in Electrical
Impedance Tomography... 337
    Stefania Russo, Nicola Carbonaro, Alessandro Tognetti,
    and Samia Nefti-Meziani

Wearable Augmented Reality Optical See Through Displays Based
on Integral Imaging... 345
    Emanuele Maria Calabrò, Fabrizio Cutolo, Marina Carbone,
    and Vincenzo Ferrari

Emerging Experiences into Receiving and Delivering Healthcare Through Mobile and Embedded Solutions

Interference Between Cognitive and Motor Recovery in Elderly Dementia
Patients Through a Holistic Tele-Rehabilitation Platform   359
   Alberto Antonietti, Marta Gandolla, Mauro Rossini, Franco Molteni,
   Alessandra Pedrocchi, and The ABILITY Consortium

Supporting Physical and Cognitive Training for Preventing the Occurrence
of Dementia Using an Integrated System: A Pilot Study   367
   Mauro Marzorati, Simona Gabriella Di Santo, Simona Mrakic-Sposta,
   Sarah Moretti, Nithiya Jesuthasan, Andrea Caroppo,
   Andrea Zangiacomi, Alessandro Leone, Marco Sacco,
   and Alessandra Vezzoli

A New Personalized Health System: The SMARTA Project.   375
   Massimo W. Rivolta, Paolo Perego, Giuseppe Andreoni,
   Maurizio Ferrarin, Giuseppe Baroni, Corrado Galzio, Giovanna Rizzo,
   Marco Tarabini, Marco Bocciolone, and Roberto Sassi

Advances in Personalized Healthcare Services, Wearable Mobile Monitoring, and Social Media Pervasive Technologies

Identification of Elders' Fall Using the Floor Vibration   383
   Marco Bocciolone, Filip Gocanin, Diego Scaccabarozzi,
   Bortolino Saggin, and Marco Tarabini

The Role of Design as Technology Enabler: A Personalized Integrated
Predictive Diabetes Management System   392
   Venere Ferraro and Venanzio Arquilla

Detecting Elderly Behavior Shift via Smart Devices and Stigmergic
Receptive Fields   398
   Marco Avvenuti, Cinzia Bernardeschi, Mario G.C.A. Cimino,
   Guglielmo Cola, Andrea Domenici, and Gigliola Vaglini

A Pilot Study of a Wearable Navigation Device with Tactile Display
for Elderly with Cognitive Impairment.   406
   Rosalam Che Me, Venere Ferraro, and Alessandro Biamonti

Author Index   415

Technological Development for m-Health Application

Self-Powered Implantable Electromagnetic Device for Cardiovascular System Monitoring Through Arterial Wall Deformation

Grigorios Marios Karageorgos[1], Christos Manopoulos[2],
Sokrates Tsangaris[2], and Konstantina Nikita[1(✉)]

[1] Biomedical Simulations and Imaging Laboratory, and Mobile Radiocommunications Laboratory, School of Electrical and Computer Engineering, National Technical University of Athens, 15780 Athens, Greece
knikita@ece.ntua.gr
[2] Biofluid Mechanics and Biomedical Engineering Laboratory, Fluids Section, School of Mechanical Engineering, National Technical University of Athens, 15780 Athens, Greece

Abstract. In this paper, we present the potential of a device, originally designed for energy harvesting, to form a self-powered medical implant that monitors critical parameters of the cardiovascular system. The original design consists of a coil that deforms with an artery inside magnetic field applied by two permanent magnets. We fabricated the device, and developed appropriate experimental setup that simulates blood flow and arterial wall pulsation with adjustable frequency and pressure. The voltage and power of the moving coil, as well as the pressure inside the tube simulating the pulsating artery were measured at different frequencies. In-vitro experiments and theoretical analysis showed that the voltage induced across the coil's terminals can provide information on blood pressure, heart rate, arterial wall deformation and velocity.

Keywords: Self-powered · Implantable devices · Cardiovascular system · Arterial wall deformation · Blood pressure monitoring · Energy harvesting

1 Introduction

Blood pressure monitoring is of utmost importance for the prognosis and treatment of various diseases. High Blood Pressure (HBP) has no specific symptoms, but it can cause serious damage or even death. Heart attack, aneurism, atherosclerosis, stroke, kidney damage and vision loss can be some of the consequences when HBP is left untreated [1].

Cuff-style monitors are the most common non-invasive commercial devices for blood pressure monitoring, but they usually provide intermittent measurements and their accuracy is lower than that of invasive methods [2, 3]. A cuffless, non-invasive approach to estimate blood pressure is through Pulse Transit Time (PTT), which is defined as the time of propagation of a pulse to travel in artery. However, the correlation between PTT and blood pressure can be affected by viscoactive and other drugs, thus reducing the reliability of the method [4]. Arterial catheterization is an invasive method that offers

© ICST Institute for Computer Sciences, Social Informatics and Telecommunications Engineering 2017
P. Perego et al. (Eds.): MobiHealth 2016, LNICST 192, pp. 3–10, 2017.
DOI: 10.1007/978-3-319-58877-3_1

continuous and accurate measurements, but in some cases it can cause complications such as bleeding, hematoma, nerve damage, arterial thrombosis and infection [5].

Medical implantable devices have become quite popular during the last decades, since they permit continuous and precise measurements of critical physiological parameters. CardioMEM's Champion implantable device is a commercially available pressure monitoring system. An implantable blood pressure monitor that uses MEMS capacitive sensors has been fabricated [6], while an implantable wireless device that provides pressure measurements through a Surface Acoustic Wave (SAW) resonator has also been proposed [7]. Moreover, an implantable sensor that measures blood pressure through PTT by using an accelerometer has also been developed [8].

A major issue associated with implantable devices arises from the limited lifetime of their battery, which imposes the need for the patient to undergo surgery for their replacement. To address this problem, energy harvesting devices have been developed, which exploit energy sources either in the environment or in the human body, in order to recharge or power medical implants. Among these energy sources, the cardiovascular system seems very promising, since the motion of the heart and the arteries is a continuous and periodical source of mechanical energy, which can be converted to electrical energy.

Using an energy harvesting device as a sensor would be quite beneficial to the power efficiency of a medical implantable device. A device that exploits the pulsation of aorta to produce electrical energy through a piezoelectric thin film and functions as blood pressure sensor has been recently constructed [3]. Moreover, a mechanism that harvests energy from arterial wall deformation through a coil that moves in magnetic field has been developed [9]. The purpose of our work is to demonstrate that an energy harvester based on the design proposed in [9], can be used to monitor blood pressure and other cardiovascular parameters.

2 Methods

2.1 Sensor Description

We consider an energy harvesting device which consists of two ring magnets placed in parallel through metallic holders and a flexible coil [9]. Both permanent magnets are magnetized along the artery axis. The coil is placed between the magnets and it is constructed with side loops as depicted in Fig. 1(a). The purpose of the side loops is to make the coil flexible, in order to deform freely without restraining arterial wall movement. The artery comes through the holes of the magnets and the main loop of the coil (Fig. 1(b)). The coil moves inside the magnetic field applied by the magnets, and as a result, an alternating voltage proportional to its velocity is induced.

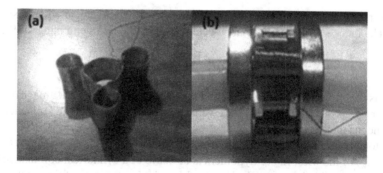

Fig. 1. (a) Flexible coil with side loops which is wound around the artery. (b) Energy harvesting device [9] used in our experiments.

2.2 Theoretical Analysis

A theoretical analysis was developed to support the scenario, according to which the energy harvesting device of Fig. 1 can operate as a pressure sensor. Figure 2 illustrates the ring magnets, the artery, and the coordinates system. The z-axis is parallel to the artery and the arterial wall deforms along the radial r-direction. Moreover, l and s denote the length of the magnets and the spacing between them, respectively, while R_{in}, R_{out} are the inner and outer radius of the ring magnets, R_0 is the artery's undeformed inner radius and d is the arterial wall's thickness.

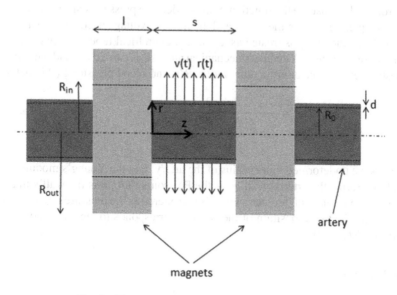

Fig. 2. Ring magnets, artery and coordinates system

The coil moves perpendicularly to z-axis, so only the z-component of the magnetic field contributes to the induced voltage. Assuming a cylindrical coil without side loops, then, the radial position r(t) and velocity v(t) of the coil are identical with those of the artery. The induced voltage V(t) can be determined by the following integral [9]:

$$V(t) = -\int_c v(t) \times B_{z2}(r(t), z)dl \tag{1}$$

where c is the curve defined by the coil and B_z is the z-component of the magnetic field. The latter (B_z) is determined in [9] for given dimensions (R_{in}, R_{out}, l) and remanent field (B_r) of the magnets.

The total resistance (R_c) of the coil depends on the resistivity (ρ_w), length (L_w) and surface (A_w) of the wire. In our hypothetical scenario of a cylindrical coil that deforms radially together with the artery, the length of the wire is a function of time and depends on its radial position r(t) [9]. Thus, the total resistance of the coil is given by:

$$R_c = \rho_w \frac{L_w(t)}{A_w} = \rho_w \frac{\pi N r(t)}{\pi d_w^2/4} \tag{2}$$

where N is the number of windings that form the coil and d_w is the diameter of the wire. The power transfer of the device is maximum when the coil is connected in parallel with a resistance equal to its own resistance and can be expressed as [9]:

$$P_{max}(t) = \frac{(V(t)/2)^2}{R_c(t)} \tag{3}$$

In order to demonstrate the function of the device as a pressure sensor, a relationship between the pressure inside the artery and the induced voltage needs to be determined. In our analysis, the artery is treated as an elastic, cylindrical tube, in which a periodic pressure pulse is applied. A detailed mechanical analysis is carried out and the following relationship between the artery's inner radius R(t) and blood pressure P(t) is obtained:

$$R(t) = \frac{R_0}{1 - \dfrac{(P(t) - P_e)}{Ed}R_0(1 - m^2)} \tag{4}$$

where R_0 is the undeformed inner radius of the artery, E is the Young's modulus of the material that forms the arterial wall, m is the Poisson's ratio, d is the wall's thickness and P_e is the environmental pressure which is considered as the pressure reference point. It is noted that the radial position of the coil r(t) corresponds to the outer radius of the artery (r(t) = R(t) + d).

2.3 Fabrication

Sensor

We used Neodymium ring magnets with inner and outer radius of R_{in} = 7.5 mm and R_{out} = 20.5 mm, respectively, and length l = 10 mm. Both magnets are magnetized along their length and their remanent magnetic field is B_r = 1.2 T. Non- magnetic, stainless steel screws were used as holders to place the magnets in parallel and at constant spacing. The coil was constructed using enamelled copper wire with diameter $d_w = 0.2$ mm. For the above given parameters, an analytical model of the energy harvesting device was developed using Matlab. From our simulations, we determined that the power generation is maximum when the spacing between the magnets is $s = 2$ cm, and selected this value for our in-vitro experiment.

Experimental Setup

In order to test the energy harvesting device, an experimental setup was constructed to simulate the arterial wall pulsation. An elastic tube made of platinum cured silicon rubber with $R_0 = 6$ mm undeformed inner radius, $d = 1$ mm wall thickness and $E = 1.97$ MPa Young's modulus was used to simulate the artery. An open loop was formed by connecting the elastic tube to a rigid tube made of Plexiglas, as depicted in Fig. 3(a). A catheter was then inserted to the latter through a thin hole on its wall, and the loop was filled with water. An Edwards Truwave pressure disposable transducer integrated in a sterile pressure monitoring kit was used to receive pressure measurements inside the open loop through the catheter. The elastic tube was placed inside the energy harvesting device. Both ends of the open loop, the connection between the elastic and rigid tube, as well as

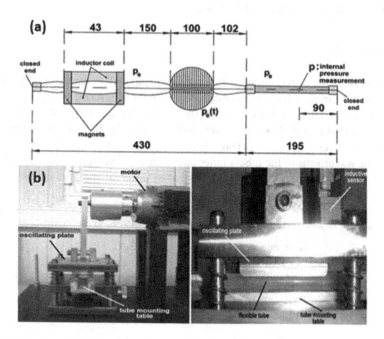

Fig. 3. (a) Representation of the open loop and the experimental set up. The elastic tube comes through the energy harvesting device and is connected to a rigid tube, where a catheter is inserted. A pressure pulse is applied through partial compression and decompression of an elastic tube's segment. (b) Motor-based compression mechanism. The elastic tube is inserted in the tube mounting table and is compressed and decompressed through an oscillating plate with adjustable compression rate. The motor drives the plate with controlled frequency.

the hole where the catheter was placed, were air tightly sealed. Moreover, all the air inside the loop was removed through a valve connected to its one end.

Blood flow and arterial wall deformation were reproduced by applying a periodic pressure pulse inside the tube, through a motor-based compression device, as shown in Fig. 3(b). A 10 mm long segment of the elastic tube was placed in the tube mounting table of the compression device and was periodically partially compressed and decompressed by a reciprocating flat plate. The latter moves due to the motor's rotation and the compression-decompression frequency can be controlled through the velocity of the motor. Special care is taken so that the latter is parallel to the tube axis and as a consequence the compression is applied uniformly along the tube. The device also contains a mechanism so that both the flexible tube mounting table and the reciprocating flat plate can be moved in small steps up and down, adjusting the compression of the elastic tube. The amplitude of the pressure pulse was adjusted in order to achieve a physiological arterial wall deformation, which is typically 10% of the artery diameter [9].

The time waveform of the pressure measured by the Edwards Truwave pressure disposable transducer was obtained by HBM QuantumX MX440A Analog to Digital Converter (ADC). An instrumentation amplifier was used to amplify the voltage induced in the coil and its output was sampled by a microcontroller Arduino Uno. The output power was measured by connecting a resistor of 8.2 Ω to the coil's terminals, which is approximately equal to the coil's resistance.

3   Results

Table 1 shows the peak open circuit voltage of the coil, as well as the mean output power at four different frequencies corresponding to a different heart rate (sleep, rest, tachycardia and exercise). Figure 4 demonstrates the internal pressure P (Fig. 4(a)), the elastic tube's inner radius R (Fig. 4(b)) and wall velocity dR/dt (Fig. 4(c)), as well as the coil's denoised open circuit voltage V_{oc} (Fig. 4(d)) over time, at a rate of 119 bpm (tachycardia). The waveforms of the tube's inner radius and wall velocity were derived from our pressure measurements, by using Eq. (4) and by differentiating the radius.

Table 1. Peak open circuit voltage and mean output power for frequencies corresponding to typical heart rates of a person at the states of sleep, rest, tachycardia and exercise

Heart rate (bpm)	V_{peak} (mV)	P_m (nW)
52.7	2.3	19.1
82.2	2.4	28.1
119	2.5	52.2
139.1	2.7	68.5

From Fig. 4(c) and (d), we can see that the waveforms of tube's wall velocity and the output voltage have similar shape, as expected, given that the induced voltage is proportional to the velocity of the coil, which deforms along with the elastic tube. Given that the velocity of the arterial wall v(t) is the first time derivative of the radius R(t) (v(t) = dR(t)/dt), blood pressure can be derived from the output voltage of our sensor

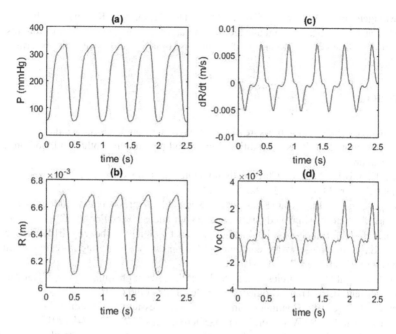

Fig. 4. Time waveforms of (a) internal pressure, (b) elastic tube's radius, (c) elastic tube's wall velocity, (d) open circuit voltage of the deforming coil

and vice versa through Eqs. (1) and (4). We also note that all the quantities presented in Fig. 4 have the same frequency, which in our experiments corresponds to the heart rate. Moreover, the produced power and voltage increases with increasing frequency of the pressure pulse. This can be attributed to the fact that the tube deforms faster at higher rates.

4 Conclusion

In vitro experiments and theoretical analysis indicate that the output voltage of the coil can be used to estimate cardiovascular parameters such as blood pressure, heart rate, arterial wall deformation and velocity. The next steps of our research would be to further study the voltage variation as a function of the desired bio-parameters by running the experiment for different values of pressure and construct a prototype with smaller dimensions for in vivo experimentation. Its biocompatibility is also a matter that needs to be investigated. Furthermore, an appropriate packaging would be necessary to prevent possible interaction with other implantable electromagnetic devices, or electromagnetic interferences from external sources. Though there are several issues that need to be addressed prior to its in vivo application, the presented energy harvesting method has the potential to form an implantable medical device that offers continuous monitoring of the cardiovascular system and simultaneously produces electrical energy to power itself.

Acknowledgements. We would like to thank Dr. Alexandros Karagiannis, Postdoctoral Researcher at Mobile Radiocommunications Laboratory, for his contribution to this research through useful discussions. Moreover, the help of Maria Angelika with the experiments is acknowledged.

References

1. Mayo Clinic, High blood pressure dangers: Hypertension's effects on the body. http://www.mayoclinic.org/diseases-conditions/high-blood-pressure/in-depth/high-blood-pressure/art-20045868
2. Yu, L., Kim, B.J., Meng, E.: Chronically implanted pressure sensors: challenges and state of the field. Sensors **14**(11), 20620–20644 (2014)
3. Cheng, X., et al.: Implantable and self-powered blood pressure monitoring based on a piezoelectric thinfilm: simulated, in vitro and in vivo studies. Nano Energy **22**, 453–460 (2016)
4. Nikita, K.S. (ed.): Handbook of Biomedical Telemetry. Wiley, Hoboken (2014). Chapter 4
5. Chung, E., et al.: Non-invasive continuous blood pressure monitoring: a review of current applications. Front. Med. **7**(1), 91–101 (2013)
6. Chow, E.Y., et al.: Fully wireless implantable cardiovascular pressure monitor integrated with a medical stent. IEEE Trans. Biomed. Eng. **57**(6), 1487–1496 (2010)
7. Murphy, O.H., et al.: Continuous in vivo blood pressure measurements using a fully implantable wireless SAW sensor. Biomed. Microdevices **15**(5), 737–749 (2013)
8. Theodor, M., et al.: Subcutaneous blood pressure monitoring with an implantable optical sensor. Biomed. Microdevices **15**(5), 811–820 (2013)
9. Pfenniger, A., et al.: Design and realization of an energy harvester using pulsating arterial pressure. Med. Eng. Phys. **35**(9), 1256–1265 (2013)

A Custom Base Station for Collecting and Processing Data of Research-Grade Motion Sensor Units

Kamen Ivanov[1,2], Zhanyong Mei[3], Huihui Li[1], Wenjing Du[1], and Lei Wang[1(✉)]

[1] Key Laboratory for Low-Cost Healthcare,
Shenzhen Institutes of Advanced Technology, 1068 Xueyuan Avenue, Shenzhen University Town, Shenzhen 518055, People's Republic of China
{kamen,hh.li,wj.du,wang.lei}@siat.ac.cn
[2] University of Chinese Academy of Sciences, Beijing 100049, People's Republic of China
[3] College of Information Science and Technology, Chengdu University of Technology,
Chengdu 610059, People's Republic of China
zhanyongm99@163.com

Abstract. In studies of human biomechanics utilizing inertial sensors, motion sensor units of type Xsens are recognized as the state-of-the-art. However, the requirement to use them with a personal computer for collecting and processing data could be a limiting factor. In the present work, we demonstrate a simple solution to using up to four Xsens MTx units with a custom portable base station. The base station is capable of obtaining data from Xsens MTx units, processing the data and saving them to an SD card. Thus, it allows the use of the units outside laboratory settings without the need of a personal computer, the capability to directly use onboard custom algorithms to process the data of several units in real time, and interconnectivity with external systems for synchronized collection of multimodal data. We demonstrate these benefits by two examples: synchronized collection of data from an Xsens MTx unit and a Footscan® plantar pressure plate, and knee angle measurement using two Xsens MTx units that we validated by synchronized recording of goniometric data.

Keywords: MTx · Xsens · Base station · Inertial sensors · Footscan

1 Introduction

In recent years, microelectromechanical sensors incorporating a triaxial accelerometer, triaxial gyroscope, and triaxial magnetometer more often take place in studies of human biomechanics. In this context, motion sensor units by Xsens are recognized as the state of the art [1–4]. Such a unit, when attached to a human body segment, provides data that allow describing the motion of that segment with respect to the Earth-fixed coordinate system. When using multiple sensor units attached to different body segments, the relative motion between body parts can be estimated. When using Xsens units, however, a personal computer is needed in close vicinity which could restrict experiments that require overcoming of distances longer than those determined by the short-range connecting links.

© ICST Institute for Computer Sciences, Social Informatics and Telecommunications Engineering 2017
P. Perego et al. (Eds.): MobiHealth 2016, LNICST 192, pp. 11–18, 2017.
DOI: 10.1007/978-3-319-58877-3_2

While many studies on human biomechanics use only a single sensor modality [2–7], advancement of sensor technologies allows for deeper insights by multimodal measurements [8, 9]. In that, precise time synchronization between the different recording devices is desired [9].

In the present work, we demonstrate the implementation of a custom low-cost base station to connect Xsens modules. It allows to capture independently, process and save data of up to four Xsens MTx sensor units and also provides features for synchronization with external systems. We describe the system design and provide two application examples. The first example demonstrates synchronized data collection of inertial data from an Xsens MTx unit and plantar data from a Footscan® plantar pressure plate. The combination of the two systems could aid the study of the movement characteristics by allowing both kinetic and kinematic analysis. The second example demonstrates knee angle measurement using two Xsens MTx units. This scenario shows the accuracy of the Xsens MTx modules when performing short-time human body joint angular measurements.

Since the communication protocol of these sensor units is open to customers, with the present work we in no way aim to replace any proprietary tools, but to confirm the flexibility of Xsens modules by demonstrating new schemes of their application.

2   Methods

2.1   Hardware Implementation of the Custom Base Station

The proposed system consists of a custom control board which supports up to four sensor modules MTx-28A53G25 (by Xsens Motion Technologies, Enschede, the Netherlands) (Fig. 1). Each sensor module contains a 3-axis accelerometer, 3-axis gyroscope, and a 3-axis magnetometer. They are connected to the host system via an RS232 interface and support baud rates of the serial interface of up to 921.6 kbps. The protocol for communication with the modules is provided by the manufacturer [10]. The sensors are capable of providing raw data and processed data. The latter include angular data and the so-called calibrated data. Calibrated data are corrected based on a physical model that reflects the response of the sensors to different external factors. For processed data, the maximum sampling frequency is 256 Hz. The range of the accelerometer is 5 g, and the range of the gyroscope is ± 1200 deg/s. Each module is provided with a synchronization input. The nominal power supply voltage of the sensor unit is 5 V with consumption of 70 mA and maximum starting current of up to 200 mA [10, 11]. The control board is based on the STM32F407 microcontroller. We chose it because it offers up to six serial ports, a reasonable amount of operational memory allowing for large communication buffers, and a hardware unit for floating point arithmetic. The system is equipped with an SD card to store acquired and calculated data. There are synchronizing output and input. Thus, the system can be synchronized with external devices for the goal of multimodal measurements. The microcontroller system requires a power supply of 3.3 V; the sensor unit rated power supply is 5 V; the voltage of four 1.5 V batteries connected in series is about 4.8–6 V and will decrease when discharging. To ensure proper power supply for each subsystem, we used voltage regulators TPS74701 and TPS61252 for the

3.3 V and 5 V power supply, respectively. A translating transceiver 74LVC4245A ensures the level shifting between the microcontroller output and MTx trigger line input, and the synchronization output. A buffer 74LVC14A ensures the level shifting between the output of external 5 V systems and the microcontroller trigger input. By jumpers, it is possible to pass the external synchronization signal directly to the synchronization input of the MTx modules or to synchronize the MTx modules by the microcontroller. The complete system is powered by a 4.8 V battery pack that ensures the operation of the system for at least one hour, depending on the particular application. The dimensions of the board are 100 mm × 120 mm.

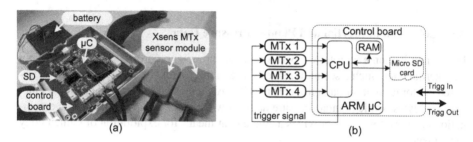

Fig. 1. Illustration of the system: (a) the developed custom board (b) simplified block diagram of the base station.

2.2   Software Implementation of the Custom Base Station

The basic task of the firmware of the control board is to configure the operating mode of the Xsens MTx modules and receive data from them. We implemented the firmware in C language. Any recorded data on the SD card were later processed using custom software routines prepared under MATLAB environment.

(1) *Communication with the sensor units:* The reception of data uses streaming mode and is based on interrupts. We implemented the protocol for communication with the sensors as described by the manufacturer [10]. The volume of data that comes from a single MTx inertial module is determined by its activated options [10, 11]. The total time to transfer and process data of a single sampling is limited by the sampling period. Thus, high speed of the serial interface is needed. In our case, the speed of the serial communication is 460 kbps, at a sensor sampling frequency of 200 Hz. The software ensures that there are no missing samples by checking the proper incrementing of the sample counter.

(2) *Recording on an SD card:* Inertial data and calculated angles obtained in real time are recorded to the SD card. The recording process should not affect time performance of data collection and any signal processing tasks. To ensure this condition, we allocated two buffers A and B for each MTx module. The data from each module are temporarily stored into one of the buffers. The capacity of a buffer allows recording for at least one second. A ping-pong operation of buffers is implemented: once a buffer becomes full, next samples are collected to the other empty buffer while the content of the first one is transferred onto the card. Later, in a similar way

the buffers are switched again. At the selected sampling frequency, the total time to record the buffer content of all connected sensor modules on the card must be shorter than the time to fill a single buffer. Another measure to minimize the time for recording on the SD card is to store the data in the same binary format as they are received from the Xsens modules.

For the experiments demonstrating the two application examples, we enrolled a total of ten young healthy volunteers (five males and five females, weight 55–75 kg, age 23–31, foot size 23.5–27 cm) from the Shenzhen Institutes of Advanced Technology, Chinese Academy of Sciences.

2.3 Collection of Inertial and Plantar Pressure Data

In this application example, we performed synchronous recording of plantar pressure and inertial data. Such a scenario makes sense in the context of a body sensor network-based exploration of human biomechanics [9]. Also, inertial sensor data allow for kinematic analysis, while plantar pressure data allow for kinetic analysis. Thus, the combination of the two systems provides a convenient means for exploration of human body movement.

For plantar pressure data collection, we used a Footscan® system (RSscan International, Olen, Belgium, 1068 mm × 418 mm × 12 mm, 8192 sensors). It supports sampling rates of up to 500 Hz, depending on the operating mode [12]. The plate was mounted in the middle of a walkway with a total length of 8 m. Inertial data were collected from a single MTx module attached laterally under the knee on the left shank segment of the subjects. We configured the Footscan® system to act as the master, providing per-frame synchronization signal which was passed directly to the MTx module. The hardware scenario is illustrated in Fig. 2. We asked each subject to walk without shoes at his/her self-selected speed over the walkway, crossing the pressure plate. The sampling frequency of the plate was set to 200 Hz. Since the plate collects data only for a short time when the subject crosses it, we considered the data from the two modalities only for the time they were simultaneously active.

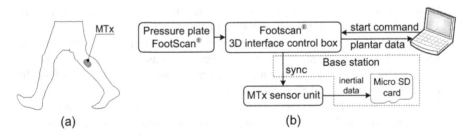

(a)   (b)

Fig. 2. Plantar pressure and inertial synchronous data collection (a) position of the inertial sensor on the left shank during data collection; (b) block diagram of module interconnections.

2.4 Knee Joint Extension Angle Evaluation

With this example, we demonstrate knee joint extension angle measurement. Such a measurement finds application when evaluating the performance of the knee joint [6]. We make use of the option for synchronized recording to prove the accuracy of knee joint angle measurement when using MTx inertial modules. The experimental setup we used is illustrated in Fig. 3a and b.

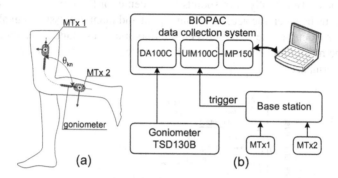

Fig. 3. Knee angle measurement scenario (a) attachment of the sensors (b) module connections.

1. *MTx sensor locations and coordinate systems:* One MTx unit was attached to the left thigh laterally, and the other one was attached to the left shank laterally. In that, we adopted the MTx sensor positions, and the definitions of the femoral, tibial, and Earth-fixed coordinate systems as they were defined in [6].
2. *Validation:* For validation, we used a goniometer device (TSD130B, Biopac) connected to a Biopac data acquisition system. An effort was made to align each segment of the goniometer in parallel with the sagittal plane.
3. *Experimental procedure:* Before each data collection, a sensor-to-body calibration procedure was performed. Each data collection started simultaneously between our system and the reference system using a cable connection for the synchronization. The subject was asked to perform full flexion-extension cycles from standing position for 120 s and also walking at self-selected speed for the same duration. Each subject performed ten trials of each kind.
4. *Angle calculation:* MTx sensors provide drift-free orientation data. For the derivation of the knee joint flexion angle we used the methodology given in [6].

3 Results

3.1 Collection of Plantar Pressure and Inertial Data

The both kinds of collected data showed a repetitive pattern. An example of this pattern is shown in Fig. 4, for the case, when the left foot was the first in the gait cycle. The main phases of the gait cycle are also denoted [13–15]. In Fig. 4, the magenta curve (the solid line) represents the magnitude of acceleration vector (also referred to as "resultant acceleration") which is defined as $a = \sqrt{a_x^2 + a_y^2 + a_z^2}$, where a_x, a_y and a_z are the components along the x, y and z axis, respectively. As to collected plantar pressure data, in Fig. 4 the blue curve (the dotted line) represents the maximum pressure for the time interval between left foot initial contact and right foot toe-off. The curve was built based on the "Entire plate roll off" export of Footscan® pressure plate software since this export provides the pressure on the entire plate while the subject feet contact the plate [12]. The blue curve actually corresponds to the center of force path [16]. From Fig. 4 timing relations between the accelerometer signal and plantar pressure signal could be observed. For example, the time between the maximum resultant acceleration at heel strike and the maximum heel pressure of the same leg can serve as an indicator for the walking performance.

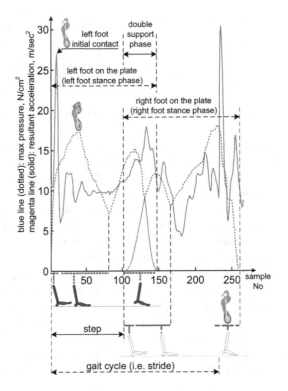

Fig. 4. An example of synchronously collected inertial and foot plantar pressure data (Color figure online)

3.2 Knee Joint Angle Derivation

The knee joint extension angle obtained using MTx sensors showed a high correlation with the one obtained from the reference system. To estimate the accuracy of the inertial sensor measurement system, we used the root mean square error (RMSE) as an objective measure. Pearson's correlation coefficient was also computed. Table 1 contains the results from the validation. Figure 5 shows an example of the angular waveforms obtained from each system during left knee flexion-extension motion. The system demonstrated a high accuracy (RMSE = 3.3570) and high correlation (p = 0.9965) with the reference.

Table 1. Results of knee joint angle measurement (representative values).

Test motion	Pearson's correlation coeff.	Root mean square error, deg
Left knee flexion/extension from standing position	0.9965	3.3570
Walking at normal speed	0.8964	6.1105

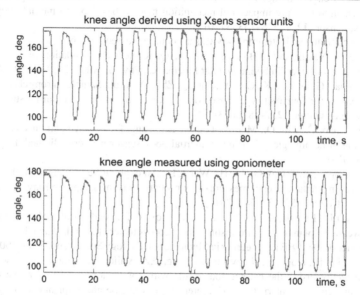

Fig. 5. Comparison between angular data of the left knee joint obtained synchronously by the proposed system and the reference during left knee flexion/extension.

4   Conclusions

In this work, we present a base station developed by us for collecting data from motion sensor units of type Xsens MTx. Since the communication protocol of these sensors is available, we demonstrate their flexibility for use with a custom system. In many cases, such an approach could simplify experimental scenarios. We provided two application examples with a focus on synchronized data collection from biomedical systems of different kinds. Options that can easily be utilized are to synchronize several base station boards if more than four MTx units are required or add a wireless module to achieve wireless synchronization.

Acknowledgments. This work was supported in part by National Natural Science Foundation of China (Grant Nos. 61401454, 71532014 and U1505251), the Key Research Program of the Chinese Academy of Sciences (KFZO-SW-202), Technology Development Program of Shenzhen (CXZZ20150401152602734), Project of Nanshan (KC2015JSJS0014A) and Major project of Guangdong Province (2014B010111008).

References

1. Seel, T., Raisch, J., Schauer, T.: IMU-based joint angle measurement for gait analysis. Sensors **14**, 6891–6909 (2014)
2. Zhao, G., Mei, Z., Liang, D., Ivanov, K., Guo, Y., Wang, Y., et al.: Exploration and implementation of a pre-impact fall recognition method based on an inertial body sensor network. Sensors **12**, 15338–15355 (2012)
3. © Xsens company website. http://www.xsens.com. Accessed 15 Sept 2016
4. Zhang, J.T., Novak, A.C., Brouwer, B., Li, Q.: Concurrent validation of Xsens MVN measurement of lower limb joint angular kinematics. Physiol. Meas. **34**, N63–N69 (2013)
5. Mei, Z., Zhao, G., Ivanov, K., Guo, Y., Zhu, Q., Zhou, Y., et al.: Sample entropy characteristics of movement for four foot types based on plantar centre of pressure during stance phase. Biomed. Eng. Online **12**, 1–18 (2013)
6. Guo, Y., Zhao, G., Liu, Q., Mei, Z., Ivanov, K., Wang, L.: Balance and knee extensibility evaluation of hemiplegic gait using an inertial body sensor network. Biomed. Eng. Online **12**, 83 (2013)
7. Mei, Z., Ivanov, K., Zhao, G., Li, H., Wang, L.: An explorive investigation of functional differences in plantar center of pressure of four foot types using sample entropy method. Med. Biol. Eng. Comput. **55**, 537–548 (2016)
8. Howcroft, J.D., Lemaire, E.D., Kofman, J., McIlroy, W.E.: Analysis of dual-task elderly gait using wearable plantar-pressure insoles and accelerometer. In: 36th Annual International Conference of the IEEE Engineering in Medicine and Biology Society, pp. 5003–5006 (2014)
9. Jarchi, D., Lo, B., Ieong, E., Nathwani, D., Yang, G.Z.: Validation of the e-AR sensor for gait event detection using the parotec foot insole with application to post-operative recovery monitoring. In: 11th International Conference on Wearable and Implantable Body Sensor Networks, pp. 127–131 (2014)
10. Xsens Technologies B.V.: MT Low-Level Communication Protocol Documentation (2010)
11. Xsens Technologies B.V.: MTi and MTx User Manual and Technical Documentation (2010)
12. RScan International: Footscan® advanced & hi-end system, user guide, v.7, gait software, footwear adviser software (2009)
13. Perry, J.: Gait Analysis: Normal and Pathological Function, 1st edn. SLACK, Vancouver (1992)
14. Lisa, J.A.D.: Gait Analysis in the Science of Rehabilitation. DIANE Publishing, Collingdale (2000)
15. Kirtley, C.: Clinical Gait Analysis: Theory and Practice. Elsevier, Amsterdam (2006)
16. Rose, N.E., Feiwell, L.A., Cracchiolo 3rd, A.: A method for measuring foot pressures using a high resolution, computerized insole sensor: the effect of heel wedges on plantar pressure distribution and center of force. Foot Ankle **13**, 263–270 (1992)

Energy-Efficient IoT-Enabled Fall Detection System with Messenger-Based Notification

Igor Tcarenko[1(✉)], Tuan Nguyen Gia[1], Amir M. Rahmani[1], Tomi Westerlund[1], Pasi Liljeberg[1], and Hannu Tenhunen[1,2]

[1] Department of Information Technology, University of Turku, Turku, Finland
{igotsa,tunggi,amirah,tovewe,pakrli}@utu.fi
[2] Department of Industrial and Medical Electronics,
KTH Royal Institute of Technology, Stockholm, Sweden
hannu@imit.kth.se

Abstract. Falls might cause serious traumas especially among elderly people. To deliver timely medical aid, fall detection systems should be able to notify appropriately personnel immediately, when fall occurs. However, as in any system, notification mechanism affects overall energy consumption. Considering that energy efficiency affects reliability, as it influences runtime of the system, notification mechanism should be energy aware. We propose an IoT-enabled fall detection system with a messenger-based notification method, which allows to obtain energy efficient solution, decrease development time and allow to reuse facilities of a popular messaging platform.

Keywords: Internet of Things · Messenger · Fall detection · Fog computing · Energy efficiency · Real-time systems

1 Introduction

Falling is a treacherous issue for elderly. It might cause serious injuries such as bone fractures or traumatic brain damages caused by head traumas for instance [1,2]. More than one third of senior people, whose age is above 65, experiences a fall each year [3]. However, only in less than half of the cases the professional aid is delivered timely. Unattended cases might very likely lead to injuries worsening, which later complicates medical treatment. Fear of falling itself, especially if the aid is not immediate, results in decreased confidence [4], which declines physical activity, lessens social contacts, and eventually leads to depression [5,6]. Thus, there exists an apparent demand for systems which are capable of detecting falls and notifying appropriate personnel.

Internet of Things (IoT), whose application area has been rapidly expanding, provides efficient means for solving variety of problems. In principle, an IoT architecture comprises edge sensor nodes for collecting data, a fog layer [7] for data pre-processing and local decision making as well as a cloud layer for data analysis and storage. All these make IoT a convenient leverage to solve a wide range of

© ICST Institute for Computer Sciences, Social Informatics and Telecommunications Engineering 2017
P. Perego et al. (Eds.): MobiHealth 2016, LNICST 192, pp. 19–26, 2017.
DOI: 10.1007/978-3-319-58877-3_3

health-care related problems [8,9] and offer means for monitoring and predicting patients' condition autonomously and remotely. Combined with miniaturized
wearable devices that collect patient's health- and activity-related parameters,
an IoT-based solution helps to preserve patients' independent lifestyle. Offering
several valuable features, wearable's battery-operated nature is one of its main
barrier affecting the battery operation time which can result in a limited overall reliability. Reliability is of paramount importance in e-health applications;
therefore, we utilise the fog layer that resides in a gateway in our IoT-based fall
detection system. Stationary nature of the gateway implies unconstrained power
supply, and thus the computational load can be redistributed among the fog and
the wearable devices optimizing energy efficiency of the latter.

Notification mechanism is vital for IoT systems such as fall detector. Often an
optimal and most promising solution appears as a combination of technologies.
As messengers (with over 1 billion monthly active users [10]) are believed to be
the next revolutionary communication media after the social networks era, the
exploitation of their facilities can reduce the cost of IoT solutions and ease their
integration into society.

In this paper, taking advantage of the IoT fog layer, we first built an energy
efficient fall detection system. We then amalgamate and consolidate the concepts
of IoT and evolutionary mobile messaging to present a messenger-based notification mechanism for our IoT-based fall detection system in order to reduce the
implementation cost and enhance wide spread use of the system.

The remainder of the paper is organized as follows. In Sect. 2, we discuss
related work and draw the motivation of the work. In Sect. 3, we present the system architecture, after which the system implementation is described in Sect. 4.
Section 5 presents experimental results, and finally we conclude in Sect. 6.

2   Related Work and Motivation

Existing approaches for developing fall detection systems can be conventionally
categorized into camera-, accelerometer-, gyroscope-based and hybrid solutions.
In [11,12], hybrid (Kinect depth camera and accelerometer) and accelerometer-
based systems are presented with reported accuracies of 87.29% and 95.71%,
respectively. In [13], authors proposed a solution, built on a smartphone utilizing
accelerometer measurements with the accuracy of over 93%. In these works, accuracy is in the main focus, leaving energy consumption a secondary role. However,
as mentioned, power efficiency is an important component of overall reliability of
the solution, and therefore it should be primarily considered in designing the system. Considering all the upsides of the mentioned solutions, such as utilization of
widespread platforms and sophisticated analysis algorithms, we, however, uphold
the view that the system architecture should stay simple though providing sufficient degree of accuracy. In other words, the solution should avoid unnecessary
components which are power hungry. Hence, our approach has an accelerometer-
based wearable at its core, because as shown, it can provide sufficient degree of
accuracy. Operating in the scope of IoT, in particular in conjunction with the

fog layer computing unit, the wearable device can be computationally offloaded, leaving to a sensor node a function of transmitting the measured data.

System's capability to notify appropriate personnel about a fall is essential. Pervasive nature of mobile networks provides a convenient leverage to implement a notification mechanism. A GPRS module, attached to a wearable, represents a viable fall detection system with a pervasive notification method [14]. However, as any part of a system, a notification mechanism affects overall energy efficiency and, therefore, should be considered.

To build energy efficient, yet ubiquitous notification mechanism, we propose to use messengers' bots [15]. Bots approach is an emerging trend in instant messaging technologies. Such bots are basically software-operated messenger users that can resign in a remote or a local network server. Thus, the bots provide an opportunity to leverage messenger's facilities, such as servers and client side applications, for building distributed systems.

Putting all together, the rationale behind this work is to build a reliable and energy efficient fall detection system with a messenger-based notification mechanism, capable of working autonomously for a long period of time.

3   System Architecture

The overall system architecture is shown in Fig. 1. It consists of a wearable device working as a sensor node at the edge layer, a smart gateway with the developed messenger bot at a fog layer, and a messenger server located in a cloud (in our system, we use Telegram Messenger [16]). A fall signal, which indicates that the fall has occurred, is sent to the server from the bot. After receiving the fall notification, the messenger server sends a push notification to the Telegram Messenger client application.

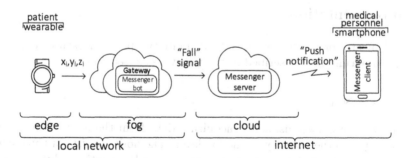

Fig. 1. The system consists of the wearable device, smart gateway with the messenger bot, and messenger server in a cloud. Push notification, triggered by an active fall signal, is sent to a remote smartphone.

Among the fall detection acceleration-based algorithms [14,17–20], we exploit the one which relies on the prototypical acceleration curve of a forward

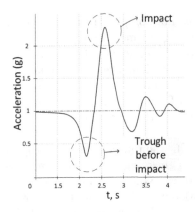

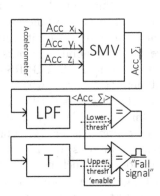

Fig. 2. Prototypical acceleration curve of a forward fall. The pit depicts the falling phase, whereas the peak reflects the impact from hitting the surface.

Fig. 3. The block diagram of the algorithm. The algorithm filters the input raw data and searches for the pit and peak.

real-world fall, depicted in Fig. 2. The block diagram of the algorithm includes the calculation of the signal magnitude vector (as a square root of sum of squares of accelerations along X,Y,Z axis), low pass filtering and comparing the result with the lower and higher thresholds in order to draw the final decision (Fig. 3). Hence, the wearable's accelerometer provides acceleration measurements (along three orthogonal axis X,Y,Z) that are sent to the gateway and processed by the aforementioned algorithm (Fig. 2) to draw the final decision about a the occurrence of a fall.

4   Implementation

The implementation of the system is divided into two parts, the sensor node and the fog computing unit, described in the following subsections.

4.1   Sensor Node

The sensor node is responsible for acquiring data from the accelerometer and transmitting it to the gateway in the fog layer. The node consists of three components: a microcontroller, an accelerometer, and a Bluetooth module. For our experiment, we use ATMega328 (microcontroller), ADXL345 (accelerometer), BLE Micro (bluetooth interface). The implemented node is shown in Fig. 4.

The core component is ADXL345 [21]. It is a 3-axis high resolution accelerometer with I2C and SPI communication interface. This chip features an ultra-low power consumption mode, providing measurements at a rate of 200 Hz or 400 Hz, while current consumption is only 90 μA.

ATMega328 (8 MHz), embedded into a tiny (diameter of 50 mm) LilyPad development board, serves as a node's processing unit [22]. It is a low power 8-bit AVR microcontroller. Operating at a speed of 1 MHz, the microcontroller consumes as little as 0.2 mA. The microcontroller has USART and two SPI communication interfaces. The microcontroller receives measurements over SPI interface, whereas the USART is used for communicating with the Bluetooth module.

BLE Micro [23] is an ultra-low power Bluetooth module, which is used for transmitting accelerometer data from the sensor node to the gateway. Operating at 3.3 V, BLE Micro consumes 2 μA in idle mode and around 10 mA when transmitting data at a rate of 1 Mbps (2 Mbps is the maximum data rate). The module's small size (13.0 mm × 18.5 mm × 2.3 mm) makes it suitable for our use case.

4.2 Fog Computing Unit and Client Side Application

The fog layer comprises a computing unit, realized on Raspberry Pi 3 (Fig. 5) with installed Linux-based operating system Raspbian Jessie. The unit plays two roles. First, it serves as a gateway, which connects the lower edge layer with the Telegram server, located in the cloud, by the means of the developed Telegram bot. Second, it processes the received acceleration measurements to detect falls. Communication with the wearable is carried out over the Bluetooth 4.1, whereas the Internet connection is held via Wi-Fi 802.11n.

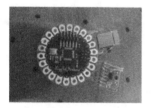

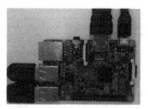

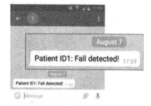

Fig. 4. A wearable sensor node is attached to the patient to detect falls.

Fig. 5. Fog computing unit, with developed bot is realized on Raspberry Pi 3.

Fig. 6. A client side Telegram messenger has received a notification about the fall.

The unique token, which is used for Fog-Cloud communication, ensures the exclusive identification of the developed bot - this makes the approach scalable. This means that the fog units can be spread in different locations to cover larger area, where each unit will be easily accessed and controlled. Client side application for receiving notifications is a Telegram Messenger android application (Fig. 6).

5   Experimental Results and Demonstration

In order to demonstrate functionality of our fall detection system, the fall detection system was experimented by several volunteers whose heights are between 165–175 cm and weights 60–75 kg. Each volunteer's sensor node is powered by 1100mah Li-Ion battery. The volunteers were monitored while imitating falls at arbitrary times. In the experiment, we estimate energy consumption of the wearable, using the following equation [24]:

$$E = V \times I(w) \times (t(w) - t(o)) + V \times I(o) \times t(o) \tag{1}$$

where E is the total energy consumption (mJ); V is the applied voltage supply; $I(w)$ is an average current consumption while the system is idle (mA); $I(o)$ is an average current consumption when the system is operating (mA); $t(w)$ is waiting time (s) and $t(o)$ is operating time (s).

We compare our approach with an implemented GPRS-based solution, consisting of ATmega328V microcontroller, ADXL345 accelerometer and a SIM900 GPRS module. We use a fall detection algorithm described in Figs. 2 and 3. A notification about a fall is sent via a mobile network as an sms message to a smartphone.

Figure 7a shows energy cost of gathering and transmitting different number of samples for the sensor node, operating in the proposed system. As seen in Fig. 7b, the solution with the GPRS-based notification mechanism requires more energy to realize the same functionality.

Samples	I(mA)	V	E(mJ)
50	29.17	3.3	97.8
100	29.28	3.3	98.1
200	29.39	3.3	98.5

(a) Energy consumptions of a node, operating in the proposed system.

MCU	I(mA)	V	E(mJ)
ATmega328 (16MHz)	104.3	5	521.5
ATmega328 (8MHz)	88.4	3.3	291.72

(b) Energy consumptions of a node with a GPRS-based notification mechanism.

Fig. 7. Experimental results of energy consumption of the proposed solution and the GPRS-based approach.

The results in Fig. 8 demonstrate that the Messenger-based notification mechanism, providing the same coverage as the GPRS-based approach, requires 3 times less energy. In addition, our approach allowed to reuse messenger's client application and servers - this accelerated and simplified development process.

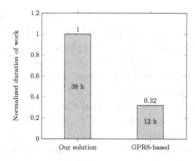

Fig. 8. Comparison of normalized durations of work of the proposed and GPRS-based solutions. Numbers on the bars represent duration of work of the sensor nodes, powered from 1100 mAh battery.

6   Conclusions

Energy efficient fall detection system with a small wearable device at its core was proposed. By leveraging the advantages of the fog computing and messengers' bot platform, the wearable's energy consumption decreased 3 times, compared to the GPRS-based approach. The total operating time of the wearable was 38 h (using a 1100 mAh battery). Combination of IoT and Messengers technologies allowed to address the cost of the solution and its development time. Notification mechanism, which relies on the popular messaging platform, delivers immediate notices to responsible personnel to provide timely aid to the user of the device.

References

1. Sterling, D.A., O'Connor, J.A., Bonadies, J.: Geriatric falls: injury severity is high and disproportionate to mechanism. J. Trauma Acute Care Surg. **50**(1), 116–119 (2001)
2. Stevens, J.A., Corso, P.S., Finkelstein, E.A., Miller, T.R.: The costs of fatal and non-fatal falls among older adults. Inj. Prev. **12**(5), 290–295 (2006)
3. CDC-Centers for Disease control and prevention: Important facts about falls, January 2016. http://www.cdc.gov/homeandrecreationalsafety/falls/adultfalls. html. Accessed Jul 2016
4. Friedman, S.M., Munoz, B., West, S.K., Rubin, G.S., Fried, L.P.: Falls and fear of falling: which comes first? J. Am. Geriatr. Soc. **50**(8), 1329–1335 (2002)
5. Scheffer, A.C., et al.: Fear of falling: measurement strategy, prevalence, risk factors and consequences among older persons. Age Ageing **37**(1), 19–24 (2008)
6. Igual, R., Medrano, C., Plaza, I.: Challenges, issues and trends in fall detection systems. Biomed. Eng. Online **12**(1), 1 (2013)
7. Bonomi, F., Milito, R., Zhu, J., Addepalli, S.: Fog computing and its role in the internet of things. In: Proceedings of the 1st edition of the MCC Workshop on Mobile Cloud Computing, pp. 13–16. ACM (2012)
8. Gia, T.N., et al.: Fog computing in healthcare internet of things: a case study on ECG feature extraction. In: 2015 IEEE International Conference on Computer and Information Technology (CIT), pp. 356–363. IEEE (2015)

9. Natarajan, K., Prasath, B., Kokila, P.: Smart health care system using internet of things. J. Netw. Commun. Emerg. Technol. (JNCET) **6**(3) (2016). www.jncet.org
10. Statista. Number of monthly active WhatsApp users. http://www.statista.com/statistics/260819/number-of-monthly-active-whatsapp-users/
11. Kepski, M., Kwolek, B.: Embedded system for fall detection using body-worn accelerometer and depth sensor. In: 2015 IEEE 8th International Conference on Intelligent Data Acquisition and Advanced Computing Systems: Technology and Applications (IDAACS), vol. 2, pp. 755–759. IEEE (2015)
12. Kostopoulos, P., et al.: Increased fall detection accuracy in an accelerometer-based algorithm considering residual movement. In: International Conference on Pattern Recognition Applications and Methods (2015)
13. Casilari, E., Oviedo-Jiménez, M.A.: Automatic fall detection system based on the combined use of a smartphone and a smartwatch. PloS One **10**(11), e0140929 (2015)
14. Tang, A.Y.C., Ong, C.-H., Ahmad, A.: Fall detection sensor system for the elderly. Int. J. Adv. Comput. Res. **5**(19), 176 (2015)
15. Telegram.org. Telegram bot platform. https://telegram.org/blog/bot-revolution
16. Telegram.org. Telegram. https://telegram.org/
17. Li, Y., et al.: Accelerometer-based fall detection sensor system for the elderly. In: 2012 IEEE 2nd International Conference on Cloud Computing and Intelligence Systems, vol. 3, pp. 1216–1220. IEEE (2012)
18. Nguyen, T.T., Cho, M.-C., Lee, T.-S.: Automatic fall detection using wearable biomedical signal measurement terminal. In: 2009 Annual International Conference of the IEEE Engineering in Medicine and Biology Society, pp. 5203–5206. IEEE (2009)
19. Li, Q., et al.: Accurate, fast fall detection using gyroscopes and accelerometer-derived posture information. In: 2009 Sixth International Workshop on Wearable and Implantable Body Sensor Networks, pp. 138–143. IEEE (2009)
20. Odunmbaku, A., et al.: Elderly monitoring system with sleep and fall detector. In: International Conference on IoT Technologies for HealthCare (2015)
21. Analog Devices: Adxl345-digital accelerometer, January 2016. http://www.analog.com/media/en/technical-documentation/data-sheets/ADXL345.pdf. Accessed Jul 2016
22. Leah and SparkFun: Lilypad arduino mainboard, January 2016. https://www.arduino.cc/en/Main/ArduinoBoardLilyPad. Accessed Jul 2016
23. Seeed Studio: Ble micro, January 2016. http://www.seeedstudio.com/wiki/BLE_Micro. Accessed Jul 2016
24. Gia, T.N., et al.: Fog computing in body sensor networks: an energy efficient approach. In: IEEE International Body Sensor Networks Conference (BSN 2015) (2015)

Promotion for Healthy Lifestyle

A Mobile Adviser of Healthy Eating by Reading Ingredient Labels

Man Wai Wong, Qing Ye, Yuk Kai Chan Kylar, Wai-Man Pang[✉],
and Kin Chung Kwan

School of Computing and Information Sciences,
Caritas Institute of Higher Education, Tseung Kwan O, N.T., Hong Kong
wmpang@ieee.org

Abstract. Understanding ingredients or additives in food is essential
for a healthy life. The general public should be encouraged to learn more
about the effect of food they consume, especially for people with allergy
or other health problems. However, reading the ingredient label of every
packaged food is tedious and no one will spend time on this. This paper
proposed a mobile app to leverage the troublesome and at the same time
provide health advices of packaged food. To facilitate acquisition of the
ingredient list, apart from barcode scanning, we recognize text on the
ingredient labels directly. Thus, our application will provide proper alert
on allergen found in food. Also it suggests users to avoid food that is
harmful to health in long term, like high fat or calories food. A preliminary user study reveals that the adviser app is useful and welcomed by
many users who care about their dietary.

Keywords: Healthy dietary · Food ingredient · Text recognition ·
Health suggestion · Mobile health

1 Introduction

As a metropolitan nowadays, we are busy at every moment for our work or
study. We get used to choose food based on their flavor or common sense, but
we seldom think about if its ingredients are good to our health or not. While
there is a huge number of new food products to the market every day, it is
somehow risky to simply choosing them based on previous knowledge. However,
reading the information from food packages can be tedious and require specific
knowledge in judging whether certain food had positive or negative effects to
our health. Hence, probably no one is willing to spend time on reading them.

Our health is directly affected by what we consumed in both short or long
term. For instance, people with food allergy can have fatal reactions to certain
food after food intake shortly or instantly. According to a recent study, there
are about 5% of children and 4% of adults allergic to one or more kinds of
food. 90% of their allergic responses are caused by common foods such as cow's

© ICST Institute for Computer Sciences, Social Informatics and Telecommunications Engineering 2017
P. Perego et al. (Eds.): MobiHealth 2016, LNICST 192, pp. 29–37, 2017.
DOI: 10.1007/978-3-319-58877-3_4

milk, peanuts, and eggs. For long term health, high fat or calories food can accumulate in the body and cause artery diseases, diabetes and other illnesses. Some studies also believe that food additives and preservatives can increase hyperactive behavior in young children. Thus, it is important to be aware of the food in-taken in a daily manner.

Our project comes into the place to help people who suffer from food allergies to select their food safely, as well as the general public in understanding more on their daily dietary. We developed a mobile application to relieve the difficulties in learning food ingredients in packaged food and provide alerts or suggestions for a healthy dietary. Our system provides ways in identifying the ingredients of food products from barcode scanning to direct recognizing the ingredient label. By associating with an ingredient database, suggestions can be provided automatically. As a result, when a user is going to buy a packaged food, he/she can scan the barcode or the text printed on the package to understand the ingredients as in Fig. 1(a).

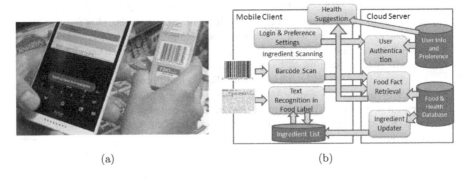

(a)   (b)

Fig. 1. (a) A usage scenario of our mobile app: a user can easily understand more on the ingredients of a food product by simple scanning. (b) An overview of our system.

There are two main technical challenges in this project: text recognition in ingredient label and automatic health suggestion. Although text recognition or optical character recognition (OCR) had reported many successful results from the literature, existing mobile OCR engines may not perform well especially when the recognition is done under poor lighting conditions. Thus, we employed several image processing techniques to reduce effect caused by poor lighting, and incorporating approximate matching to our ingredient database in order to improve the recognition outcome. Moreover, providing health related suggestions purely based on the elements listed on the ingredient list is insufficient. It is because some ingredients are correlated and contains similar effects after consumption. Naïvely providing suggestions may generate tons of duplicated messages and easily overwhelm users. So, we proposed a method to consolidate and better organize the suggestions.

A number of users are invited for testing our app. Most of them are satisfactory to the functionality provided and think the health suggestion are helpful for choosing food products. With our system, the ingredient label becomes more meaningful to everyone. The public can understand more about what they eat and eat wisely. We believe that this application will promote the awareness of healthy eating habits as well as to help people with food allergy to regain certain pleasures of eating in their life.

2   Related Works

In recent years, many systems for mobile health (mHealth) have been developed and widely accepted by the public. Most of them are common in exploiting the ubiquitous nature of mobile applications in order to provide monitoring or tracking of physiological status [7,8,10,12].

Among all these examples, food monitoring or logging system is a popular kind of mHealth applications. These food monitoring systems mainly target to analyze the food habit of users and provide suggestions or alert for the diet program of the users. SapoFitness [11] is a mHealth application for dietary assessment. This application provides a list of food for user to input the calories intake. Unlike our system, this kind of application usually cannot help the users in choosing a new product before they make a purchase.

MyFitnessPal [9] obtains the nutritional values of food by scanning the barcode and suggests users how to keep fit. Image-based food monitoring systems [2,5] recognize the foods by analyzing food photos. This allows the user to learn the food ingredients or nutrition by simply taking photo. Available works for people with food allergy [1,4] allow the user to check the existence of food allergens by barcode scan of package labels. However, these systems all require the products to be registered in the database for their system. In contrast, our system can read the ingredients label and find out food allergens even if the product is not found in the database.

3   System Overview

Our system is mainly divided into 3 major components, they are the ingredient scanning module, health suggestion module and food & health database. Figure 1(b) illustrates the relations between components in the system.

The ingredient scanning module enables the user to identify food product and related ingredient quickly with barcode scanning, as well as text recognition of ingredient label when the food product is not available in the food database. The health suggestion module relies on the food & health database on the server, together with the user's preferences stored with his/her user account which is managed by the user authentication module. The food & health database stores updated information about food products including its product name, ingredient, manufacturer, health suggestion, and etc.

4   Implementation

Following the standard of mobile apps nowadays, the interface is designed to be simple and user friendly enough for daily use. Figure 2 shows a number of screenshots of our mobile app. To enable personalization and support user preferences, user has to login (Fig. 2(a)) to our system. The user preferences include selection of allergic ingredients to give alert (Fig. 2(b) and (c)).

4.1   Barcode Scanning and Food Database

Almost all packaged food products are printed with barcode labels, but it is designed for sale purposes. It is seldom for the barcode to associate with food ingredient information or even health related suggestions. Thus, many databases are developed to include barcode-ingredient relation. However, most of these databases are proprietary, except the open food facts [14], or they do not fully cover enough food product entries.

Taking open food facts as an example, it contains 50,000 entries of food products from 134 countries, but most of them are from Europe. The database stores many useful product related data, including the generic name, category, list of ingredients, nutrition facts and etc. Thus, we directly make use of these existing entries for a preliminary retrieval of ingredients. While, we also have our own database which is built to tailor for local food products. Thus, whenever an entry does not exist in the open database, we will rely on our own. Figure 2(e) shows the food ingredient retrieval result by scanning the barcode.

However, most of the food database contains only manufacturing and nutrition information of the food product. No health related information is included. Our food & health database therefore serves this purpose by associating health recommendations to ingredients. The major effective component in the ingredients are factored out so as to produce useful and tidy suggestions in time. For example, many food ingredients like gluten, wheat, and rye, they may cause

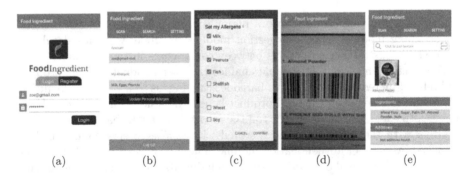

(a)   (b)   (c)   (d)   (e)

Fig. 2. The user interface of our mobile application, including (a) user login page, (b) account settings, (c) allergen selection, (d) scanning of barcode, and (e) result of barcode scanning.

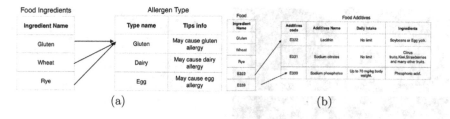

Fig. 3. Relationship between food ingredients and health suggestions.

the same gluten allergy, because all of them contains gluten which is the actual source of allergy. Thus, the recommendations are associated with the actual source gluten only but not the ingredient as in Fig. 3(a).

Similarly, some additives are made of other ingredients which further causes other health problems. Like Fig. 3(b), additive E322 is made from soybeans and egg yolk. Thus, additive E322 should produce similar health suggestions to soybeans and egg yolk. This decomposition of ingredient to effective components can avoid repeated suggestions which overwhelm the user.

4.2   Text Recognition in Ingredient Labels

One way to identify the food ingredient is to read the ingredient list printed on the package of food. This ingredient list can be easily found on many packaged food products as it is required by the safety regulation of many countries. However, reading all the ingredient lists of every food one-by-one is tedious and sometimes difficult. Some ingredients, like additives, are either not well-known to the general public or written in scientific names. For instance, not many people know that "Mandelona" and "Enchilada sauce" are two ingredients which contain peanuts.

As a result, our mobile app allows users to scan the label, and analyze the ingredients. To accomplish this, we rely on OCR techniques with improvements in speed and accuracy by means of text region extraction, adaptive thresholding, and approximate matching.

Text Region Extraction. Before recognition, our method tries to locate text regions in image. Thus, we employ MSER (Maximally Stable Extremal Regions) [3] algorithm for fast region detection as shown in Fig. 5. It will extract regions (in red) which have high chance containing text. Hence, later processing like image enhancement and OCR will only involve these extracted regions. This speeds up a lot as irrelevant regions are ignored. Moreover, we can effectively reduce noise generated from OCR as non-text parts are filtered out before the recognition.

Adaptive Thresholding. Most of the text recognition engines begin with a grayscale conversion of image and followed by a thresholding to produce a binary

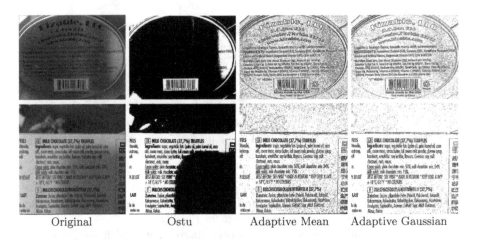

| Original | Ostu | Adaptive Mean | Adaptive Gaussian |

Fig. 4. Comparison of different thresholding methods.

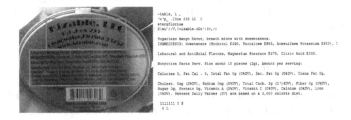

Fig. 5. Left: Text region detection. The red colored box indicates the detected regions containing character. Right: the corresponding scrambled OCR results. (Color figure online)

image. In our implementation, we use Tesseract-OCR engine [13] which preforms thresholding with Otsu approach. However, the Otsu method does not work well under extreme lighting conditions, like environment containing regions that are too bright and too dark.

We, therefore, try to improve thresholding with the use of adaptive approaches, including the Adaptive Mean and Adaptive Gaussian Thresholding. Figure 4 shows the results with different methods. Otsu thresholding always fails to handle changes of brightness across text regions. Shadow regions will completely turn into black, seriously ruins the recognition. Both adaptive methods generate more reasonable binary results useful for subsequent recognitions.

Approximate Matching. Directly performing recognition with Tesseract-OCR engine does not always provide acceptable results in practice. One reason is that the thresholding result always contains noise. Thus, the recognized text outcome usually looks scrambled or incorrect as shown in Fig. 5 or Fig. 6(b). It often returns paragraphs of text with extra punctuations or irrelevant digits (Fig. 5) and some spelling of words are wrong (underlined in Fig. 6(b) in red).

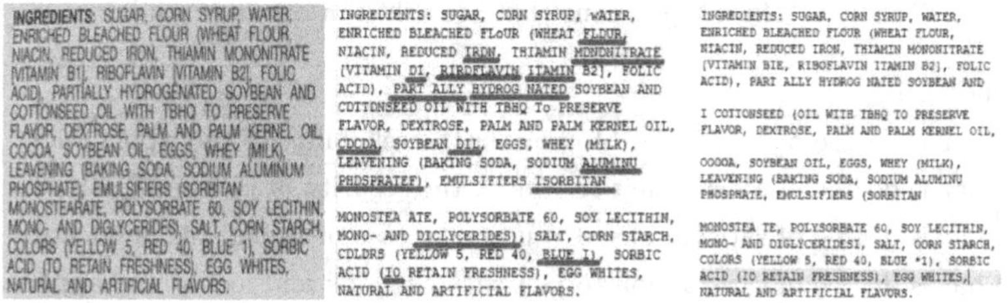

(a) Original food label   (b) Result directly from OCR   (c) Result tidied up

Fig. 6. Recognition accuracy improved with use of approximate matching with the ingredient list. (Color figure online)

Moreover, we would like to extract only words that are ingredients, and remove those irrelevant like product name, weight or manufacturer name.

To tidy up the results, our idea is to remove or correct them based on our ingredient list. That means only words that are certain or likely to be ingredient will be extracted. Currently, we have implemented a full text search with criteria to approximate match strings that are smaller than half word length of the ingredient name. A simple approximate string distance measure based on the Levenshtein algorithm [6] is employed with a quick pruning when the word length difference is more than double. Figure 6(c) demonstrates an example of applying approximate matching after OCR. We can find that many of the wrongly recognized words in Fig. 6(b) are now corrected with the use of ingredient list.

5   Preliminary Result

To evaluate the effectiveness of the developed mobile application and obtain useful user opinions for further improvements, a small scale user study is carried out. A total of 20 subjects are asked to make a trial to our app using an Android phone with Qualcomm snapdragon 615 CPU and 2GB RAM, followed by completing 12 questions listed in Table 1.

Some of the responses to the questions are shown in Fig. 7. We can find that the satisfactions to different aspects of our application are slightly satisfied in general, with nearly no unsatisfied or totally satisfied. Most of the users think ease of use is one of the best parts in our application, while barcode scan is also another part which they like most. Regarding to the speed of OCR, over half of them think it is slow, this may be caused by the low-end android device and the preprocessing is not optimized yet. It is also the reason why only 5% of them think OCR is the best part in the mobile app. In contrast to speed of OCR, over 90% of the users will prefer to have better accuracy in the text recognition which is the focus of enhancement we made in the current prototype.

Besides the above responses, the interviewees further provide us some useful suggestions. For example, they suggest that the app should support more languages and localization. They also suggest that we can extend to other allergens

Table 1. The 12 questions that are asked in our user study.

No.	Question
1	What is degree of satisfaction to you on the reliability of this application?
2	What is degree of satisfaction to you on the security of this application?
3	What is degree of satisfaction to you on the ease of use of this application?
4	What is degree of satisfaction to you with the look and feel of this application?
5	What is degree of satisfaction to you with the account setup experience?
6	Choose the best in the app from (UI/layout; ease of use; barcode scan; OCR)
7	Choose the worst in the app from (UI/layout; ease of use; barcode scan; OCR)
8	Do you think the health suggestion are helpful?
9	What else do you think the health suggestion function should provide?
10	What do you think about the speed of OCR function?
11	Which is more important to you about the OCR function? Speed or accuracy?
12	Please provide further comments or suggestion to improve the application

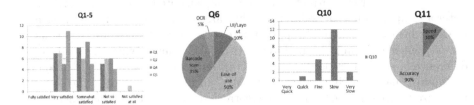

Fig. 7. Responses from our user study.

such as metal, animal skin tissue, dust mites etc. Some of them want the app to include additional information to the users; for instance, the first aid guide about suffered from allergen by mistake.

6   Conclusions

We presented a prototype of a food ingredient analysis mobile app which can scan the barcode or ingredients label on packaged food products to obtain included ingredients and provide proper health suggestions. A preliminary user study reveals that our application is ease to use and potentially helpful to promote healthy dietary to the general public. The prototype should be further improved with the speed of scanning ingredient labels and multiple languages support. This enables users to identify the potential allergens and additive for imported ingredient labels written in a foreign language.

Acknowledgment. The work described in this paper was fully supported by a grant from the Research Grants Council of the Hong Kong SAR, China (Ref. No. UGC/FDS11/E03/15).

References

1. Adelmann, R.: Mobile phone based interaction with everyday products-on the go. In: The 2007 International Conference on Next Generation Mobile Applications, Services and Technologies (NGMAST 2007), pp. 63–69. IEEE (2007)

2. Ahmad, Z., Khanna, N., Kerr, D.A., Boushey, C.J., Delp, E.J.: A mobile phone user interface for image-based dietary assessment. In: IS&T/SPIE Electronic Imaging, pp. 903007-1–903007-9. International Society for Optics and Photonics (2014)

3. Donoser, M., Bischof, H.: Efficient maximally stable extremal region (MSER) tracking. In: 2006 IEEE Computer Society Conference on Computer Vision and Pattern Recognition (CVPR 2006), vol. 1, pp. 553–560, June 2006

4. Gaßner, K., Vollmer, B., Prehn, M., Fiedler, M., Ssmoller, S.: Smart food: mobile guidance for food-allergic people. In: Seventh IEEE International Conference on e-Commerce Technology (CEC 2005), pp. 531–534 (2005)

5. Kawano, Y., Yanai, K.: FoodCam: a real-time mobile food recognition system employing fisher vector. In: Gurrin, C., Hopfgartner, F., Hurst, W., Johansen, H., Lee, H., O'Connor, N. (eds.) MMM 2014. LNCS, vol. 8326, pp. 369–373. Springer, Cham (2014). doi:10.1007/978-3-319-04117-9_38

6. Levenshtein, V.I.: Binary codes capable of correcting deletions. Insertions and reversals. Sov. Phys. Dokl. **10**, 707 (1966)

7. Nam, Y., Kim, Y., Lee, J.: Sleep monitoring based on a tri-axial accelerometer and a pressure sensor. Sensors **16**(5), 750 (2016)

8. Poon, G., Kwan, K.C., Pang, W.M., Choi, K.S.: Towards using tiny multi-sensors unit for child care reminders. In: 2016 IEEE Second International Conference on Multimedia Big Data (BigMM), pp. 372–376, April 2016

9. Rebedew, D.: Myfitnesspal. Fam. Pract. Manage. **22**(2), 31–31 (2014)

10. Sama, P.R., Eapen, Z.J., Weinfurt, K.P., Shah, B.R., Schulman, K.A.: An evaluation of mobile health application tools. JMIR mHealth uHealth **2**(2), e19 (2014)

11. Silva, B.M., Lopes, I.M., Rodrigues, J.J.P.C., Ray, P.: Sapofitness: a mobile health application for dietary evaluation. In: 2011 13th IEEE International Conference on e-Health Networking Applications and Services (Healthcom), pp. 375–380. IEEE (2011)

12. Silva, B.M.C., Rodrigues, J.J.P.C., de la Torre Díez, I., López-Coronado, M., Saleem, K.: Mobile-health: a review of current state in 2015. J. Biomed Inform. **56**, 265–272 (2015)

13. Smith, R.: An overview of the tesseract OCR engine. In: Proceedings Ninth Internatioal Conference on Document Analysis and Recognition (ICDAR), pp. 629–633 (2007)

14. The Open Food Facts Team: The open food facts (open food products database)

Investigating How to Measure Mobile User Engagement

Stefano Carrino[✉], Maurizio Caon, Omar Abou Khaled, and Elena Mugellini

HumanTech Institute, University of Applied Sciences and Arts Western Switzerland (HES-SO),
Fribourg, Switzerland
{stefano.carrino,maurizio.caon,omar.aboukhaled,
elena.mugellini}@hes-so.ch

Abstract. User Engagement is a keyword employed by software companies, researchers, and developers designing user-centred applications. Indeed, designing digital experiences to engage users is a goal that is becoming increasingly important for several disciplines such as education, marketing, information systems, and much more. Since opinions concerning the definition of user engagement greatly vary, the question comes up whether it is possible to provide a universal set of metrics to equally measure the engagement in any kind of application and in mobile applications in particular. Starting from results in the literature, this paper provides a simple definition of user engagement and a related set of metrics. Such metrics will be evaluated in a pilot study with more than 300 teenagers in four European countries.

Keywords: Mobile engagement · Web engagement · Mobile analytics · Web analytics · User engagement metrics

1 Introduction

For the case of mobile technology, successful technologies are not simply usable but they should engage users [16]. However, there is not consensus on what engagement is and how to measure it. In the past few years, web sites and web applications are the kind of applications in which more studies have been conducted to define and measure user engagement. Websites need to be engaging in order to achieve their purpose, which might be sharing knowledge, selling advertisement, providing customer support, etc. Independently from the specific purpose, if the website is not engaging, it is probably not achieving its goal [14]. Very similar goals and issues are present in the world of mobile applications. Our research project provides an ecosystem of apps and services, the definition and metrics of user engagement that we are seeking should be scalable and distributed (having multiple and variated sources of data) but nevertheless be summarized by a unique score.

Several definitions of user engagement exist. This variability is due to the difficulty in limiting this concept to a specific domain. In fact, user engagement ranges from psychology to marketing, from technology to services. In the marketing context, user engagement is often referred to as customer engagement.

© ICST Institute for Computer Sciences, Social Informatics and Telecommunications Engineering 2017
P. Perego et al. (Eds.): MobiHealth 2016, LNICST 192, pp. 38–44, 2017.
DOI: 10.1007/978-3-319-58877-3_5

2 Background – User Engagement Definitions

A simple definition can be found in [5], in which Chapman describes the engagement as something *"that attracts and holds our attention"*. A more complex and widely used definition is based on the research of O'Brien and Toms [16] and reads *"Engagement is a category of user experience characterized by attributes of challenge, positive affect, endurability, aesthetic and sensory appeal, attention, feedback, variety/novelty, interactivity, and perceived user control."* Quite similar are the conclusions of Attfield et al. [2], whose definition is based on existing literature concerning user engagement: *"User engagement is the emotional, cognitive and behavioural connection that exists, at any point in time and possibly over time, between a user and a resource."* Our project grounds part of its behavior change techniques on serious games and gamified applications [4]. In this domain, engagement is frequently related to the *flow state*, defined as *"an experience in which interactions cause intrinsic pleasure while an individual is involved in an activity"* and users are completely absorbed and immersed in the activity as presented in [6, 15]. However, as stated by Jennett et al. [9], in games and gamification user engagement can be associated to *immersion,* which can be a less intense experience than flow. In particular, Brown and Cairns [3] consider engagement as the first level of immersion (being engrossment and total immersion the deepest ones). These definitions present the concept of user engagement highlighting its different facets. However, our approach is based on operative and measurable definitions. Haven and Vittal [8] provide a more operative definition if compared to the strictly psycho-physiological approaches. Authors aim to provide a business-centred framework in which engagement can be described as: *"the level of involvement, interaction, intimacy, and influence an individual has with a brand over time."* Ensuing from this definition, Haven and Vittal provide a simple framework called the *4 I's*. While the study provides very useful and simple measures, they have been designed for businesses and marketing purposes and focusing in the web app field. Hence, the type of engagement may differ from the one found in mobile and pervasive applications.

Again in the domain of web apps, Peterson and Carrabis in [17] focus on websites and their visitors, and define engagement as follows: *"Visitor Engagement is a function of the number of clicks, the visit duration, the rate at which the visitor returns to the site over time, their overall loyalty to the site, their measured awareness of the brand, their willingness to directly contribute feedback and the likelihood that they will engage in specific activities on the site designed to increase awareness and create a lasting impression."* In contrast to the previously mentioned definitions of engagement, this approach is based on web metrics only. Tools like Google Analytics and others can be used to simply gather visitor data and derive their engagement while browsing a web service. Nowadays, the same tool and other very similar tools (e.g., Amazon Mobile Analytics [1]) can be used to measure similar parameters for mobile applications.

Finally, to the best of our knowledge, the only research papers that exclusively focus on mobile user engagement are [10] (authored by Kim et al.) and the work by Tomaselli et al. [18]. In their study, Kim et al. build a model to describe mobile user engagement (focusing on smartphone engagement) categorized into the three dimensional stages of human attitude: Cognitive stage, Affective stage and Conative stage. They try to define mobile user engagement via four different factors: Mobile engagement motivation (classified into three groups: Functional/Utilitarian motivation, Social motivation and Hedonic motivation), Perceived value, Satisfaction, and Engagement intention. Unfortunately, as in most of the previous definitions, authors do not provide operative measures that can be automatically acquired simply using an application as our project requires. Therefore, we propose our metrics in this paper.

3 Measure User Engagement

Starting from the previous definitions. We have realized a small survey on the different metrics that have been adopted so far for technological applications. The measure of user engagement appears in various forms. Depending on the aim that a company or research team is targeting, the metrics and the measuring approaches to capture user engagement clearly differ from each other. We base our taxonomy on the works of Lehmann et al. [12] and Lalmas et al. [11]. Summarizing their findings, the approaches to measure user engagement can be divided into three main approaches. **Self-reported Engagement.** In this group the way of capturing user engagement is by reporting the individual's perceptions, which can be done with questionnaires, interviews and think-aloud protocols. **Cognitive Engagement.** This approach uses task-based methods in combination with physiological measures to evaluate the cognitive engagement; in other words, this approach uses tools, such as heart rate monitors, eye trackers, etc. while a user is completing a predefined task. This approach is typically more objective than the former group, and can provide emotional and attentional information, which are not available in the conscious awareness. However, due to the complex setup needed, this method is not applicable in large-scale. **Interaction Engagement.** The preferred approach to measure user engagement is to exploit (web) analytics tools indicating information about the user's behaviour on a website. Such tools measure the user engagement based on a predefined set of metrics, e.g., the number of clicks, time spent on a site, return rate, etc. Although these metrics cannot explain why users engage with a service, it can be used to collect objective data from millions of users over a long period of time. Since this scenario is close to our needs, this paper focuses on this approach.

3.1 Measuring Metrics

According to Lehmann et al. [12], the engagement of a user strictly depends on the online services at hand and thus cannot be used for all kinds of web applications, e.g., the engagement of a user on a news portal differs from that on a search engine. On the contrary, Peterson and Carrabis [17] claim that the engagement measure can be unique otherwise this is like saying that *"every car will need a different measure of velocity or fuel consumption"*. In our opinion, both views might be right: we can define one set of metrics that can be used in different applications, but we need to interpret the engagement based on the type of the application, e.g., comparing a search engine with a gaming site indicates large differences regarding the dwell-time; but a short dwell-time on a search site does not imply low engagement; on the other hand, a gaming site with long dwell-times does not imply high engagement when it has a small number of visitors. The most widely used web analytics tool on the Internet is Google Analytics, a service that generates detailed statistics about the visits to a website [19]. Among a variety of metrics, which can be used by site owners for retrieving various kinds of visitor information, it provides three metrics that are commonly used to compute the engagement: *Page Views Per Session, Average Session Duration, and Bounce Rate* [7]. Once visitors come to a website, they will either read the page, click to more pages linked on the site, or leave the website. Previous, engagement metrics focus on the actions visitors are taking, and how good the website is at keeping the visitors there [4]. Other commonly known metrics used as measures of engagement are *Visits Per Visitor* and *Customer Satisfaction*. However, also these metrics have some limitations and can be inappropriate for use [17]. Under the assumption that a visitor will be considered engaged as long as she/he is paying attention to a website, Peterson and Carrabis [17] provide the following formula to calculate the engagement:

$$\sum (C_i + D_i + R_i + L_i + B_i + F_i + I_i)/7. \tag{1}$$

Each of these component indices represents a metric that is calculated based on a predefined threshold. Such thresholds are strictly depending on the corresponding website to be measured. In order to demonstrate the diversity of user engagement, authors analysed a large number of online sites of various types, and then derived models of engagement by clustering the sites against the criteria 'user type' and 'temporal aspect'. As proxy for online user engagement they measured the web usage assuming the higher and the more frequent the usage, the more engaged the user. The considered metrics to measure the user engagement cluster in three groups that reflect the *popularity, activity,* and *loyalty* of users. Therefore, a highly engaging site is one with a high number of visits (popular), where users spend lots of time (active), and return frequently (loyal). In order to effectively measure user engagement, authors propose of eliminating metrics that are too correlated. Their results show that metrics of the same groups mostly correlate, whereas metrics from different groups correlate only weakly or even not at all. Based on their results, Lehmann et al. claim that *Users, Click-Depth, DwellTimeA,* and *ActiveDays* are the most significant metrics that can be combined to obtain different models for different web applications.

4 Mobile Engagement

So far we have seen which metrics are widely used to measure user engagement in web applications. As the goal of this paper is to investigate the engagement in mobile applications, and as the topic of mobile user engagement is young, and therefore no profound investigative knowledge is available, we try to gain some new insights. In order to derive mobile engagement from web engagement, we first need to point out the differences between mobile and web usage. Based on these differences we then try to assess what metrics, which we defined for web engagement, can be used in mobile applications to measure user engagement. According to Isensee [13], the difference between mobile and web usage is in their concepts: while the mobile world follows the concept of users, the web world focuses on the concept of a visitor. The user concept states that the mobile phone is ubiquitous, much more personal than a PC which entails that if we want to measure the engagement of a certain mobile user we only need to know the device ID since mobile devices, in particular the mobile phone, are not shared among different people. However, this is not the case with PCs since they can be used in workstations, coffee shops, or shared with other family members. Hence, to figure out which person is behind the computer screen, we need to authorize the user, such as with a login, or in case the site does not provide authorization, just look to the IP address, which is often not easy. Another difference between mobile and web is that in web applications we can open several tabs in a browser, or even use multiple browsers simultaneously. This problem entails that we cannot know to which site the user behind the screen is really focusing its attention on. Even if we use a browser function that notifies us that the user switched the browser tab, we still cannot prove whether the user is consuming the open site or if it is doing something else, like cooking or talking on the phone. In contrast to this, in mobile applications there is the restriction that only one application can be launched at a time. If the mobile user is not focusing its attention to the mobile phone and does not interact with it, the screen would turn off within seconds.

5   Recommendations

As we stated in the Background Section, the metrics to measure user engagement must be based on the definition of engagement. In this section, we try to provide a set of metrics, which can be used to measure the user engagement in mobile applications based on the definition that *a user is engaged as long as he/she is actively paying attention to the application.* As this definition can be considered as a general mobile user engagement definition, it allows us to provide a set of metrics that has a universal character. This entails that our set of metrics is applicable to any kind of mobile application, regardless the definition of the user engagement. A mobile application owner who differently defines user engagement, only needs to change the weights of single metrics, e.g., in a news app the number of screen views typically must be more weighted than in a search engine app. Therefore, we propose the following metric:

$$ScreenView = \frac{\#Visit_i(Screens_i \geq T_{sv})}{\#TotalVisit_i}, \tag{2}$$

$$VisitDuration = \frac{\#Visits_i(Duration_i \geq T_{vd})}{\#TotalVisit_i}. \tag{3}$$

$$UserLoyality = \frac{\#Days_i \geq T_{ul}}{\#TestDays_i}, \tag{4}$$

Where: n = *number of users of the app;* i = *user-index;* M = *metric.*

Equation 2 Rationale. *ScreenView* computes the number of screens viewed by user i, which were over the threshold T_{sv} divided by the total number of visits by user i. Consider the following example: Customer sets threshold to $T_{sv} = 3$. The mobile user visits 3 times the app: visit 1: 3 screen views; visit 2: 8 screen views; visit 3: 2 screen views. As result *ScreenView* $= (1 + 1 + 0)/3 = 67\%$.

Equation 3 Rationale. *VisitDuration* computes the number of visits by user i, which lasted at least T_{vd} minutes, divided by the total number of visits by user i. Consider the following example: Customer sets threshold to $T_{vd} = 5$. The mobile user visits 4 times the app: visit 1: 4 min; visit 2: 5 min; visit 3: 100 min; visit 4: 2 min. As results *Visit-Duration* $= (0 + 1+1 + 0)/4 = 50\%$.

Equation 4 Rationale. *UserLoyalty* computes the number of days on which user i at least visited the app T_{ul} times, divided by the number of days of the considered timeframe for measuring the engagement. Again, consider the following example in which a customer sets the threshold to $T_{ul} = 2$. On a timeframe of 30 days, the mobile user visits every day the app, but only on 10 days it is visited more than once. As result, we obtain *UserLoyalty* $= 10/30 = 33\%$.

If each metric is equally weighted, we have an Engagement of $User_i = (67 + 50 + 33)/3 = 50\%$.

The above equations represent the user engagement in the per-user-scope. In order to compute the engagement in the per-app-scope, we propose Eq. 4, which averages the results over n users for a certain metric M:

$$EngagementPerApp_M = \sum_{i=1}^{n} \frac{M_i}{\#users}. \tag{5}$$

Where: $n = $ *number of users of the app; $i = $ user-index; $M = $ metric.*

6   Conclusion

This paper provides recommendations for measuring user engagement in mobile applications following the interaction measuring approach. We have investigated different definitions of user engagement and related metrics. Based on differences between web and mobile application nature and usage, we have defined our own set of metrics, which should be able to measure the user engagement in mobile applications. In addition to our recommendations for mobile metrics, we also have pointed out an important issue that asks whether it is possible to measure user engagement with a universal formula, or does every application need to be measured differently. These metrics will be evaluated in a pilot study involving 400 teenagers in four European countries (England, Italy, Scotland, and Spain).

References

1. Amazon Mobile Analytics. https://aws.amazon.com/mobileanalytics/. Accessed May 2016
2. Attfield, S., Kazai, G., Lalmas, M., Piwowarski, B.: Towards a science of user engagement (Position Paper). In: WSDM Workshop on User Modelling for Web Applications (2011)
3. Brown, E., Cairns, P.: A grounded investigation of game immersion. In: CHI 2004, pp. 1279–1300. ACM Press (2004)
4. Carrino, S., Caon, M., Abou Khaled, O., Andreoni, G., Mugellini, E.: PEGASO: towards a life companion. In: Duffy, V.G. (ed.) DHM 2014. LNCS, vol. 8529, pp. 325–331. Springer, Cham (2014). doi:10.1007/978-3-319-07725-3_32
5. Chapman, P.: Models of engagement: intrinsically motivated interaction with multimedia learning software (1997)
6. Csikszentmihalyi, M.: Beyond Boredom and Anxiety: Experiencing Flow in Work and Play. Jossey-Bass, San Francisco (1975)
7. Google Developers - Analytics Core Reporting API. https://developers.google.com/analytics/devguides/reporting/core/dimsmets#cats=session. Accessed Nov 2015
8. Haven, B., Vittal, S.: Measuring engagement. Marketing (2008)
9. Jennett, C., Cox, A.L., Cairns, P., Dhoparee, S., Epps, A., Tijs, T., Walton, A.: Measuring and defining the experience of immersion in games. Int. J. Hum.-Comput. Stud. **66**(9), 641–661 (2008)
10. Kim, Y.H., Kim, D.J., Wachter, K.: A study of mobile user engagement (MoEN): engagement motivations, perceived value, satisfaction, and continued engagement intention (2013)
11. Lalmas, M., O'Brien, H.L., Yom-Tov, E.: Measuring user engagement. Tutorial presented at the WWW Conference, Rio de Janeiro, Brazil, 13 May 2013
12. Lehmann, J., Lalmas, M., Yom-Tov, E., Dupret, G.: Models of user engagement. In: Masthoff, J., Mobasher, B., Desmarais, M.C., Nkambou, R. (eds.) UMAP 2012. LNCS, vol. 7379, pp. 164–175. Springer, Heidelberg (2012). doi:10.1007/978-3-642-31454-4_14
13. Localytics - Key Differences Between Mobile and Web Analytics. http://info.localytics.com/blog/. Accessed July 2016
14. Megalytic - Measuring Engagement with Google Analytics. https://megalytic.com/blog/measuring-engagement. Accessed Nov 2015
15. Nakamura, J., Csikszentmihalyi, M.: The concept of flow, in handbook of positive psychology. In: Snyder, C.R., López, S.J. (eds.) p. 829. Oxford University Press, New York (2002)
16. O'Brien, H.L., Toms, E.G.: What is user engagement? A conceptual framework for defining user engagement with technology. J. Am. Soc. Inform. Sci. Technol. **59**(6), 938–955 (2008)
17. Peterson, E.T., Carrabis, J.: Measuring the immeasurable: visitor engagement. Web Analytics Demystified **14**, 16 (2008)
18. Tomaselli, F., Sanchez, O., Brown, S.: How to engage users through gamification: the prevalent effects of playing and mastering over competing (2015)
19. W3 Techs - Web Technology Surveys. http://w3techs.com/technologies/overview/traffic_analysis/all. Accessed May 2016

Personalised Guidance Services for Optimising Lifestyle in Teen-Agers Through Awareness, Motivation and Engagement – PEGASO: A Pilot Study Protocol

Fulvio Adorni[1(✉)], Federica Prinelli[1], Chiara Crespi[1], Elisa Puigdomènech[2], Santiago Felipe Gomez[2], Espallargues Carreras Mireia[2], Castell Abat Conxa[2], Brian McKinstry[3], Anne Martin[3], Lucy McCloughan[3], Alexandra Lang[4], Laura Condon[4], Sarah Atkinson[4], Rajeeb Rashid[5], and On Behalf of the PEGASO Consortium

[1] Institute of Biomedical Technologies-National Research Council Segrate (MI), Segrate, Italy
{fulvio.adorni,federica.prinelli,chiara.crespi}@itb.cnr.it
[2] Agència de Qualitat i Avaluació Sanitàries de Catalunya, Barcelona, Spain
{epuigdomenech,sgomez,mespallargues,conxa.castell}@gencat.cat
[3] The University of Edinburgh, Edinburgh, UK
{Brian.McKinstry,Anne.Martin,lucy.mccloughan}@ed.ac.uk
[4] University of Nottingham, Nottingham, UK
{Alexandra.Lang,Laura.Condon,Sarah.Atkinson}@nottingham.ac.uk
[5] NHS Lothian, Edinburgh, UK
rajeeb.rashid@nhs.net

Abstract. Adolescence is a vulnerable stage in which the development of certain unhealthy behaviours can occur. The prevalence of overweight and obesity among European teenagers is rapidly increasing and may lead to both short- and long-term health complications. The fast development of the ICT, and in particular mobile technologies, together with their increasing diffusion among the EU populations offers an important opportunity for facing these issues in an innovative manner introducing the possibility of a new technological framework to re-design the healthcare system model. The PEGASO project relies on a mobile-and-cloud-based ICT platform to set up a system of new healthcare services targeted to teens for obesity prevention. The present paper describes the protocol of a six-month Pilot Study that will be carried out on 525 adolescents in four different European sites (Italy, Catalonia, England, Scotland), aiming to evaluate the PEGASO system usability and effectiveness in promoting healthy lifestyles.

Keywords: ICT · Lifestyles habits · Adolescents · Awareness · Motivation

1 Introduction

Adolescence is a vulnerable stage in which the development of certain unhealthy behaviours can occur, such as the adoption and maintenance of maladaptive lifestyles [1].

© ICST Institute for Computer Sciences, Social Informatics and Telecommunications Engineering 2017
P. Perego et al. (Eds.): MobiHealth 2016, LNICST 192, pp. 45–52, 2017.
DOI: 10.1007/978-3-319-58877-3_6

The adoption of and the adherence to healthy lifestyles amongst the young population is a crucial issue in order to: (a) improve the health, as well as physical and mental well-being of teenagers [2–5]; (b) maintain a healthy lifestyle during adulthood; and, (c) prevent sedentary behaviour, overweight and obesity and other chronic diseases related to a unhealthy lifestyle, like cardiovascular diseases or cancer [6].

In particular, healthy dietary habits [7], regular physical activity [8], and good sleeping behaviour [9] during adolescence play an important role as protective factors in the development of both short- and long-term chronic diseases, also including overweight and obesity during adulthood [10, 11]. According to the World Health Organization (WHO), more than 50% of the European adult population is overweight, more than 20% are obese, and the prevalence of overweight among European 13-year-olds is about 27% [12, 13]. Taking into account these data and the fact that overweight adolescents are at higher risk to be overweight in adulthood [12], the promotion of healthy lifestyles among adolescents is a major issue from a public health perspective.

Concurrently, the rapid development of the information and communication technologies (ICTs) – and in particular mobile technologies – together with their increasing diffusion among the EU populations (>60 millions of person only in EU-5), offers an important opportunity for facing overweight and obesity issues in an innovative manner, and also introduces the possibility to re-design the healthcare system model on the basis of a new technological framework.

Teenagers live in a highly technological world and are considered to be technology natives. In fact, ICTs – and especially those linked to mobile phones/smartphones, tablets, electronic bracelets, intelligent clothing and other devices – are being rapidly extended amongst adolescents. Digital platforms allow teenagers to go beyond mere face-to-face contact, to be connected online and to have access to information included in social media and networks, independently from the socioeconomic or familial strata [14]. In this context, public health authorities have a great opportunity to spread key messages for adolescents to promote habits of healthy life in a creative and innovative way [15].

2   Objectives

The PEGASO (Personalised Guidance Services for Optimising lifestyle in teen-agers through awareness, motivation and engagement) project aims to develop an ICT based system to motivate behavioural changes towards healthier lifestyles in adolescents. The specific objectives of the present Pilot Study are to test the PEGASO system in real life conditions in Lombardy, England, Scotland and Catalonia, as well as to assess changes in teenagers' awareness and lifestyles as a result of the use of PEGASO system. Specifically, we aim to:

(1) Test the usability of PEGASO platform.
(2) Test the effectiveness of the system to promote:
     (a) increase of knowledge/awareness about healthy habits
     (b) behavioural change in lifestyle, and specifically on target behaviours.

3   Subjects and Methods

3.1   Study Design

A multi-centre quasi-experimental controlled pilot study will be undertaken to evaluate the PEGASO System from October 2016 to March 2017.

3.2   Study Population

Approximately a total of 525 voluntary adolescents aged 13–16 years old (gender balanced) will be enrolled in selected high schools belonging to the four different sites, including Lombardy (Italy), Catalonia (Spain), England and Scotland (UK). Participants will be allocated to the intervention or comparative group in a 2:1 ratio. Therefore, about 350 participants will test the PEGASO platform, whilst 175 will be included in the comparative group. Sample selection will be carried out in two stages: in the first phase, schools with medium-low socioeconomic level will be selected by convenience sampling; in the second phase classes will be selected for participation in each school in agreement with schools principals/head teachers. Classes of students at each school considered suitable to take part in the study will be identified. Study information will then be disseminated to parents and students so that individuals can voluntarily 'opt in' and take part in the study.

The approval from the research Ethics Committee (EC) of the participant pilot sites will be asked. Students and their parents will be required to sign the informed consent prior to inclusion in the study, in accordance with the Declaration of Helsinki. The confidentiality of the recruited subjects will be ensured at all times in accordance with the provisions of current legislation on personal data protection.

3.3   PEGASO Ecosystem

The development of the PEGASO system is guided by the comprehensive Behaviour Change Wheel (BCW) framework [16] and in particular by the Capability-Opportunity-Motivation-Behaviour (COM-B) system. The highly innovative key component of the PEGASO system is the behaviour recognition system that allows detection and evaluation of participants' real-time behaviour (collected through other components of the PEGASO system. The lifestyle behaviours targeted (Table 1) by the PEGASO system include known potential modifiable risk factors for obesity development in adolescents.

PEGASO comprises seven different components (Fig. 1). The Companion is the main application of the platform that integrates all the apps developed in the PEGASO system and provides a seamless and unique experience to the participant. Companion is a Personal Digital "Friend" acting as a daily-life guide for coaching, caring for, and empowering the participants in their activities toward healthy habits. The Companion includes:

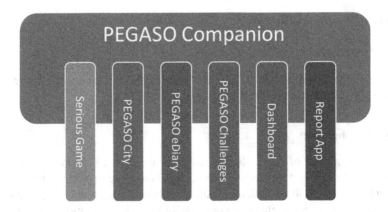

Fig. 1. PEGASO ecosystem

Table 1. Target behaviours definitions

Target behaviours	Cut-off definition
Diet	Fruit consumption of ≥2 servings (250–375 g)/day of at least two different types
	Vegetable consumption of ≥2 servings (300–450 g)/day of at least two different types
	Reduced intake of sugar-sweetened beverages
	Breakfast consumption including intake of food from more than two food groups
	Reduced intake of fast food
	Reduced sweet and salty high-energy snack intake
Physical activity and Sedentariness	60 min of daily physical activity in moderate-to-vigorous intensity
	12.000 steps/day
	Daily active transport to and from school (walking, cycling, skateboarding)
	<45% of after-school time daily spent in sedentary activities (<1.5 MET)
Sleep	Daily sleep duration of at least 8 h
	≥95% of bed time spent sleeping (i.e. sleep quality/efficiency)

(i) The *eDiary* app is an application that collects dietary habits entered by the users and provides feedback about the healthy eating habits and suggestions for improving their dietary behaviours;

(ii) The *Challenge* app allows users to challenge themselves and other users in a competitive or collaborative way.

(iii) The *City* app is a bridge between the digital world of the PEGASO system with the physical world: helps teenagers to find places that are part of the PEGASO

Stakeholder Ecosystem and provides the teenagers a set of possible interactions and actions that contribute to the gamification process and the rewarding system.

(iv) The *Dashboard* app allows visualizing all the data acquired (steps and minutes of activities, sleep time, type of activities) by the PEGASO system. The smart garments measure heart rate (ECG) and physical activities (accelerometer) whereas the bracelet monitors physical activities and sleep.

(v) The *Serious Game* serves a central role as the motivational component of PEGASO. As such, it needs to entertain and engage the player, whilst using the PEGASO ecosystem to capture information about lifestyles and encourage positive health behaviour changes.

(vi) The *Web Portal* allows participants to socially interact and learn via training module; two (technological): aggregate data and services across the whole PEGASO platform (images, video, blog materials, activities data, n° of steps, n° of km).

(vii) The *Report App* represents a connection between the PEGASO ecosystem and the personal health folder. The BRIDGE allows extracting health data collected and elaborated into the PEGASO ecosystem and to create a report to be shared with physicians into the personal health folder (PHF). This functionality will only be available in Lombardy and Catalonia.

3.4 Procedures

Schools and participants of both intervention and comparative group will be given information about the purpose of the study at a single face-to-face session held by the field researchers. The students allocated to the intervention group will be provided with a smart phone (android, version 5.0), two smart garments, a smart garment sensor and an activity bracelet (Fig. 2) for the duration of the Pilot Study (6 months). The smart phones will have all apps of the PEGASO ecosystem installed.

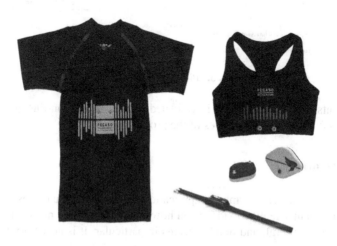

Fig. 2. Smart garments and bracelets sensors

In addition, participants will be asked to join the PEGASO community by signing in to the PEGASO Portal (https://portal.pegasof4f.eu/web/others/sign-in).

Those students assigned to the comparative group will be asked to continue their routine daily physical and educational activities related to leading a healthy lifestyle.

PEGASO framework will provide the tools to evaluate the groups in three time points during the pilot study (Fig. 3):

- *Baseline evaluation*: assessment of users' profile regarding the pre-specified indicators before the use of the platform (i.e., socio-demographic characteristics, anthropometric measurements, lifestyle behaviours, motivation, knowledge);
- *Mid-pilot evaluation (month 3)*: mid-term evaluation will be focused on teenagers' feelings and perceptions of the platform (i.e., usability, satisfaction, emotional response, motivation);
- *Final evaluation (month 6)*: at the end of the intervention we will compare teenagers' progresses against the identified targets and both the initial and the mid-pilot evaluation (i.e., usability, satisfaction, emotional response, trusting technology, anthropometric measurements, lifestyle behaviours, motivation, knowledge).

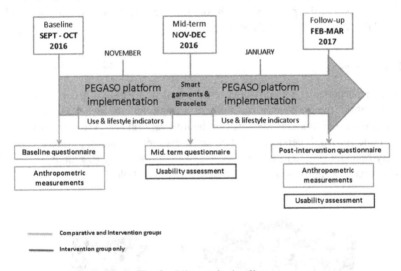

Fig. 3. Pilot study timeline

Participants will be asked to fill in validated and/or 'ad *hoc*' on-line questionnaires in order to assess the main objectives of the project.

4   Discussion

The vast development of smartphone applications in health care and lifestyles fields is lacking of sufficient scientific evidence on how applications can improve the health of the population in general, and in adolescents in particular. It is necessary to pilot and conduct experimental studies to obtain sufficient scientific evidence of the possible usefulness of these tools.

With the present Pilot Study we expect to test the effectiveness that regular use of the PEGASO platform will have on the improvement of lifestyles (in terms of dietary behaviour, physical activity and sedentary and sleeping behaviours) among adolescents, over a period of six month. Hence, the results of this study could lead to a strategy based on the incorporation of mHealth solutions among teenagers, would result in healthier lifestyles.

Acknowledgements. The European Commission under the 7th Framework Programme funds the PEGASO project. The authors of the paper wish to thank all the partners of the PEGASO Consortium for their contribution to the work.

References

1. Moreno, L.A., Gottrand, F., Huybrechts, I., Ruiz, J.R., González-Gross, M., DeHenauw, S.: HELENA study group: nutrition and lifestyle in European adolescents: the HELENA (Healthy lifestyle in Europe by nutrition in adolescence) study. Adv. Nutr. **5**, 615S–623S (2015)
2. Sawyer, S.M., Afifi, R.A., Bearinger, L.H., Blakemore, S.-J., Dick, B., Ezeh, A.C., et al.: Adolescence: a foundation for future health. Lancet **379**, 1630–1640 (2014)
3. Black, M.M., Hurley, K.M.: Investment in early childhood development. Lancet **384**, 1244–1245 (2014)
4. Dick, B., Ferguson, B.J.: Health for the world's adolescents: a second chance in the second decade. J. Adolesc. Health **56**, 3–6 (2015)
5. World Health Organization (WHO): Adolescent Development (2015). http://www.who.int/maternal_child_adolescent/topics/adolescence/development
6. Diethelm, K., Jankovic, N., Moreno, L.A., Huybrechts, I., De Henauw, S., De Vriendt, T., González-Gross, M., Leclercq, C., Gottrand, F., Gilbert, C.C., Dallongeville, J., Cuenca-Garcia, M., Manios, Y., Kafatos, A., Plada, M., Kersting, M.: HELENA study group: food intake of European adolescents in the light of different food-based dietary guidelines: results of the HELENA (Healthy lifestyle in Europe by nutrition in adolescence) study. Public Health Nutr. **15**, 386–398 (2012)
7. Ambrosini, G.: Childhood dietary patterns and later obesity: a review of the evidence. Proc. Nutr. Soc. **73**, 137–146 (2014)
8. Rauner, A., Mess, F., Woll, A.: The relationship between physical activity, physical fitness and overweight in adolescents: a systematic review of studies published in or after 2000. BMC Pediatr. **13**, 19 (2013)
9. Fatima, Y., Doi, S.A., Mamun, A.A.: Longitudinal impact of sleep on overweight and obesity in children and adolescents: a systematic review and bias-adjusted meta-analysis. Obes. Rev. **16**, 137–149 (2015)
10. Pate, R.R., O'Neill, J.R., Liese, A.D., Janz, K.F., Granberg, E.M., Colabianchi, N., Harsha, D.W., Condrasky, M.M., O'Neil, P.M., Lau, E.Y., et al.: Factors associated with development of excessive fatness in children and adolescents: a review of prospective studies. Obes. Rev. **14**, 645–658 (2013)
11. Biro, F.M., Wien, M.: Childhood obesity and adult morbidities. Am. J. Clin. Nutr. **91**, 1499S–1505S (2010)

12. World Health Organization. Country profiles on nutrition, physical activity and obesity in the 53 WHO European Region Member States. Methodology and summary (2013). https://issuu.com/whoeurope/docs/country_profiles_on_nutrition_53_me/6847445
13. Gallus, S., Lugo, A., Murisic, B., Bosetti, C., Boffetta, P., La Vecchia, C.: Overweight and obesity in 16 European countries. Eur. J. Nutr. **54**, 679–689 (2015)
14. Wong, C.A., Merchant, R.M., Moreno, M.A.: Using social media to engage adolescents and young adults with their health. Healthc (Amst) **2**, 220–224 (2014)
15. Vandewater, E.A., Denis, L.M.: Media, social networking, and pediatric obesity. Pediatr. Clin. North Am. **58**, 1509–1519 (2011)
16. Michie, S., Atkins, L., West, R.: The Behaviour Change Wheel: A Guide to Designing Intervention. Silverback Publishing, UK (2014)

PEGASO Companion: A Mobile App to Promote Healthy Lifestyles Among Adolescents

Maurizio Caon[1(✉)], Stefano Carrino[1], Laura Condon[2], Antonio Ascolese[3],
Sara Facchinetti[4], Marco Mazzola[5], Paolo Perego[6], Filip Velickovski[7],
Giuseppe Andreoni[6], and Elena Mugellini[1]

[1] University of Applied Sciences and Arts Western Switzerland, Fribourg, Switzerland
maurizio.caon@hes-so.ch
[2] University of Nottingham, Nottingham, UK
[3] Imaginary SRL, Milan, Italy
[4] Lombardia Informatica SPA, Milan, Italy
[5] Neosperience SPA, Milan, Italy
[6] Politecnico di Milano, Milan, Italy
[7] Technology Centre of Catalonia, Barcelona, Spain

Abstract. Promoting healthy lifestyles can be a successful weapon in counter-fighting the epidemics of overweight and obesity. The PEGASO project aims at encouraging adolescents to become co-creators of their own health. In particular, it aims at creating an ecosystem where adolescents are motivated and supported in adopting healthy lifestyles. In this ecosystem, the PEGASO Companion, a smartphone app, plays the role of universal access to healthy services and providing personalised mechanisms to support behaviour change.

Keywords: Obesity prevention · Persuasive technology · Gamification · Behaviour change

1 Introduction

In the last few years, obesity became epidemic and a general alarm has been issued worldwide. Although many organisations, research institutes and governments took action to solve this problem, no country to date has reversed its obesity epidemic [10]. In this scenario, prevention in healthcare plays a crucial role: the aim of each national healthcare system should be shifting from the concept of "cure" to "care" emphasising also the reciprocal nature of the interaction between the environment and the individual [8]. This requires new regulatory actions from governments, to be coordinated with increased efforts from industry and civil society in order to create a new complex and multifactorial process in which technological factors, organisational strategies, and human dimensions can find the correct balance to enable the population to adopt healthy lifestyles [8].

The PEGASO project aims at developing an ecosystem where users are encouraged and facilitated in adopting healthy lifestyles through the coordinated actions of policy makers, schools, healthcare providers and other stakeholders (such as companies and

P. Perego et al. (Eds.): MobiHealth 2016, LNICST 192, pp. 53–61, 2017.
DOI: 10.1007/978-3-319-58877-3_7

associations). In this ecosystem, the multi-dimensional and cross-disciplinary ICT system plays a key role. This system includes game mechanisms, multimedia services and social activities to influence users' behaviours in order to fight and prevent overweight and obesity in the younger population by encouraging them to become coproducers of their wellness and take an active role in improving it. This complex system communicates with the young users through a smartphone application called Companion, which is able to monitor the user's lifestyle in order to empower and support him/her in improving his/her wellbeing through motivational mechanisms and tailored interventions.

In this paper, the PEGASO Companion is introduced in the frame of the vision for the application of artificial intelligence in the future of healthcare. After presenting this vision, the paper follows describing the current development of a first version of the PEGASO Companion in the frame of the current European project: in particular, the architecture, the user experience design and scientific grounding are presented and briefly discussed.

2   The Companion Vision

In the frame of the PEGASO project, the smartphone will embody the Companion to guide the user's lifestyle. However, the PEGASO Companion vision is not linked to a unique physical device but it is conceived as a ubiquitous artificial intelligence, which changes form over time to accompany the user throughout her/his life adapting to her/his evolving needs and desires [4]. The Companion will understand the user's personality and will establish with her/him a long-lasting affective relationship. The Companion will participate to the whole user's life in order to become a real life companion. Different ages and stages of maturity have different requirements and the Companion has to be able to continuously adapt to novel needs and propose appropriate activities.

Although the Companion vision comprehends a large picture depicting a future artificial intelligence being able to accompany the user's whole life, in the frame of the PEGASO project, the system has been conceived to be focused on just the adolescence. Indeed, the World Health Organization reported that over 60% of children who are overweight before puberty will be overweight in early adulthood. This implies that the adolescence is a crucial period for choices concerning the lifestyle. PEGASO aims at developing a whole ecosystem that would be able to motivate teenagers to learn and to apply a healthy life-style effortlessly in order to prevent obesity in adulthood.

3   Architecture

Many entities compose the PEGASO guidance and support system. Figure 1 presents the relationship between the different entities from a functional perspective to provide a preview of the elements that will be addressed in this document. This figure abstracts from the actual technological implementation.

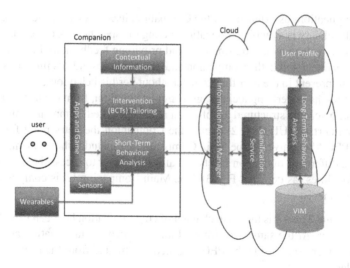

Fig. 1. Relation among the entities composing the PEGASO guidance and supporting system. (Color figure online)

The user interacts with the system via wearable sensors, sensors embedded in the smartphone, multiple apps and a serious game (in purple in Fig. 1). Such interactions allow the system to tailor the Virtual Individual Model (VIM) to the user (the VIM concept and the tailoring approach are detailed in [2, 3]). The VIM, together with the user profile, allows the long-term behaviour analysis module to suggest a healthy target behaviour and to assess the user adherence to the selected target behaviour. At the same time, the long-term module will specify to the gamification service, which personalised rewards should be created and evaluated (red blocks in Fig. 1). Then, inside the user's smartphone, contextual information, together with the events detected in the short-term behaviour analysis module, the output from the cloud long-term module and the gamification service will allow creating tailored interventions (blue blocks in Fig. 1). Such interventions will be operationalised via functions inside the app and the PEGASO serious game. All these modules are embedded in a container mobile app called Health Companion.

4   User Experience

PEGASO is composed of multiple applications and services. Most of them are related to one or multiple target behaviours that have been selected by the user with the help of the system. However, the PEGASO Companion is the main interface between the user and the PEGASO system and plays a major role in PEGASO. In fact, the role of the Companion is to unify the user experience within PEGASO. Via the Companion, the user will have the possibility to access seamlessly the different apps, which for the user will appear as a unique, modular application. Therefore, in this paper we focus on the action mechanisms present in the Companion taking into account the functionalities of the other applications as extension of the Companion itself. Consider the eDiary app as example: the eDiary is a mobile application having the specific task of dealing with the nutrition target behaviours, acquiring data and providing feedback to the user. Such an application is integrated in the Companion and, therefore, extends its functions with the possibility to present to the user the feedback about her/his behaviour.

Neglecting the underlying technological implementation, from the user perspective the Companion can be structured as follow: a main app called Companion provides the Main User Interface (UI) (Fig. 2). Being the Companion the entry point for the user inside the PEGASO universe, the Main Companion UI includes the elements that glue together the different Companion facets and allows the user to access the different apps and functionalities (as depicted Fig. 3). The Main Companion UI is composed by the following elements:

- News stream. This UI is the main channel of communication between PEGASO and the final user. At the same time, this UI allows receiving information and updates from the other users inside the PEGASO ecosystem, and from the user's friends in particular.
- Friend UI. This UI allows the user to add friends and accept friendship requests.
- App launcher. This UI allows launching the other PEGASO functions (such as applications).
- User profile. This UI presents the profile to the user showing personal information, the FitCoins balance, the level and badges.

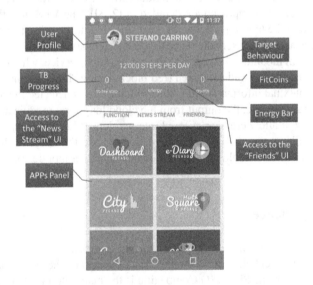

Fig. 2. Companion main User Interface.

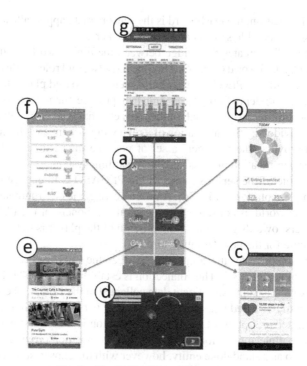

Fig. 3. The PEGASO mobile ecosystem.

Another important aspect of the Companion is that it integrates different services for Gamification (connected to a rewarding system with access to services provided by other stakeholders), and a tailored messaging system, which allows personalising the communication with the user according to her/his characteristics and preferences.

Moreover, as already mentioned, the Companion provides the possibility to access all the PEGASO services from a single point of access. In practical terms, this main access is represented by the "Function" tab, which contains all the Apps Panels, which are buttons that allow launching the associated services or applications.

The Companion applications integrated in the current version of the Companion are the eDiary, the Challenges, the Dashboard, the PEGASO City, the Mobile Serious Game, and the Report App. These apps are introduced in the next paragraph.

The **eDiary** is a new kind of food record application for smartphone explicitly designed for teenagers and able to monitor their dietary behaviours (Fig. 3b). It also is able to provide an immediate educational feedback based on dietary data patterns introduced by the users.

The **Challenges** app is another component of the PEGASO Companion allowing users to challenge themselves and the other users (Fig. 3c). Its objective is to motivate the user to achieve her/his target behaviour exploiting goal fixing and social elements.

The main goal of the PEGASO **Dashboard** is to present to the user visual feedback and suggestions about target behaviours related to physical activity, sedentariness and sleep (Fig. 3f). In addition, the Dashboard is the sensors mate app: it allows connecting with and managing wearable sensors and fitness trackers.

The PEGASO **City** creates the bridge between the digital world of the PEGASO system with the physical world (Fig. 3e). This app has a twofold role inside the PEGASO Health Companion: firstly, PEGASO City helps teenagers to find places that are part of the PEGASO Stakeholders' Ecosystem, and that provide them opportunities to act healthy and progress towards the reach of their target behaviour. Secondly, through the empowerment provided by the integration of a reviewing system and sharing functions, the application provides the teenagers a set of possible interactions and actions that contribute to the gamification process and the rewarding system.

The primary role of the **serious game** within PEGASO is to engage and motivate users of the complete platform (Fig. 3d). An immersive game environment, in this case a post-apocalyptic world, is considered as a central component of the PEGASO game to engage the users towards gameplay. The mission of the player is to help the government finding a cure for the new 'zombie' virus [7].

The **Report** App provides the connection between the PEGASO ecosystem and the personal health folder (Fig. 3g). The connection is established via the "bridge" system, which allows extracting some significant data collected in the PEGASO ecosystem and to create a report to be shared with physicians into the personal health folder.

From an architectural point of view, the Companion is a modular application that allows other compatible applications to plug in. The Companion provides a basic set of functionalities also as a standalone entity, however with the chosen solution, the user is able to select which component is more suitable for her/him. For instance, if a user does not want to use the eDiary but she likes playing the serious game or challenging her friends, she can decide to have only these modules of the PEGASO ecosystem.

5 Scientific Grounding and Main Concepts

PEGASO has developed a conceptual framework for biological, behavioural and psychosocial characterisation of adolescents, which will allow their behaviour recognition, personalised interaction and, in specific cases, the intervention for behaviour change. More in detail, PEGASO system focuses on those behaviours, pertaining to nutrition, physical activity and sleeping habits, which have been recognised to have impact on overweight/obesity prevention, and are amenable to be changed.

Their identification is based also on their detectability using the interaction with the user through the PEGASO Companion, the eDiary, the game, and also through non-invasive devices, such as mobile embedded accelerometers, sensorised bracelet and garments, which will accompany the users during their everyday life.

On the selected target behaviours, the system of PEGASO will be able to start user-specific educative/informative interaction, in order to raise users' awareness and tailor adequate actions to change them, when appropriate. Such tailored interventions are grounded on psychological theories and frameworks: the Behaviour Change Wheel framework, the Positive psychology, the Self-Determination Theory and Gamification.

5.1 Behaviour Change Wheel

The Behaviour Change Wheel framework (BCW) is a meta-framework synthesised from 19 existing frameworks of human behaviour change [9]. At the centre of the BCW is the COM-B behaviour system involving three essential components of human behaviour: Capability, Opportunity, and Motivation around which are positioned nine intervention functions aimed at addressing deficits in one or more of these components. The strength of this framework is the easiness to design tailored interventions for a specific user associating the sources of behaviours to specific intervention functions. In particular, PEGASO will tailor the intervention using a complementary tool the COM-B questionnaire. This self-assessment questionnaire provides an indication of the user self-awareness related to a specific target behaviour for each of the three components of the COM-B behaviour system that contribute to motivate the user to adhere to the target behaviour.

5.2 Positive Psychology

Positive psychology focuses on positive subjective experience, positive personality traits, and improving quality of life to prevent the negative consequences (i.e., negative mental and physical health consequences) of living an empty and unfulfilling life [13]. At the subjective level, it is concerned with valued personal experiences: well-being, contentment, and satisfaction (in the past); hope and optimism (for the future); and flow and happiness (in the present). Finally, at the group level, it is about the civic virtues and the institutions that move individuals toward better citizenship: responsibility, altruism, civility, moderation, tolerance, and work ethic.

- Autonomy means to be the first responsible of the actions of one's one life
- Competence means to gain mastery (via experience) in a specific task.
- Relatedness refers to the innate desire for interpersonal attachments: interacting, being connected and caring for the others [1].

Motivational mechanisms argue that social-contextual events can increase the feelings of autonomy, competence and relatedness. For example, a simple badge provided when achieving a goal can affect the feeling of competence.

5.3 Self-Determination Theory

The Self-Determination Theory (SDT) is a theory of motivation concerned with supporting behaviours that are natural and intrinsic in the human being (and, therefore, self-motivated and self-determined) [5, 11]. SDT states that there are three universal, innate, psychological needs: need for autonomy, competence and psychological relatedness [12]. The satisfaction of these needs lead to an enhanced self-motivation and mental-health.

5.4 Gamification and Serious Games

The user will follow the strategies for behaviour change only if the system is successful to engage her/him. Therefore, the user motivation plays a crucial role for the functioning of PEGASO (it is not just a chance that motivation is one major component of the COM-B model). PEGASO directly tackles this aspect via the use of two different persuasive mechanisms: gamification and serious gaming. It is important to distinguish these two close approaches:

- **Gamification.** The definition of Gamification consists of the use of game design elements in non-game contexts [6].
- **Serious Game.** The Serious Game describes the design of full-fledged games for non-entertainment purposes [6].

From these definitions, we can see that the boundary between the two approaches can be blurred and the actual approach will be subjective and dependent on how the user plays or uses an application. In PEGASO, we are developing a serious game and different gamified applications that are gamified, but that are not games.

6   Conclusion

In this paper, the PEGASO project has been presented. In particular, the focus was on the role of the Companion in providing access to innovative services and for the use of personalised mechanisms to motivate teenagers to adopt healthy lifestyles in order to promote obesity prevention.

Acknowledgment. The PEGASO project is co-funded by the European Commission through the 610727 FP7 project grant under the 7th Framework Programme.

References

1. Baumeister, R.F., Leary, M.R.: The need to belong: Desire for interpersonal attachments as a fundamental human motivation. Psychol. Bull. **117**(3), 497 (1995)
2. Caon, M., Carrino, S., Guarneri, R., Andreoni, G., Lafortuna, C.L., Abou Khaled, O., Mugellini, E.: A persuasive system for obesity prevention in teenagers: A concept. In: Proceedings of the Second International Workshop on Behavior Change Support Systems (BCSS 2014), Padova, Italy, May 2014
3. Carrino, S., Caon, M., Angelini, L., Mugellini, E., Khaled, O.A., Orte, S., Vargiu, E., Coulson, N., Serrano, J.C., Tabozzi, S., Lafortuna, C.: PEGASO: A personalized and motivational ICT system to empower adolescents towards healthy lifestyles. In: Innovation in Medicine and Healthcare (2014)
4. Carrino, S., Caon, M., Khaled, O.A., Andreoni, G., Mugellini, E.: PEGASO: Towards a life companion. In: Duffy, V.G. (ed.) International Conference on Digital Human Modeling and Applications in Health, Safety, Ergonomics and Risk Management. LNCS, pp. 325–331. Springer, Cham (2014). doi:10.1007/978-3-319-07725-3_32

5. Deci, E.L., Vansteenkiste, M.: Self-determination theory and basic need satisfaction: Understanding human development in positive psychology. Ricerche di Psicologia (2004)
6. Deterding, S., Sicart, M., Nacke, L., O'Hara, K., Dixon, D.: Gamification using game-design elements in non-gaming contexts. In: CHI 2011 Extended Abstracts on Human Factors in Computing Systems, pp. 2425–2428. ACM, May 2011
7. Dunwell, I., Dixon, R., Morosini, D.: A mobile serious game for lifestyle change: Conveying nutritional knowledge and motivation through play. In: 2015 International Conference on Interactive Mobile Communication Technologies and Learning (IMCL), pp. 259–263. IEEE (2015)
8. Guarneri, R., Andreoni, G.: Active prevention by motivating and engaging teenagers in adopting healthier lifestyles: In: Duffy, Vincent G. (ed.) DHM 2014. LNCS, vol. 8529, pp. 351–360. Springer, Cham (2014). doi:10.1007/978-3-319-07725-3_35
9. Michie, S., van Stralen, M.M., West, R.: The behaviour change wheel: a new method for characterising and designing behaviour change interventions. Implementation Sci. **6**(1), 1 (2011)
10. Roberto, C.A., Swinburn, B., Hawkes, C., Huang, T.T., Costa, S.A., Ashe, M., Zwicker, L., Cawley, J.H., Brownell, K.D.: Patchy progress on obesity prevention: Emerging examples, entrenched barriers, and new thinking. Lancet **385**(9985), 2400–2409 (2015)
11. Ryan, R.M., Deci, E.L.: Intrinsic and extrinsic motivations: Classic definitions and new directions. Contemp. Educ. Psychol. **25**(1), 54–67 (2000)
12. Ryan, R.M., Deci, E.L.: Self-determination theory and the facilitation of intrinsic motivation, social development, and well-being. Am. Psychol. **55**(1), 68 (2000)
13. Seligman, M.E., Csikszentmihalyi, M.: Positive psychology: An introduction, pp. 279–298. Springer, Netherlands (2014)

Device for m-Health

SmartMATES for Medication Adherence Using Non-intrusive Wearable Sensors

A.H. Abdullah$^{(\boxtimes)}$ and T.H. Lim

Universiti Teknologi Brunei, Tungku Highway, Gadong, Brunei Darussalam
thlim73@gmail.com, lim.tiong.hoo@utb.edu.bn

Abstract. According to the National institute on Aging, 8% of the world's population is over 65 or older. There is a need for a long term care and a remote home-care environment for the aging population using smart technologies as this number expected to double by 2050. With the advancement of embedded sensing technologies, wireless sensing technologies have been used to monitor user's activities and maintain a healthy lifestyle. In this paper, we develop a Smart Medication Alert and Treatment Electronic Systems (SmartMATES) using a non-intrusive wearable sensor system to detect and prevent a home-based patient from missing his or her medication. The sensor collects and processes both the accelerometer and radio signal strength measurement on the left and right wrist. Based on the data collected, SmartMATES correlates the left and right wrist accelerometer reading to model the action of taking medication. If SmartMATES detects the patient is not taking the medication within a time-frame, it will be send an alert to the mobile phone to remind the users to take their medication. We have evaluated the SmartMATES on 9 participants. The results show that the Smart-MATES can identify and prevent missing dosage in a less intrusive way than existing mobile application and traditional approaches.

Keywords: Medication adherence · Body sensor networks · Activities recognition · Hand gesture

1 Introduction

Medication adherence is known to be a problem for patients especially elderly who experience forgetfulness and suffers from a number of medical conditions that require different medications. Studies have shown that 26% of the hospitalization were caused by non-adherence of medicine therapy which involved elderly patients above 75 years of age due to fall, postural hypotension, heart failure and delirium [1]. According to the World Health Organization [2], medication adherence is defined as "the degree to which the person's behavior corresponds with the agreed recommendations from a healthcare provider". When the patients begin to deviate from their recommended prescription, it is known as non-adherence. There are two types of non-adherence namely primary and non-persistence [2]. Primary non-adherence occurs when healthcare providers

© ICST Institute for Computer Sciences, Social Informatics and Telecommunications Engineering 2017
P. Perego et al. (Eds.): MobiHealth 2016, LNICST 192, pp. 65–70, 2017.
DOI: 10.1007/978-3-319-58877-3_8

prescribe the medicine but is never filled or started. Non-persistence occurs when the patients accidentally miss or stop taking medication after starting it without the advice from a doctor. Non-persistence is usually unintentional and occurs when there is a misunderstanding between the patients and healthcare providers. It may also happen for elderlies who suffer from a decline in functional abilities, such as cognitive, vision and/or hearing impairment, that prevent them from executing their decisions to follow treatment [3]. Hence, there is a need for an assisted Internet based technology to detect and alert the patient to take miss dosage or realignment of medication adherence.

Advancement in electronic technologies and smart mobile applications have helped in medication adherence. Electronic monitoring chip, such as the Medication Event Monitoring Systems (MEMS) [4], has been inserted into medication bottle cap to record the date and time the patient opens and closes the bottle. This system can detect single opening and closing for a single dose but may result in inaccuracy for multiple doses [4]. The device also only records the prescription intake and does not provide any reminder or alert for missing dosage. It is necessary to alert the patients to take the missing doses using device such as CompuMed [5] and mHealth [6]. CompuMed is a medication dispenser that emits an audible tone to remind the patients. It can be programmed at regular to alert the patients to take their medication, with an option to call the patient. Although experimental results from Winland and Valiente have shown fewer missed doses with CompuMed compared to MEMS pill box [5], constantly sending alert at regular interval can be very annoying to the patients. There is also a probability that the patients may miss their medication when they are outdoor as they cannot take the CompuMed with them. The price of CompuMed is also significantly higher than MEMS pill box.

In this paper, we develop a non-intrusive wearable Smart Medication Alert and Treatment Electronic Systems (SmartMATES) and test SmartMATES on 15 participants. SmartMATES uses two 3-axis accelerometer to track the left and right hand gestures and identify the motion of taking a medicine from its packaging and consuming it. Based on the measurement of the accelerometers and the radio signal between the left and right wrists, SmartMATES will detect and only alert the user if he or she forgets misses a medicine prescription. Existing smart phone applications use pre-defined interval to remind the user to take the medication. However, constantly sending alarm to the users can be intruding when the users have already taken the medication. The main contributions of the paper are:

- A real time smart medicine adherence systems system only alert the user if they have not taken the medicine within the prescription time.
- An non-intrusive wearable sensor system that can identify and differentiate between the action of taking medication from other Activities of Daily Life (ADL). These sensor systems can be attached to cardigan or other clothing materials.

The remaining of this paper is structured as follows. In Sect. 2, we present the architecture of the system and the component of the SmartMATES. We describe the experimental scenario to analysis SmartMATES in Sect. 3. The results from the experiment are discussed in Sect. 4. The paper concludes by highlighting the future works in Sect. 5.

2   System Design

Fig. 1 shows the overall architecture of SmartMATES consisting of three units namely: M-App (A mobile Application), Left MATES Sense (LMS) and Right MATES Sense (RMS).

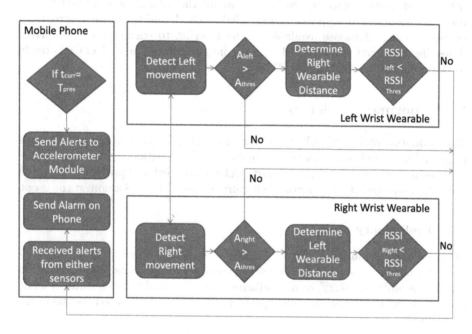

Fig. 1. SmartMATES system architecture

SmartMATES operates on the assumption that *medication intakes generally occur within the same time of day or at a recommended interval*. This assumption is usually true for most medications such as hypertension medication or antibiotics. In SmartMATES, an accelerometer sensor is attached to patient's wrist to monitor the ADL and identify the action of consuming a medication when it is time for a patient medication. Accelerometer is commonly used for gait analysis to detect walking pattern [7] and fall detection [8] using Wireless Sensor Networks [9]. Using the same approach, SmartMATES uses accelerometer to detect non-medication adherence by applying gait analysis on the accelerometer x, y, z to determine the specific pattern feature of consuming the medication. The algorithm used to detect the pattern is an extension of our previous work in [10]. The system generates an alert on the user's mobile phone if the feature is not observed within the time frame.

The LMS and RMS track the hand movement using the FLORA Accelerometer/Compass Sensor (LSM303) and a bluetooth module. The M-App is a medication management and alerting application installed on the mobile phone. M-App manages and stores the patient medication history and schedule information. When an user first installs the SmartMATES, he or she needs to enter his or her personal and medications details including user name, age, weight, drug name, type, strength, frequency of doses per day, doses intake times, number of doses per intake, and before or after meals. Currently, M-App does not verify the prescription instructions and assumes that all the information entered by the users are accurate. M-App can be extended to check and verify the instructions against a drugs database available in the Internet to ensure that the correct doses are consumed. Once the M-App is configured, the SmartMATES is ready to communicate with LMS and RMS.

3   Experimental Setup

The evaluation of SmartMATES consists of two stages: (i) Identifying the groups of participants and (ii) Deploying in homes with real patients. Our main goal is to demonstrate the reliability of SmartMATES to detect and prevent medication non-adherence and the non-intrusive feature of SmartMATES amongst the users.

3.1   Preliminary Study

We conducted an online survey to identify users had problem in adhering medication schedule. From 155 online participants, 86 respondents have medication adherence problem. 87.2% of non-adherence were caused by forgetfulness while the remaining 13.8% had disability problems that hinder them to take the medicines on time.

3.2   SmartMATES Case Study

From the preliminary study, we randomly selected 9 participants from the 86 respondents. Each participant wore a wrist strap, attached with an accelerometer sensor, on the left and right wrists to track the movement of the hands as illustrated in Fig. 2. The LMS and RMS began to sample the accelerometers at a sampling rate of 100 Hz when the systems received a notification from the mobile phone M-App via the bluetooth. The M-App is configured to trigger the tracking systems on the LMS and RMS five minutes before the patient medication time.

The participants were divided into 3 groups for three experiments. The first experiment was the control group where the participants did not use any tool and rely on oneself to take the medications. To check if the participants missed a medication, a carer was assigned to call and check on the participants remotely daily, five minutes after the prescription time for the patient. In the second

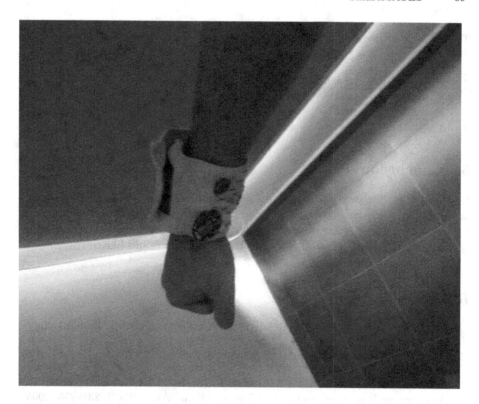

Fig. 2. A wearable accelerometer to track movements RMS

experiment, the participants were asked to install the PillBox, a medication and pill reminder mobile application to help the patients to tracks and reminds their medications. The third and final group of participants wore and used the SmartMATES. The experiment ran for 3 days continuously. The participants were given the prescription to take the medication three times a day.

4   Results

As shown in Table 1, SmartMATES and PillBox have managed to prevent the patients from missing their medication and have achieved 100% adherence compared to manual intervention. In manual, one of the patients has forgotten to take his medication within the five minutes interval after the prescription time and was requiring reminder from the carer to take the medicine in day 3 (Table 1). Although the Mobile App and SmartMATES have achieved 100% adherence, SmartMATES had only triggered an alert to the patient as he has forgotten to take the medication on time (Table 2). Users with SmartMATES have also reported they felt less intrusive as SmartMATES did not raise any alarm if the user have taken the medication compared to PillBox.

Table 1. Medicine adherence for 3 days

Group	SmartMATES	My Pillbox	Manual
Day 1	100%	100%	100%
Day 2	100%	100%	100%
Day 3	100%	100%	50%

Table 2. Number of alerts

Group	SmartMATES	My Pillbox	Manual
Day 1	0	3	2
Day 2	0	3	3
Day 3	1	3	1

5   Conclusion

In this paper, we developed and tested a non-intrusive wearable medication adherence systems, SmartMATES. Although SmartMATES has only been tested for a small sample in short duration, SmartMATES had achieved the same reliability rate with a mobile application. In the future, we would like to test Smart-MATES for long term clinical used.

References

1. Chan, M., Nicklason, F., Vial, J.: Adverse drug events as a cause of hospital admission in the elderly. Intern. Med. J. **31**(4), 199–205 (2001)
2. Sabaté, E.: Adherence to Long-term Therapies: Evidence for Action. World Health Organization, Geneva (2003)
3. MacLaughlin, J., Raehl, C.L., Treadway, K., Sterling, L., Zoller, D., Bond, C.: Assessing medication adherence in the elderly. Drugs Aging **22**(3), 231–255 (2005)
4. Urquhart, J.: The electronic medication event monitor. Clin. Pharmacokinet. **32**(5), 345–356 (1997)
5. Winland-Brown, J., Valiante, J.: Effectiveness of different medication management approaches on elders' medication adherence. Outcomes Manage. Nurs. Pract. **4**(4), 172–176 (1999)
6. Gandapur, Y., Kianoush, S., Kelli, M., Misra, S., Urrea, B., Blaha, J., Graham, G., Marvel, F., Martin, S.: The role of mHealth for improving medication adherence in patients with cardiovascular disease: A systematic review. Eur. Heart J. Qual. Care Clin. Outcomes **2**(4), 237–244 (2016). qcw018
7. Lim, T., Weng, T., Bate, I.: Optimistic medium access control using gait anaysis in body sensor networks. In: EAI 4th International Conference on Wireless Mobile Communication and Healthcare (Mobihealth), pp. 308–311 (2014)
8. Zhu, L., Zhou, P., Pan, A., Guo, J., Sun, W., Chen, X., Wang, L., Liu, Z.: A survey of fall detection algorithm for elderly health monitoring. In: 2015 IEEE Fifth International Conference on Big Data and Cloud Computing (BDCloud), pp. 270–274. IEEE (2015)
9. Lim, T.H., Lau, H.K., Timmis, J., Bate, I.: Immune-inspired self healing in wireless sensor networks. In: Coello Coello, C.A., Greensmith, J., Krasnogor, N., Liò, P., Nicosia, G., Pavone, M. (eds.) ICARIS 2012. LNCS, vol. 7597, pp. 42–56. Springer, Heidelberg (2012). doi:10.1007/978-3-642-33757-4_4
10. Lim, T.H., Abdullah, A.H.: Real-time adaptive medium access control protocol to improve transmission efficiency in body sensor networks. In: Proceedings of the 5th EAI International Conference on Wireless Mobile Communication and Healthcare. ICST (Institute for Computer Sciences, Social-Informatics and Telecommunications Engineering), pp. 249–252 (2015)

Paradigm-Shifting Players for IoT: Smart-Watches for Intensive Care Monitoring

Francesca Stradolini[1(✉)], Eleonora Lavalle[1,2], Giovanni De Micheli[1], Paolo Motto Ros[3], Danilo Demarchi[2], and Sandro Carrara[1]

[1] Laboratory of Integrated Systems, EPFL, Lausanne, Switzerland
francesca.stradolini@epfl.ch
[2] Department of Electronics and Telecommunications,
Politecnico di Torino, Turin, Italy
[3] Istituto Italiano di Tecnologia,
Center for Sustainable Futures (CSF@Polito), Turin, Italy

Abstract. Wearable devices, *e.g.* smart-watches, are gaining popularity in many fields and in wellness monitoring too. In this paper we propose an IoT application to alert the medical doctor assigned to a critical unit by using a smart-watch. The wearable device improves the efficacy of monitoring patients at risk in hospital units allowing the medical doctor to access information at any time and from any place. A network was built to wirelessly connect bio-sensing platforms, which measure metabolites concentration in patients' fluids (*e.g.* blood), with a dedicated application running on the smart-watch. In case of anomalous measured values, incoming alert notifications are received to ask urgent medical intervention. The main advantage of this new approach is that the doctors, or in general the caregivers, can freely move in the hospital other structures and perform other tasks meanwhile simultaneously and constantly monitoring all the patients thanks to the technology on their wrist.

Keywords: Remote continuous monitoring · IoT · Biomedical devices · Wireless network · Android wear

1 Introduction

Wearable Technology is considered as the revolution in the area of *Internet of Things* (IoT) [1]. Indeed, IoT satisfies the increasing request of always-connected devices to provide information accessible at any time and from any place [2]. In this context, wearable devices, *e.g.* smart-watches, can be highly exploited also for wellness monitoring or real medical applications thanks to their small-size, low-cost, easy-to-use, and multiple functionalities [3]. Even if smart-watches and *Goggle Glasses* have been introduced in the market only few years ago, these advanced devices have been already considered for patient monitoring scenarios [4, 5].

F. Stradolini and E. Lavalle contributed equally to this work.

© ICST Institute for Computer Sciences, Social Informatics and Telecommunications Engineering 2017
P. Perego et al. (Eds.): MobiHealth 2016, LNICST 192, pp. 71–78, 2017.
DOI: 10.1007/978-3-319-58877-3_9

Most of the wearable applications are developed for patients' smart-watches to detect their body-motion, body-temperature, physical exercises and amount of sleep [6]. Otherwise, monitoring systems are also used in specialized medical applications, as for the home monitoring in dementia care [7] or for patients with specific illness [8, 9].

Continuous monitoring concept is extremely impor-

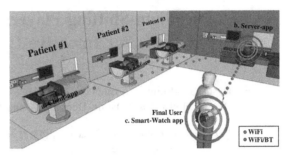

Fig. 1. IoT monitoring scenario: (*a*) Client-Android app gathers data from each patient's biosensor, (*b*) Server-Android app redirects data to a (*c*) Watch-AndroidWear app to keep the medical doctor continuously connected.

tant and beneficial in hospital environment too, especially for critical patients in *Intensive Care Units* (ICUs) [10] or during surgery under anesthesia [11]. To address the necessity of keeping constantly under control vital parameters, some solutions have been proposed. A Nurse-Watch with vital sign monitoring and checklist reminders has been proposed to assist nurses with their daily responsibilities [12]. Although, this system does not allow nurses to freely move in the hospital without both the phone and the smart-watch. Indeed, the connection between these two devices relies on Bluetooth technology that can support only short-range distances. To overcome this limitation, we propose a system, shown in Fig. 1, where the smart-watch becomes the only center of a monitoring network for hospital environments. Indeed, it is connected via Wi-Fi to a series of independent bedside monitoring systems connected to each patient. The monitoring system consists of bio-sensing platforms able to detect different endogenous and exogenous metabolites in patient's fluids [13, 14] plus an Android device to display the measured data. In this way, a flexible and personalized monitoring is performed. The medical doctor or the caregiver, wearing the smart-watch, is able to remotely monitor, with different levels of responsibility, multiple molecular parameters of many different patients at the same time. Incoming alert notifications are received on the smart-watch in case of anomalous values that requires medical support. It is important to underline that another strength of our system is its flexibility in measuring different endogenous/exogenous metabolites by properly functionalizing the biosensors.

The paper is organized as follow: *Sect.* 2 describes the system architecture; *Sect.* 3 collects the solutions developed for realizing the system. The validation of the network is presented in *Sect.* 4, and, finally, *Sect.* 5 concludes the paper.

2 Network Architecture

Figure 1 sketches the proposed scenario based on three main building blocks: (*a*) a *Client Android^{TM} interface*, running on a bedside tablet, that continuously receives and displays all the data measured by the biosensing platform on the patient, (*b*) an *Android intermediary Server-side,* running on a tablet/smart-phone in a central workstation, that collects data from different clients and enable the bidirectional communication with them, and (*c*) a *Smart-Watch application* on the doctor watch device. The *Android intermediary Server-side* is unavoidable to enable the multi-patients monitoring from the *Smart-Watch* since the wearable can be paired, by default, to only one device. Hereafter, a detailed description is provided separately for each system component.

2.1 Client Android Interface

The client Android application collects data from several hardware biosensors that directly measure metabolites of each patient. In this way, the concentrations of the most critical biomolecules measured by the sensors are available to be immediately displayed on a tablet placed near patient's bed. The aim is to offer the same potentialities of the already largely used patient monitors. Filtering options on incoming raw data are provided to reduce noise and to ensure smooth traces of the measured concentrations.

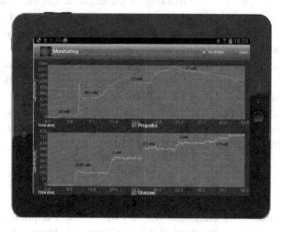

Fig. 2. Measure values displayed on bedside Client tablet. Monitored parameters are: endogenous glucose and exogenous propofol anesthetic.

Moreover the acquired values are stored in files on the memory of the device to allow *a-posteriori* consulting. The connection between the biosensors and the Android interface exploits Bluetooth® technology because it provides a standard, reliable, economic, wireless and secure method for the exchange of data via a short-range radio frequency. Moreover it does not interfere with medical equipment if fully certified [15].

Figure 2 shows an example of monitored values displayed on the bedside client-tablet interface. Starting from an application previously developed and validated by our group [16], the updated client-Android app offers new functionalities based on a Wi-Fi protocol for the communication with the intermediary-server. Thus, security mechanisms must be in place to prevent malicious attacks since sensible personal data are transmitted [17]. Securing the Wi-Fi connection is an important element of protecting the exchanged data. Basic points to be implemented are: to change the network name (*Service Set IDentifier* - SSID) from the default one and to adopt *Wi-Fi Protected Access* (WPA) security protocol [18].

2.2   Android Intermediary Server-Side

The server-side application is a completely new part of the present system we have realized to the aim of this paper. It gathers the monitored data from all the patients that, now on, could be seen as the clients connected by the network. In this way, it is possible to overcome the limitations of having the smart-watch connected to only one patient at time and one patient to a single doctor/caregiver. The intermediate server acts as a bridge between the doctor/caregiver application on the smart-watch and the patient applications on the client tablets. Indeed we wanted to maintain a bedside tablet near each patient to show the real-time trend of all the metabolite concentrations in time and for *a-posteriori* consulting of patient data. On the other side, the smart-watch receives data *on-demand* or alert without saving the received values in order to keep lightened the wearable app. To enable this scenario, the intermediate server pushes data to the smart-watch *on-demand* and, moreover, sends automatic messages to the doctor/caregiver in case of anomalies in recorded values. All these messages exchanged between the server and the smart-watch contain explicitly the patient identifier and the parameter-of-interest. Both the connections server–to-clients and server-to-SmartWatch adopt Wi-Fi communication. Indeed, we also assessed the implementation of the network through a Bluetooth® *piconet*, but the distance restriction would be too limiting in the final application [19].

2.3   Smart-Watch Application

Finally, we have also realized the Android application that runs on the smart-watch. The main advantage is that it allows the doctor to freely move in other areas of the hospital and to perform different tasks in parallel without leaving the constant and simultaneous monitoring of all the critical patients under his responsibility. In other words, the critical values of all the patients connected to the network are constantly taken under control even if the doctor is not physically present in the same room. The bidirectional communication between smart-watch and intermediate server could be both via Wi-Fi or Bluetooth depending on the convenience. Indeed, normally the smart-watch prefers to communicate with the server tablet via Bluetooth to save battery enabling reliable data transmission, but in case of far distances Wi-Fi is necessary and automatically adopted.

3   Proposed System

3.1   Communication Protocol

As already explained, three are the main peers that interact in the proposed system: (*a*) the *Client Android interface* for patient monitoring, (*b*) the *Android Server* running on a tablet that can be placed in any room of the ward, and (*c*) the *Smart-Watch application* for doctors/caregivers (*final users*). Figure 3 shows the communication protocol based on two main processes: *requesting* data (the blue process on the top of

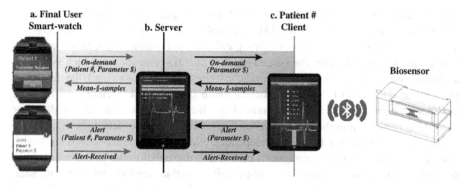

Fig. 3. Wi-fi Communication protocol: (*a*) Client – Patient #, (*b*) Server and (*c*) SmartWatch – Final User. Bluetooth data transmission is adopted between Client and sensing platform. (Color figure online)

Fig. 3) and *alerting* user in case of anomalies in recorded values (the purple process on the bottom of Fig. 3).

The *requesting process* allows the user to query a specific client in order to obtain the value of a parameter. A message containing the selected patient and the requested parameter (*On-demand (Patient #, Parameter $)*) is sent to the server from the smart-watch. Therefore, the server re-directs this query to the # client asking for the $ parameter (*On-demand (Parameter $)*). When the client # receives the request, the mean of the last § samples is algorithmically evaluated and sent back to the server (*Mean-§-samples*), which re-transmit to the smart-watch.

The *alerting process* occurs when there is an out-of-safe-range parameter. The involved client # sends a message to the server explicating the parameter (*Alert (Parameter $)*). The server, on its side, pushes the warning to the smart-watch (*Alert (Patient #, Parameter $)*). The notification on the smart-watch occurs as a strong vibration and with a pop-up that shows the number of the involved client (*Patient #*) and the anomalous value (*Parameter $*).

In order to face Internet unavailability, the alert/messages are sent several times until the smart-watch notifies the correct receiving through a broadcast message (*Alert-Received*). In this way we ensure to not lose any alert/message since when the Internet connection is re-established the data transmission is successfully accomplished.

3.2 Compatible Hardware

Given the flexibility and portability of our system, any Android application can be connected via Wi-Fi to the proposed network as client. This means that any type of monitoring sensor and/or biosensor that provides wirelessly the measured data can be connected at the central server thanks to a dedicated Android application. In this way the remote monitoring through the smart-watch is enabled and correctly assured. In order to test the portability of the realized network, we adopted as client both the application described in [13, 14]. Both the hardware prototypes mount a RN42 fully certified Bluetooth 2.1 module by Roving [20] that reaches a max transmission rate of 240 Kbps (in slave modality). In [13] a portable wireless system for measuring key metabolites (*e.g.* glucose, lactate, bilirubin, calcium, potassium, temperature, and pH) in ICUs is presented. Briefly, the system consists of a 3D-printed case, which integrates a fluidic system for patient body-liquids, a series of biosensors and the hardware platform to read those biosensors. The hardware platform also includes a Bluetooth module to transmit data to a mobile Android interface installed on a tablet. On the other hand, [14] presents a portable multichannel potentiostat able to detect simultaneously different blood molecules thanks to independent electrochemical biosensors on board. The system aims to provide continuous monitoring during surgeries in order to help in delivering anesthesia compounds. With this portable multichannel potentiostat, propofol (an anesthetic), paracetamol (an analgesic) and etoposide (an anti-cancer compound) have been actually detected. Even in this case, a Bluetooth module on board enables the transmission of acquired data to an Android application on a tablet.

We have integrated these two Android systems with the new protocol here proposed to make possible the communication with the server. This communication handles messages from the server and sends values-*on-demand*, meanwhile alerts are automatically transmitted to the server if any monitored parameter exceeds its physiological range.

4   Network Validation

4.1   Methods

All the interfaces were developed in *Android Studio 2.1* using Android and Android Wearable SDK Tools. Three tablets were used for the network: a *Galaxy Note pro 12.2 in* with Android 4.4.2 KitKat, a *Galaxy Tab 2* with Android 4.2.2 Jelly Bean both connected as clients and a Nexus 7 with Android 5.0.2 Lollipop as server. The smart-watch worn by the final user is a *Sony Smartwatch 3*. The server requires a minimum Android version 4.3 to be paired with the smart-watch. The pairing is enabled by the dedicated Android Wear application downloadable in *Google Play Store*. The other connections (client-to-server and client-to-biosensors) are provided by our developed applications.

4.2   Validation

The system has been validated by creating a network with two tablets as client units, one tablet as server and one smart-watch worn by the final user. Adopting this architecture, we tested all its functionalities:

- The clients simultaneously connect to the server via Wi-Fi and to the monitoring biosensors via Bluetooth. We have modified and tested both applications described in [13, 14] to that aim.

- The server connects multiple clients storing their IP addresses. Every time a new client is paired, a *Spinner List* on the smart-watch is automatically updated. The doctor handles/allows the client connection and disconnection.
- The smart-watch queries the server for receiving parameter $ from client #. In few seconds, the user receives the desired parameter from the correct patient. We tested the Internet transmission latencies by connecting to a personal hotspot obtaining less than 2 s for *on-demand* queries and less than 3 s for alerts receiving. Of course, these delays may vary accordingly to the Internet connection available.
- The alarm message is sent to the smart-watch if x values received from the monitoring biosensor exceed the physiological threshold. The threshold varies depending on the parameter and the number of acquired samples (x) to be averaged for the comparison with the threshold. This x value changes depending upon the desired medical application.
- The correct receiving of alert notifications on smart-watch also in case of Internet unavailability. The alarm is sent as soon as the connection is re-established and a notification is properly broadcast from the smart-watch.

5 Conclusions

In this paper we designed and tested a new IoT application to be used in medical critical-environments. The system is based on a network that allows doctors and caregivers in charge to monitor continuously and simultaneously key parameters of several critical patients thanks to a dedicated smart-watch application. The wearable device enables the request for metabolite concentrations and the reception of alerts in case of anomalous values. The short latencies for data/messages transmission ensure rapid medical interventions in case of incoming alert notifications. Thanks to the proposed system, the doctor is then able to freely move in the hospital area and to perform different tasks in parallel without loosing the control on the patients under his responsibility. Future work will be to carry out the usability of the network in medical daily practices and to further investigate on the security of the wireless communications.

Acknowledgments. The authors wants to thank Marcello Munari for having drawn the first image, Andrea De Gaetano, Ioulia Tzouvadaki and Tuğba Kiliç for their tips and Flavia Basilotta for the biosensor picture in *Fig.* 3. This work was supported by the CoMofA project (#325230 157139), with grant from the Swiss National Science Foundation.

References

1. Cuartielles Ruiz, D., Göransson, A.: Android wearables. Vrox (2015)
2. Murar, M., et al.: Monitoring and controlling of smart equipments using Android compatible devices towards IoT applications and services in manufacturing industry. In: AQTR. IEEE (2014)

3. Rawassizadeh, R., et al.: Wearables: has the age of smartwatches finally arrived? Commun. ACM **58**, 45–47 (2014)
4. SmartWatch (© *SmartMonitor*, San Jose, CA, 2016)
5. Zhang, Y.S., et al.: Google glass-directed monitoring and control of microfluidic biosensors and actuators. Sci. Rep. **6** (2016)
6. Subramaniam, S.: Smartwatch with multi-purpose sensor for remote monitoring of a patient, U.S. Patent No. 20,150,238,150 (2015)
7. Boletsis, C., McCallum, S., Landmark, B.F.: The use of smartwatches for health monitoring in home-based dementia care. In: Zhou, J., Salvendy, G. (eds.) DUXU 2015. LNCS, vol. 9194, pp. 15–26. Springer, Cham (2015). doi:10.1007/978-3-319-20913-5_2
8. De Lara, E., et al.: Feasibility of using smartwatches and smartphones to monitor patients with COPD. Am. J. Respir. Crit. Care Med. **193**, A1695 (2016)
9. Embrace Watch (© *Empatica Inc.,* Milan, Italy, 2016)
10. Sutter Health CPMC, What is the ICU (Intensive Care Unit)? (2014)
11. Brown, J.M., et al.: Improving operating room productivity via parallel anesthesia processing. Internat J. Health Care Qual. Assur. **27**(8), 697–706 (2014)
12. Bang, M., et al.: The nurse watch: design and evaluation of a smart watch application with vital sign monitoring and checklist reminders. In: Proceedings of the AMIA Symposium (2015)
13. Basilotta, F., et al.: Wireless monitoring in intensive care units by a 3D-printed system with embedded electronic. In: BioCAS. IEEE (2015)
14. Stradolini, F., et al.: Simultaneous monitoring of anesthetics and therapeutic compounds with a portable multichannel potentiostat. In: ISCAS. IEEE (2016)
15. Wallin, M.K., Wajntraub, S.: Evaluation of bluetooth as a replacement for cables in intensive care and surgery. Anesth. Analg. **98**(3), 763–767 (2004)
16. Stradolini, F., et al.: Wireless monitoring of endogenous and exogenous biomolecules on an Android interface. IEEE Sens. J. **16**(9), 3163–3170 (2015)
17. Ng, H.S., et al.: Security issues of wireless sensor networks in healthcare applications. BT Technol. J. **24**(2), 138–144 (2006)
18. Wi-Fi Alliance, Discover Wi-Fi: Security (2016). http://www.wi-fi.org/discover-wi-fi/security
19. Friedman, R., et al.: On power and throughput tradeoffs of wifi and bluetooth in smartphones. IEEE Trans. Mob. Comput. **12**(7), 1363–1376 (2013)
20. Roving, Bluetooth module RN42 datasheet. http://ww1.microchip.com/downloads/en/DeviceDoc/rn-42-ds-v2.32r.pdf

Toward an Open-Source Flexible System for Mobile Health Monitoring

Mathieu Bagot$^{(\boxtimes)}$, Pascale Launay, and Frédéric Guidec

Université de Bretagne Sud, Laboratoire IRISA, BP 573, 56017 Vannes Cedex, France
{mathieu.bagot,pascale.launay,frederic.guidec}@univ-ubs.fr

Abstract. Project SHERPAM (Sensors for HEalth Recording and Physical Activity Monitoring) aims to provide an open-source, flexible, customizable system to monitor the health condition of patients affected by chronic diseases during their day to day activities at home or out of home, while detecting and reacting to anomalies automatically. This paper presents the architecture of the flexible system that is being developed in the context of this project, and illustrates how this system could be used through a realistic use case.

Keywords: M-health · Sensors · Monitoring · Mobile

1 Introduction

Quantified-Self (QS) applications and software development kits have flourished during the last few years. With such systems data acquired by wearable sensors (e.g., smartwatches, digital armbands, heart rate monitors, etc.) can be transferred to the cloud, where they can remain indefinitely, while being accessible for authorized users.

There are several reasons why such solutions can hardly be used in the medical field. (a) Most of the sensors available for QS applications are not approved for medical use [1]. (b) Each vendor distributes a model of sensor with its own dedicated application, which is usually unable to interact with any other kind of sensor. Developing a system capable of interacting simultaneously with different kinds of sensors is therefore a challenge. (c) Most applications can only upload data to a single, predefined remote site [2]. Users must therefore inherently trust the owner of this site, assume that their data will be safe on that site, and will not be shared without their authorization. (d) Most of QS applications can only display nice curves or statistics based on the data they collect, with very little or no advanced processing (e.g., pattern recognition). The medical field shows higher expectations regarding health data collection and processing. A system involving wearable sensors should be versatile (i.e., capable of interacting with various sensors, and running various analysis algorithms), extensible (i.e., capable of accepting new types of sensors and algorithms as and when needed), safe (i.e., preventing data alteration, data loss, and the fraudulent disclosure of data), and dependable (i.e., usable anywhere and at any time).

© ICST Institute for Computer Sciences, Social Informatics and Telecommunications Engineering 2017
P. Perego et al. (Eds.): MobiHealth 2016, LNICST 192, pp. 79–82, 2017.
DOI: 10.1007/978-3-319-58877-3_10

Some of these requirements have already been addressed in the works presented in [3], but to the best of our knowledge no open-source, flexible, customizable system has ever been designed that can meet all these requirements at the same time. Developing such a system is one of the aims of project SHERPAM[1].

2   Use Case

Project SHERPAM's prime motivation is to allow patients affected by chronic diseases to perform their day to day activities, at home or out of home, with little or no restriction. A typical example is illustrated in Fig. 1. In this example, a patient is equipped with a wearable kit *(WK)* that includes sensors and a smartphone. The smartphone serves simultaneously as a controller for the equipped sensors, as a front-line data processing unit (data can be processed directly by local algorithms in order to trigger instant notifications to the patient when an anomaly is detected), and as a bridge between the patient and the aggregation server *(AS)*. Medical staff can review and analyse the data stored in the AS. In this scenario we assume that the AS is part of a hospital's private datacenter *(DC)*, but it could actually be deployed anywhere in the cloud. The AS stores the data it collects from patients, and it can additionally forward selected data feeds to specialized processing units. Resource-greedy algorithms that couldn't run directly on smartphones can thus be executed on dedicated units. If an anomaly is detected in the data received from a patient, visual and audible notifications can be addressed to that patient, and a warning is issued to medical personnel.

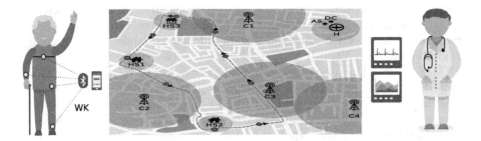

Fig. 1. Use case of the SHERPAM system

The transmission of data from the patients to the AS can rely on a combination of common wireless technologies, such as Wi-Fi and mobile data networks (i.e., 2.5G/3G/4G). Special attention is paid to tolerating networking disruptions without ever losing data. A Wi-Fi hotspot *(HS1)* is usually available at the patient's home, and this can provide a stable and continuous connection when the patient is at home. During the patient daily activities this connectivity turns out to be inconsistent and it becomes necessary to rely on another

---

[1] Sherpam: Sensors for HEalth Recording and Physical Activity Monitoring.

wireless connection to ensure the transmission. In an urban environment, free Wi-Fi hotspots *(HS2* and *HS3)* are often available, and mobile phone networks *(C1, C2* and *C3)* provide extensive coverage. However "white areas" (where no wireless connectivity is available) remain. To ensure that no data is lost when a patient moves in such areas, disruption-tolerant networking techniques have been integrated in the system. The data collected from the sensors are stored locally on the smartphone into "bundles" before being transferred to the AS when network connectivity is available. However, network operations (scanning, establishing connections, transferring data, etc.) may be power consuming and as the device used as a gateway has limited resources, special attention must be paid to the way network technologies are chosen and data are transmitted, balancing the continuity of the data transmissions with the system availability over time.

3   Architecture of the SHERPAM System

The main software components of the SHERPAM system are presented in Fig. 2. On the client side lies the application deployed on the wearable kit, and on the server side are several sub-systems dedicated to data aggregation, visualization, and processing.

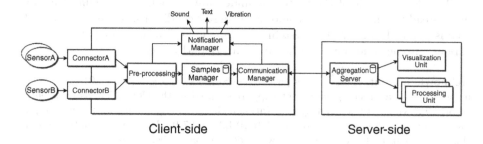

Fig. 2. General architecture of the system

On the client side, the data generated by the sensors enter the SHERPAM system via dedicated connectors. A connector is a software component that can drive a specific kind of sensors, and each connector is *plugged in* the application as and when needed. Extending the application for a new type of sensor mostly comes down to implementing a new connector module. Data processing algorithms can be embedded in the pre-processing unit. Data filters and compressors can thus be used to reduce the amount of data that must be transmitted to the AS, and pattern recognition algorithms to detect anomalies and trigger notifications to the patient locally. These are processed by the notification manager, which can warn the patient through audible or visual signals. After being pre-processed, the data samples are forwarded to the sample manager. They are then assembled in bundles, encrypted, and stored locally in the smartphone until they can be sent to the AS. Communication with the AS is managed by the network manager, which is responsible for selecting the most appropriate radio technology (e.g., Wi-Fi, 2.5G, 3.75G, 4G) at any time, based on criteria such as network availability, power consumption, and transmission needs (i.e., nature and importance of the data to be transmitted).

On the server side, the AS receives bundles, and stores them in a database. Specialized subsystems can be deployed in the cloud to access this database through a dedicated API. Visualization subsystems can thus be used by medical staff to browse the database online, using a standard Web browser. Advanced pattern recognition algorithms can also be deployed on data processing subsystems, so as to process selected data feeds in real-time, and to send warnings to a patient and/or medical staff when an anomaly is observed.

4   Conclusion and Future Work

The SHERPAM project aims to provide a flexible, customizable, open-source system capable of monitoring the health condition of patients affected by chronic diseases during their day to day activities. This system combines wearable sensors (for data acquisition), an Android application (for data gathering and preprocessing), and cloud-based units (for data storage and advanced analysis).

The development of the system is under way, although the main elements have already been implemented, and tested in real conditions. A one-year medical trial is planned in 2017. The system will thus be used to monitor patients with various chronic conditions (cardiopathy, arteriopathy, etc.).

Acknowledgment. This work is part of the SHERPAM project (2014–2018). As such it has received a French government support granted to the COMIN Labs excellence laboratory, which is managed by the National Research Agency in the *"Investing for the Future"* program under reference ANR-10-LABX-07-01. Further information about this project can be found at http://www.sherpam.cominlabs.ueb.eu/.

References

1. Schoenfeld, A.J., Sehgal, N.J., Auerbach, A.: The challenges of mobile health regulation. J. Am. Med. Assoc. **176**(5), 704–705 (2016)
2. Till, C.: Exercise as labour: quantified self and the transformation of exercise into labour. Societies **4**, 446–462 (2014)
3. Hende, A., Cem, E.: Wireless sensor networks for healthcare: a survey. Comput. Netw. **54**(15), 2688–2710 (2010)

Smart Applications for Clinical Care

A System for Hypertension Management Assistance Based on the Technologies of the Smart Spaces

Alexander Borodin$^{(\boxtimes)}$, Tatyana Kuznetsova, and Elena Andreeva

Petrozavodsk State University (PetrSU), Petrozavodsk, Russia
aborod@cs.petrsu.ru, eme@sampo.ru, elena-andreeva00@mail.ru

Abstract. Affecting up to 40% of the world's population, arterial hypertension results in high economic and social burden. Long-term treatment period along with the necessity of personal lifestyle changes lead to the low adherence to the treatment among the patients. As a consequence, the hypertension-related complications can be gradually developed between visits to the doctor, among them are heart attack, heart failures, strokes and even sudden cardiac death. In the proposed integrated approach, the mobile personal monitoring system, constructed on the principles of smart spaces, is used to address the problem of low adherence. Both continuous monitoring of the vital signs and the questionnaire-based regular health status audit are used for the assessment of the complication risk. Health parameters and evaluated risk markers are published in the semantic-driven information storage, and the personalized recommendation service, aimed at the increasing the adherence to the treatment among hypertensive patients, is constructed based on cooperation of distributed software agents.

Keywords: Mobile healthcare · Smart spaces · Hypertension management · Patient adherence

1 Introduction

Approximately 30–40% of the world's population suffers from increased arterial pressure (arterial hypertension). According to the World Health Organization report, arterial hypertension is the most essential preventable risk factor of premature death [1]. Prevention and treatment of arterial hypertension heavily rely on behaviour change, moreover, for the majority of patients, a substantial modification of their lifestyle has prime significance [2]. Therefore, the therapy is time-consuming and it demands a self-discipline from the patient. It is shown that in a six months period more than a third, and in a year more than a half of the patients, stop the appointed treatment, and about 10% of the patients forget to accept medicines daily [3,4]. Thus, there is a problem of low adherence of the hypertensive patients to prevention and treatment, i.e., of the readiness for strict observance of the instructions appointed by the doctor both at medicines

© ICST Institute for Computer Sciences, Social Informatics and Telecommunications Engineering 2017
P. Perego et al. (Eds.): MobiHealth 2016, LNICST 192, pp. 85–90, 2017.
DOI: 10.1007/978-3-319-58877-3_11

intake and at the behaviour change (e.g., of the recommendations to intensify the physical activity, stick to a healthy eating plan, etc.)

The solution of this problem can be built on an integrated approach to hypertension management including the use of the background intellectual environment to supervise the patient by means of the systems of personal recommendations (intellectual assistants). Aforesaid personalized medicine systems are considered to be a promising way to open the adaptation opportunities of a human being and to increase the duration of his active life, and research and development initiatives in the area of personalized medicine are supported by governmental programs [5]. From the other hand, personalized medicine demands support of mobility of the patient, realization of complex collecting and the analysis of personal data and a context information, and also "smart" decisions on the basis of personalisation, a context, and recommendation systems [6].

This paper presents the architectural approach to the design of the hypertension management assistance system aimed at the increasing of the adherence to the treatment among hypertensive patients. In the proposed approach, health-related data are gathered from multiple sources and are stored in semantic-driven storage for the further construction of personalized recommendations. The remote patient is equipped with wearable electrocardiogram recorder and fitness wristband that transfer health-related data to the personal mobile device. Also, the patient provides the regular questionnare-based health log. History of past medical events, individual contraindications, etc., are received from the electronic health record (EHR). The system is composed from the set of communicating agents that provide the data and consume them to produce the recommendations. Thus, the proposed solution is significantly banks on the recent advances in mobile healthcare, smart environments and cloud computing. This approach leads to minimization of risk of complications due to improvement of prevention, early diagnostics, forecasting of development of the disease.

The paper is organized as follows. In the Sect. 2, an overview of the results of recent related studies is given. Section 3 describes the sources of the gathered data. Section 4 introduces the architecture of the hypertension management system and discusses the construction of the personalized recommendation service. Section 5 concludes the study.

2   Related Work

Due to the advances in wearable technology, continuous registration of the vital signs became possible, providing the opportunity of the biosignal processing either on the local hardware, or in the cloud. For this reason, the efforts of researches are directed to the adoption of health sensors in the healthcare services.

A number of electrocardiogram analysis algorithms are developed in our previous work within a CardiaCare project that is aimed at continuous monitoring of heart function in real-time and analyzing electrocardiograms on a smartphone [7–9]. Within the CardiaCare project the efforts are concentrated on timely detection of rhythm abnormalities. Despite the fact that the arrhythmias are harmless in general, they can pose serious threat of complications against chronic diseases such as hypertension or diabetes. Thus, continuous heart rhythm monitoring provides the possibility to detect the deterioration of heart function and even to save the life, and these results form the base of our current work.

This paper significantly utilizes the concept of smart healthcare service discussed by Korzun et al. [10] and follows the idea of the smart service construction as the result of knowledge reasoning over a shared information. The ontology for hypertension management proposed by Steichen et al. [11] was adapted for representing data statements and relationships in machine-processible form.

3   Health Data Sources for Recommendation Construction

Recommendations for the patient are constructed on the base of analysis of continuously or regularly registered vital signs and personal health log. During the monitoring, the electrocardiograms and physical activity data are recorded automatically. Also, the patient manually records the results of independent measurements of the blood pressure and logs drug intakes. This allows to evaluate the blood pressure variability depending on many factors (ECG parameters, drug schedule, day time, etc.) between visits to the clinic.

There are a lot of possible ECG parameters that are considered to be the cardiovascular risk markers. The following ECG parameters are monitored: (1) heart rhythm disturbances such as arterial fibrillation, premature ventricular contraction and others; (2) heart blocks; (3) heart rate; (4) P wave duration; (5) P wave amplitude; (6) P wave morphology, in particular, two-phase shape; (7) PQ interval duration; (8) QT dispersion; (9) Q width; (10) R amplitude; (11) S amplitude; (12) QRS width; (13) QT duration; (14) T wave amplitude; (15) T wave alternation; (16) T wave width and "T peak-to-end" parameter; (17) ST elevation; (18) ST decrease; (19) rhythm turbulence; (20) heart rate variability.

To increase the adherence, the mobile app provides a simplified questionnaire for the regular log of complaints (including experiencing headaches, chest pain, interruptions in work of heart or heartbeat, breathing difficulties, physical activity interruptions in connection with an illness, sleep disorders, proper taking the medications, etc.) and analysis of their connections with hypertension and drug treatment. At the whole, the log gives the life quality assessment that defines the adherence of the patient to the treatment plan.

The application allows the patient to send the alarm notification in the emergency case in order to timely address to the doctor and obtain the further guideline (e.g., call the ambulance or to take medications independently). The patient is able to attach the list of complaints to the alarm notification.

4   Hypertension Management System Architecture

In the proposed hypertension management assistance system, the smart spaces approach is applied to achieve the high system scalability in IoT environments.

From the one hand, the market of m-Health applications with health parameter monitoring experiences the explosive growth due to the progress of IoT technology and the advances in wearable medical devices development. For this reason, the developed system should provide a way of facile integration of the new sensor hardware. From the other hand, the development of the proposed service should support effective integration of the existing healthcare services provided by hospital information systems, in particular, the electronic health records, and to enhance them up to the level of smart services [12]. Therefore, the designed smart space-based system architecture of personalized assistance services should consider the system composed from the many components, focusing on component functionality reuse instead of reinvention.

In [10], the reference scenarios of personalized assistance and their smart space-based implementations were discussed on the example of the service aimed at the increasing the efficiency of the first aid in medical emergencies. Following the same approach, we construct the smart services for hypertensive patients.

In general, a smart space provides means for many networked devices to participate by cooperatively sharing information and other resources. Each device hosts so-called knowledge processor (KP), which acts as a software agent interacting with users, sensor equipment, and other KPs. The data produced by one KP can be shared with other KPs by means of semantic information broker (SIB). The latter provides storage for shared information collection and querying mechanism. SIB and its storage can be considered as a semantic knowledge base over multiple and dynamic data sources, similarly as it happens in the Semantic Web. That is, the knowledge base and its KPs form a computing system environment that we call a smart space. According to this definition of a smart space, we propose the architecture of smart system for hypertension management assistance, as it is shown in Fig. 1.

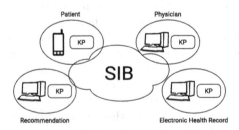

Fig. 1. Multi-agent smart hypertension management assistance system.

In the proposed system, the ontology-oriented approach is adopted for representation of the shared information in machine-processible manner as a semantic network that relates a variety of heterogeneous data sources and their consumers. Data sources and consumers are represented by KPs as well as some KPs are responsible for reasoning over the data.

Consider a part of the scenario of hypertension management in remote patient. The patient is equipped with the personal mobile device running the

KP and portable sensor devices. The mobile device has positioning capabilities, therefore, the location of the patient is also known.

The interaction of KPs resulting in service construction is shown in Fig. 2. A service is constructed due to cooperative activity of KPs participating in the same smart space. The Patient KP shares the location, questionnaire answers and health data (along with the results of its processing) in the smart space. The patient is able to use the "panic button" also. The Electronic Health Record KP updates the EHR and also publishes some data in the SIB, e.g. contraindications. Recommendation KP integrates the current health status and the data from EHR and produces recommendations to the patient.

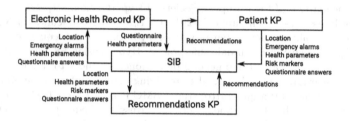

Fig. 2. Construction of the service as a cooperative activity of knowledge processors

The discussed above smart space-based hypertension assistance service provides a high level of scalability without the need of redesign of the system at whole in case of modification of individual components.

5   Conclusion

This paper proposed the system for decreasing of the hypertension-related risk and addressing the low adherence problem based on concepts of m-Health and smart spaces. The multi-agent architecture of the offered system was described and construction of the personalized digital assistance services for remote hypertensive patients was discussed.

According to the proposed approach, the prototype of the system was implemented based on the Smart-M3 platform. The mobile applications that are intended to monitor hypertensive and prehypertensive patients, to assess the risks and to track their adherence to the treatment were developed for Android OS and Sailfish OS.

For the forthcoming analysis of advantages of the approach up to the 300 hypertensive patients were selected for control group on the base of Petrozavodsk Hospital of Emergency Care. The examination included the natural history analysis, the assessment of usual risk factors, identification of subclinical asymptomatic organ damage (ultrasound scanning of carotid arteries, microalbuminuria, left ventricle hypertrophy, coronary calcium index), identification of cardiovascular or renal diseases, blood pressure variability between visits, adherence to treatment according to existing indexes and questionnaires.

Acknowledgments. This research is financially supported by the Ministry of Education and Science of the Russian Federation within projects #14.574.21.0060 (RFMEFI57414X0060) of Federal Target Program "Research and development on priority directions of scientific-technological complex of Russia for 2014–2020" and #16-07-01289 of Russian Foundation for Basic Research.

References

1. World Health Organization report, Global Health Risks. Mortality, burden of disease attributable to selected major risk. http://www.who.int/healthinfo/globalburdendisease/GlobalHealthRisks_report_full.pdf
2. Recommendations of the European Society of Hypertension. http://www.esh2013.org/wordpress/wp-content/uploads/2013/06/ESC-ESH-Guidelines-2013.pdf
3. Corrao, G., et al.: Cardiovascular protection by initial and subsequent combination of antihypertensive drugs in daily life practic. Hypertension **58**, 566–572 (2012)
4. Gale, N.K., et al.: Patient and general practitioner attitudes to taking medication to prevent cardiovascular disease after receiving detailed information on risks and benefits of treatment: a qualitative study. BMC Family Pract. **12**(1), 59 (2011)
5. The order of the Government of the Russian Federation of December 28, 2012 of N 2580-p. About the confirmation of Strategy of development of medical science in the Russian Federation for the period till 2025. http://www.rosminzdrav.ru/documents/5413-rasporyazhenie-pravitelstva-rossiyskoy-federatsii-ot-28-dekabrya-2012-g-n-2580-r
6. Demirkan, H.: A smart healthcare systems framework. IT Prof. **15**(5), 38–45 (2013)
7. Borodin, A.V., Zavyalova, Y.V.: The cross-platform application for arrhythmia detection. In: Proceedings of 12th Conference on Open Innovations Association FRUCT, Oulu, Finland, 5–9 November 2012, pp. 26–30 (2012)
8. Borodin, A.V., Pogorelov, A., Zavyalova, Y.V.: CardiaCare. Mobile system for arrhythmia detection. In: Proceedings of 13th Conference on Open Innovations Association FRUCT, Petrozavodsk, Russia, 22–26 April 2013, pp. 14–19 (2013)
9. Borodin, A.V., Zavyalova, Y.V., Zaharov, A., Yamushev, I.: Architectural approach to the multisource health monitoring application design. In: Proceedings of 17th Conference on Open Innovations Association FRUCT, by ITMO University, Yaroslavl, Russia, 20–24 April 2015, pp. 16–21 (2015)
10. Korzun, D.G., Borodin, A.V., Timofeev, I.A., Paramonov, I.V., Balandin, S.I.: Digital assistance services for emergency situations in personalized mobile healthcare: smart space based approach. In: Biomedical Engineering and Computational Technologies (SIBIRCON), pp. 62–67 (2015)
11. Steichen, O., Daniel-Le Bozec, C., Jaulent, M.-C., Charlet, J.: Building an ontology of hypertension management. In: Bellazzi, R., Abu-Hanna, A., Hunter, J. (eds.) AIME 2007. LNCS, vol. 4594, pp. 292–296. Springer, Heidelberg (2007). doi:10.1007/978-3-540-73599-1_39
12. Paramonov, I.V., Vasilyev, A., Timofeev, I.A.: Communication between emergency medical system equipped with panic buttons and hospital information systems: use case and interfaces. In: Proceedings of the AINL-ISMW FRUCT, Saint-Petersburg, Russia, 9–14 November 2015

Enhancing the Early Warning Score System Using Data Confidence

Maximilian Götzinger[1(✉)], Nima Taherinejad[2], Amir M. Rahmani[1],
Pasi Liljeberg[1], Axel Jantsch[2], and Hannu Tenhunen[1]

[1] Department of Information Technology, University of Turku, Turku, Finland
{maxgot,amirah,pakrli,hannu.tenhunen}@utu.fi
[2] Institute of Computer Technology, TU Wien, Vienna, Austria
{nima.taherinejad,axel.jantsch}@tuwien.ac.at

Abstract. Early Warning Score (EWS) systems are utilized in hospitals by health-care professionals to interpret vital signals of patients. These scores are used to measure and predict amelioration or deterioration of patients' health status to intervene in an appropriate manner when needed. Based on an earlier work presenting an automated Internet-of-Things based EWS system, we propose an architecture to analyze and enhance data reliability and consistency. In particular, we present a hierarchical agent-based data confidence evaluation system to detect erroneous or irrelevant vital signal measurements. In our extensive experiments, we demonstrate how our system offers a more robust EWS monitoring system.

Keywords: Early Warning Score · Self-awareness · Data confidence · Consistency · Plausibility · Hierarchical agent-based system

1 Introduction

Early Warning Score (EWS) systems are common practice in hospitals with the goal of detecting and predicting patients' health deterioration. In 1997, Morgen *et al.* proposed this system for the first time [1], covering vital signals such as heart rate, respiratory rate, body temperature, blood pressure, and blood's oxygen saturation. These signals are monitored and added up to derive the EWS. However, not everyone whose condition is deteriorating is already in the hospital. Therefore, portable devices and ubiquitous systems utilizing Internet-of-Things are needed for monitoring vital signals and calculating the EWS [2].

It is of key importance to provide these systems with an acceptable level of reliability. In other words, EWS systems always need to monitor vital signals accurately. Azimi *et al.* propose a system that calculates a self-aware EWS through changing the classification of the various vital signals based on the patient's activities [2]. This self-aware property is essential because the values of vital signals change when a patient is sleeping or running. Knowledge of different situations and circumstances improves the decision-making ability of the

© ICST Institute for Computer Sciences, Social Informatics and Telecommunications Engineering 2017
P. Perego et al. (Eds.): MobiHealth 2016, LNICST 192, pp. 91–99, 2017.
DOI: 10.1007/978-3-319-58877-3_12

system [3]. However, they assume that the measured data is always correct and relevant. Noisy or erroneous vital signals can lead to a wrong calculation of the EWS, which can result in false or missing alarms. Hence, EWS systems need to be robust and aware of the reliability of input data.

In this paper, we propose a modified EWS (MEWS) system by exploiting a customized data confidence enhancement technique. Our method is inspired by the concept of self-awareness enabling the system to - adaptively - correct the sensory data in case of faulty readings.

2   System Architecture

In an agent-based modular architecture (Fig. 1(a)), each sensor is connected to a dedicated module which we call an "Agent" [4]. It processes the sensory data and reports to a higher level agent, which is the "Body Agent". Each agent consists of an Abstraction-, a History-, a Confidence Validator-, and a Binding Module. The role of each module in an agent is as follows:

- *Abstraction*: To change the representation of the input data to the appropriate format of the output. The purpose is to provide the higher level agents with more compact and only relevant information [5].
- *History*: To save recent data, track changes, and establish a stable baseline for the data when possible. This unit also smooths the data via weighted averaging to eliminate the noise in the signal.
- *Confidence*: To assess the trustability of the input data and provide the output data with a confidence tag, that allows the higher levels to have a better understanding of the data and their validity. This topic is discussed in more details in Sect. 3.
- *Binding*: To bind several input data, relate or compare them, and perform necessary operations on them. This module is specifically useful when an agent has multiple inputs, as is the case with the Body Agent. We note that this process is more complicated than a simple mapping of the values as done in the Abstraction module.

To enhance the functionality of our system, we have incorporated some of the concepts of self-awareness. Self-awareness is a well-known concept which can be traced back to 1960s in psychology [6] and late 1990s in computing [7]. It provides several advantages to the system such as the ability to cope with changing environments [6] or changing goals [8], and to optimize resource utilization [9]. As the basis for our self-aware system design, we use an Observe-Decide-Act (ODA) loop [7,8] as illustrated in Fig. 2(a). For better modularity and simpler implementation we use a mini ODA loop inside each agent, as shown in Fig. 2(b). That is, each agent monitors its own behavior, decides about certain actions, and acts accordingly. Self-awareness covers a wide range of aspects in the system design under each of the chains of the ODA loop. All of which could provide the system with certain abilities and advantages. In this work, we specifically concentrate on the role of the confidence aspect of observation as elaborated in [5]. We then analyze its effect on the overall performance of our EWS system.

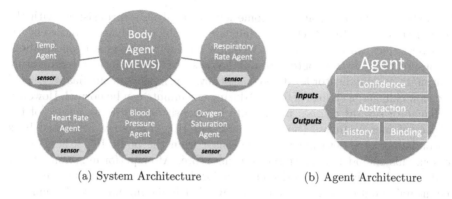

(a) System Architecture   (b) Agent Architecture

Fig. 1. System Architecture; (a) Constituting agents (modules) of the system, and (b) Constituting units of the agents.

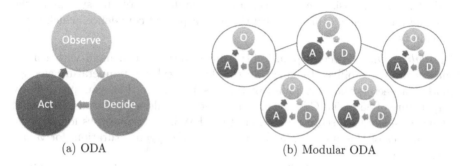

(a) ODA   (b) Modular ODA

Fig. 2. Observe-Decide-Act (ODA) loops implemented in (a) overall system, and (b) each module.

3   Data Confidence Concepts

Data Confidence is meta-data and builds on Data Reliability (which consists of accuracy and precision of sensory data [5]). It provides another level of understanding regarding the validity of the data which is beyond that of the sensors. For example, in the context of the EWS, if the sensor is not attached to the body of the subject, the temperature data provided by the sensor may still be accurate and precise. However, it is not valid in the context of the application. Therefore, although the data is reliable, the system should not consider such a value. Assessing Data Confidence based on the context and the application can be very challenging [5]. Among the identified potential solutions are consistency and plausibility control as well as redundant verification [5]. Since the latter requires redundant hardware and implies additional costs and our objectives include cost as well as energy efficiency, in this work we focus on the two former aspects: consistency and plausibility.

Consistency: Anomalies are - at some level of analysis - inconsistent with the normal trend of data, which could indicate a problem[1]. Hence, Consistency is an aspect that can provide insight into how confident the system can be about its observation. In the context of our EWS system, we consider temperature continuity as an indicator for data consistency. Body temperature has very small and slow changes; a change of $0.16\,°C$ during one minute can be normal. However, a change of several degrees per minute is inconsistent with the nature of the subject of measurements (body temperature) [10]. This may be caused by a sensor failure or a detachment of the sensor from the body. Regardless of the reason, this should not affect the warning score. After performing consistency analysis and finding an inconsistent behavior, by reducing the confidence tag of the incoming data, the EWS system knows that it should not take this number into consideration. We note that in some other parameters, such as respiratory rate, for example, some discontinuities might be acceptable and should not be marked as an inconsistency or decrease the confidence of the system in the incoming data. Hence comes forward the next aspect of confidence, which is the plausibility.

Plausibility: One aspect of plausibility which goes hand in hand with consistency is the plausibility of changes in the data, e.g. body temperature change. Another aspect is the plausibility of the absolute value. For example, a body temperature of 85 or $95\,°C$ is not plausible and regardless of the cause, it should not be considered for score evaluation of the EWS. The same goes for negative temperatures of this magnitude, or in the case of oxygen saturation, for values outside 0 to 100.

Another aspect of plausibility is the cross-validity or co-existence plausibility. That is, whether certain data could plausibly be valid given some other (complimentary) data and given certain conditions. For example, a body temperature of few degrees is valid only if the subject does not have any other vital signals (and is practically deceased), otherwise, it shows a discrepancy and the data cannot be trusted. Therefore, by adding such logical information regarding the co-existing situations and signals, the system can perform a cross-validity check and obtain another level of holistic awareness regarding the confidence it can invest in the observed data.

4   Impact Evaluation

In this section, we explain how we have taken advantage of the concepts discussed in previous sections to enhance the reliability of our EWS. The details of our experimental set-up and acquired results are as follows.

4.1   Experiments Set-Up

EWS Table: Because human body functions have some variance from person to person, there exist several different EWS classification tables from various studies

---

[1] We note that the consequence of an anomaly detection should be/is decided by higher levels of the system. Regardless, the observation unit needs to alert the higher levels.

Table 1. Score classification table of a set of vital signals

Vital signal score	3	2	1	0	1	2	3
Heart rate (beats/min)	<40	40–51	51–60	60–100	100–110	110–129	>129
Systolic blood pressure (mmHg)	<70	70–81	81–101	101–149	149–169	169–179	>179
Respiratory rate (breaths/min)		<9		9–14	14–20	20–29	>29
Oxygen saturation (%)	<85	85–90	90–95	>95			
Body temperature (°C)		<28	28–32	32–35	35–38		38–39.5	>39.5

[2,11,12]. In this work, as shown in Table 1, we mainly use a similar table as in
[2]. Whereas the original table showed only one possible score ($=2$) for the
hypothermia, Brown *et al.* introduced in their work [13] four different stages of
an accidental hypothermia (called HT I to HT IV). Following that approach, we
combined HT III and IV because HT III shows symptoms of weak- and HT IV
of no vital signals.

Patients' Data: The vital signal data were obtained from the experiments carried
out by Azimi *et al.* [2]. This dataset contained records of heart rate, systolic blood
pressure, respiratory rate, and oxygen saturation of a 35 years old healthy male
subject [2]. To evaluate the behavior of the system during a malfunction, instead
of the measured temperature, we introduced faulty temperature data.

Analysis Environment: For the analysis of the EWS, we used our hierarchical
agent-based model toolbox. It is developed in C++, and its agents can be configured in different ways based on the requirements.

4.2 Confidence Assessment and Results

Experiment 1: Absolute Bounds
    The first validation step is to check if a measured value is in a plausible range.
For temperature for example, according to Omics International[2], the temperature extremes in Europe are about $-58°C$ and $48°C$. Therefore, these values
can be used to define the extreme lower and upper bounds of the temperature.
The measured value will be classified as valid if it is in this range. Although this
boundary allows us to evaluate the behavior of system regarding this parameter,
we note that more accurate values will have to be chosen when the system is
used to monitor a patient's condition in real life.
    Figure 3 shows the results of the confidence validation's regarding the
absolute bounds. The body temperature was manually set to $100°C$ which is
out of the absolute bounds. Therefore, the score of the temperature is 3 for the
whole time if it is not checked regarding its confidence and 0 if it is checked.

---

[2] http://research.omicsgroup.org/index.php/List_of_weather_records, accessed on
    July 2016.

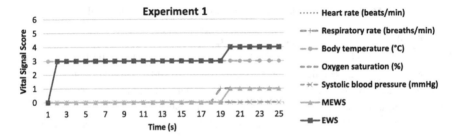

Fig. 3. Calculation of the MEWS and EWS with the same data set. Body temperature is manually set to 100 °C which is out of the absolute bounds. CCVU deactivated for showing the difference.

Experiment 2: Change Rate

Here, we concentrate on the consistency of the data based on the maximum plausible rates of change of an input signal. Regarding the body temperature, the highest cooling rates obtained from persons that got completely buried under an avalanche are between 6 °C/h to 9.4 °C/h [10, 14, 15]. Assuming that temperature of a human body cannot increase faster than it can decrease, we set the maximum possible rate of change to 10 °C/h (= 0.17 °C/min = 0.003 °C/s). The body temperature will be considered as unconfident if the rate of change is higher than the maximum allowed limit set. The input signal has to have approximately the same value (previous value ± allowed rates of change) it had before it was unconfident to get the confident status back[3].

Figure 4 shows the results of the confidence validation's regarding the change rate. The body temperature was manually set to 36 °C which is equivalent to score 0. After a short period, the temperature was decreased faster as the maximum allowed rate of change. We can see that in the absence of Confidence Validation Unit (CVU), we have false alarms which we do not observe in the enhanced system. If the CVU is deactivated, the body temperature score is unequal to zero when the associated input gets lower than 35 °C. On the other hand, the input signal is being considered as unconfident if the CVU is activated. Now to get the new data tagged as confident again, regardless of its change, its absolute value needs to go back to latest value tagged as confident ± allowed change. For example, we set the temperature signal to an unchanging value between the seconds 12 and 14 and although the input signal's rate of change is equal to zero, it is still classified as unconfident.

Experiment 3: Cross Confidence Validation

Humans' vital signals such as heart rate, blood pressure, and respiratory rate change with a body temperature when it is too high or too low [13, 16]. A mild hypothermia can come along with symptoms such as tachycardia

---

[3] We remark that to ascertain a signal's rate of change, a history is needed. As a preparatory work, history has to get smoothed before calculating the rates of change, otherwise, noise could affect this measurement.

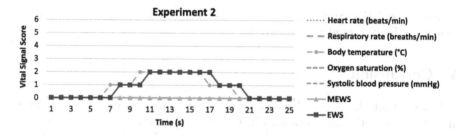

Fig. 4. Calculation of the MEWS and EWS with the same data set. Body temperature is manually set to 36 °C (score 0) and then decreased faster as the maximum allowed rates of change is set. CCVU deactivated for showing the difference.

and tachypnea, a medium hypothermia already shows signals of hypotonia and bradycardia. Henceforth, the lower the body temperature the weaker the vital signals get; until they finally stop [17]. Regarding hyperthermia, the changes of vital signals are not completely identical, but show a similar behavior; that is, general deterioration [16]. By implication, this means that body temperature cannot be injurious if all the other vital signals have a good value.

In contrast to the two steps before, the Cross Confidence Validation Unit (CCVU) needs already abstracted knowledge from different sources. Therefore, this validation is only possible at a higher hierarchical level. In our case, that is the body agent which gets the abstracted data from the different agents. The CCVU was configured to consider the measured temperature as valid if more than 50% of the vital signals (body temperature excluded) have a non-zero score in accordance to that of the temperature.

Figure 5 shows results of the confidence validation test. The body temperature was manually set to 32 °C (score 1). The other input signals are time-displaced to set their values to non-zero scores, one input after the other. It can be seen that at 17 s the MEWS is changing when more than 50% (3 out of 4) of the input variables reach a non-zero score. We can see that if the temperature sensor is included in the EWS calculation - when the CCVU is deactivated - we

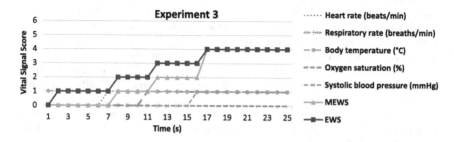

Fig. 5. Calculation of the MEWS and EWS with the same data set. Body temperature is manually set to 32 °C (score 1) and the other input signals are time-displaced (one after the other) to values where there are no score 0 present.

have a higher EWS. Such a case, nonetheless, is physiologically not possible and hence, the EWS should not be affected.

5 Conclusion

It is vital that the Early Warning Score is computed correctly at all times, in spite of potential complications in the input data stream. Otherwise, there could be false or missed alarms. In this paper, we show that it is possible to check the confidence of the input data with our modular solution based on self-awareness. Using this concept, the reliability of EWS improved in all three cases we experimented with. Thus, we demonstrated that using the data confidence validation system, the quality, and robustness of the EWS assessment can be improved.

We used a hierarchical agent-based system which allows processing both the data and their meta-data, such as the confidence assessment. Due to its modularity and a good match of the data processing flow from lower to higher abstraction levels, it is a promising architecture for EWS or similar systems.

In the future, we will extend our framework and add various features such as the ability of learning. We assume that a learning unit could help choosing better boundaries and values, based on the personalized behavior of the subject, for confidence evaluation and consequently the score calculation.

References

1. Morgan, R., Williams, F., Wright, M.: An early warning scoring system for detecting developing critical illness. Clin. Intensive Care **8**(2), 100 (1997)
2. Azimi, I., Anzanpour, A., Rahmani, A.M., Liljeberg, P., Tenhunen, H.: Self-aware early warning score system for IoT-based personalized healthcare. In: Proceedings of International Conference on IoT and Big Data Technologies for HealthCare (2016)
3. Jantsch, A., Tammemäe, K.: A framework of awareness for artificial subjects. In: 2014 International Conference on Hardware/Software Codesign and System Synthesis (CODES+ISSS), pp. 1–3. IEEE (2014)
4. Götzinger, M., Rahmani, A., Pongratz, M., Liljeberg, P., Jantsch, A., Tenhunen, H.: The role of self-awareness and hierarchical agents in resource management for many-core systems. In: Many-core Systems-on-Chip (MCSoC) (2016)
5. TaheriNejad, N., Jantsch, A., Pollreisz, D.: Comprehensive observation and its role in self-awareness; an emotion recognition system example. In: The Federated Conference on Computer Science and Information Systems (FedCSIS), September 2016
6. Rinner, B., Esterle, L., Simonjan, J., Nebehay, G., Pflugfelder, R., Fernandez Dominguez, G., Lewis, P.R.: Self-aware and self-expressive camera networks. Computer **48**(7), 21–28 (2015)
7. Dutt, N., Jantsch, A., Sarma, S.: Toward smart embedded systems: a self-aware system-on-chip (SoC) perspective. ACM Trans. Embed. Comput. Syst. (TECS) **15**(2), 22 (2016)

8. Hoffmann, H., Maggio, M., Santambrogio, M.D., Leva, A., Agarwal, A.: SEEC: a framework for self-aware computing. MIT, Technical report. MIT-CSAIL-TR-2010-049, October 2010
9. Teich, J., Henkel, J., Herkersdorf, A., Schmitt-Landsiedel, D., Schröder-Preikschat, W., Snelting, G.: Invasive computing: an overview. In: Hübner, M., Becker, J. (eds.) Multiprocessor System-on-Chip, pp. 241–268. Springer, New York (2011)
10. Pasquier, M., Moix, P.-A., Delay, D., Hugli, O.: Cooling rate of 9.4 °C in an hour in an avalanche victim. Resuscitation **93**, e17–e18 (2015)
11. Urban, R.W., Mumba, M., Martin, S.D., Glowicz, J., Cipher, D.J.: Modified early warning system as a predictor for hospital admissions and previous visits in emergency departments. Adv. Emerg. Nurs. J. **37**(4), 281–289 (2015)
12. Groarke, J., Gallagher, J., Stack, J., Aftab, A., Dwyer, C., McGovern, R., Courtney, G.: Use of an admission early warning score to predict patient morbidity and mortality and treatment success. Emerg. Med. J. **25**(12), 803–806 (2008)
13. Brown, D.J., Brugger, H., Boyd, J., Paal, P.: Accidental hypothermia. N. Engl. J. Med. **367**(20), 1930–1938 (2012)
14. Putzer, G., Schmid, S., Braun, P., Brugger, H., Paal, P.: Cooling of six centigrades in an hour during avalanche burial. Resuscitation **81**, 1043–1044 (2010)
15. Oberhammer, R., Beikircher, W., Hörmann, C., Lorenz, I., Pycha, R., Adler-Kastner, L., Brugger, H.: Full recovery of an avalanche victim with profound hypothermia and prolonged cardiac arrest treated by extracorporeal re-warming. Resuscitation **76**(3), 474–480 (2008)
16. Fauci, A.S., et al.: Harrison's Principles of Internal Medicine, vol. 2. McGraw-Hill, Medical Publishing Division, New York (2008)
17. McCullough, L., Arora, S.: Diagnosis and treatment of hypothermia. Am. Fam. Phys. **70**(12), 2325–2332 (2004)

Application of Wearable Monitoring System in Tourette Syndrome Assessment

Sofia Scataglini[1(✉)], Marcello Fusca[1], Giuseppe Andreoni[1], and Mauro Porta[2]

[1] Department of Design, Politecnico di Milano, Via Durando 38/a, 20158 Milan, Italy
{sofia.scataglini,giuseppe.andreoni}@polimi.it
[2] Department of Neurology, Tourette Centre, IRCCS "Galeazzi", Milan, Italy

Abstract. This study presents the application of a wearable monitoring system for the assessment of tic events in subjects affected by Tourette Syndrome (TS). A multifactorial analysis and validation of the proposed system is carried out collecting simultaneous and synchronized recordings of data from the wearable actigraph and from two video cameras that allowed two medical doctors with different expertise to classify the motor events as tics and their related severity scale. A dedicated software implements the algorithm for automatic tic detection and to compare this assessment with the standard video recording protocol used to discriminate and classify tic events of high intensity and tic event of low intensity (facial grimacing or vocal tics). Double blind analysis on a nine subjects allowed us to compare the variability between operators and wearable device, and conclude the system has good potential but algorithms refinement is still needed before its possible application in clinical practice. Currently it still requires the integration with a video analysis protocol if the tics are mild or are vowels giving a complete clinical frame.

Keywords: Wearable monitoring · Tourette Syndrome · Tics · Video monitoring · Automatic tic detection

1 Introduction

Tourette Syndrome (TS) is a chronic neurologic disorder characterized by the childhood onset of multiple motor and phonic tics that wax and wane over time [1]. A distinctive issue concerning the assessment of TS is the difficulty in quantifying and classifying objectively tics from clinical manifestations. Multiple variables such as frequency, number of tic-types, intensity, complexity, body distribution, supressibility, and interference with normal activities are commonly considered to assess the TS severity. The evaluation of TS is currently carried out either through a clinical examination or through patient reports based on self-assessment of tic disorder. The analysis of video-recordings is the standard reference for many TS studies but it is confined to a short and in-hospital visit: 10 min video recording in controlled environments (with and without the presence a clinical operator) and the related tic counting represents today the gold standard technique to define the choice between pharmacological or Deep Brain Stimulation (DBS) implant therapy. A longer and multifactorial monitoring should be adopted to support a

© ICST Institute for Computer Sciences, Social Informatics and Telecommunications Engineering 2017
P. Perego et al. (Eds.): MobiHealth 2016, LNICST 192, pp. 100–106, 2017.
DOI: 10.1007/978-3-319-58877-3_13

more precise and fitting to the patient intervention. Furthermore, a multifactorial assessment, e.g. including also other biosignals related to psychophysiological states (e.g. heart rate – HR and/or breathing rate - BR) that could affect the frequency of tic events, could support the identification of a more complete clinical frame that is appreciated by clinicians. For this purpose, wearables technologies (WT) are very promising. Recently our research group proposed a novel method based on WT for monitoring and quantifying motor-tics caused by the TS whose validation with respect to the standard protocol is reported in [2]. This paper discusses the further analysis of the application of this novel approach for the reliability of the systems and as a clinical decision support tool for not expert operators because it offers the opportunity to have a reliable semi-automated computation of tics also over long monitoring period and capable also to implement the different severity scale adopted in clinical practice.

2   Materials and Methods

The experimental protocol consisted in a joint video and a biosignal acquisition. The videotape protocol proposed by Goetz et al. [3] involves four sessions of about 2.5 min.

The subject was placed in a quiet room in front of a video camera. Two body views were recorded: a full frontal body and head and shoulders, both with the presence of the examiner or the absence of the examiner. An wearable device (WD) was placed through a belt on the chest of the subject for the automatic tic detection. The commercial system (PROTHEO I, SXT - Sistemi per la Telemedicina, Lecco, Italy) [5] consists of a plastic case containing a 1 ECG-lead and a 3D-acceleration sensor (LIS3L06AL, STMicroelectronics, Geneva, Switzerland), a Bluetooth transmission module, and a rechargeable Li-ion battery. The wearable device is supported by a software (HIM, Sensibilab, Politecnico di Milano, Lecco, Italy) [6] designed for collecting and managing data in applications requiring real-time biosignal monitoring (Heart Rate) and movement (3D acceleration). Two characteristics of the motor-tics were evaluated: intensity and frequency related to a 5 class scale proposed in literature [4].

According to the severity assessment proposed in the Rush Videotaping Rating Scale and revised by Bernabei et al. for the accelerometric assessment [2], we classified the motor tics into a 5-level scale: (1) barely perceptible; (2) visible; (3) some problem; (4) impaired function; (5) no function. Video analysis was carried out through an open source software (Advene, CNRS, France) providing a model and a format to share annotations about digital video documents (movies, courses, conferences…), as well as tools to edit and visualize the hypervideos generated from both the annotations and the audiovisual documents [7]. It is an easy-to-use platform with intuitive interfaces and text file output for further analysis. Video analysis was conducted by two operators: one expert, (operator 1) who was responsible for the registration; the second (operator 2) inexperienced that elaborated the data in double blind. The two operators evaluated the presence or absence of tic events and the intensity giving them a level (from 1 to 5). The third dataset is composed by tics identified by the WT system through the peaks of accelerations associated to each event. No specific on subject or self-adaptive calibration was adopted to verify a raw approach based on a simple acceleration threshold that can be related to tics. The three data were synchronized in time in the Advene platform together with their operator assessment or the classification provided by the wearable device Fig. 1).

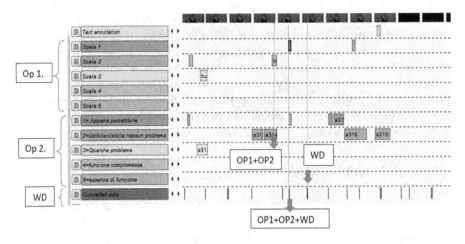

Fig. 1. The ADVENE Software suite for data synchronization and subjective assessment by the operators and correspondence analysis with automated tics computation by the WD system.

A video analysis comparison of the tics recognized by the wearable device with the tics recognized from the two operators was made. The tics can be noticed in three different ways: (a) by only the WD, (b) by the WD at least one operator, (c) by only one or two operators.

The procedure was repeated on 9 subjects without DBS implant [8] but under pharmacological treatment.

3   Results and Discussion

Table 1 shows the tics recognized and classified by both operators for typology and severity while the following columns report the tic counting carried out only by the operator no. 1 (expert neurologist). These data are assumed to be the reference in our study and they also represent the clinical gold standard.

The main goal of this study was to assess the reliability of the wearable system in measuring motor tics in TS. In Table 2 the occurrence of all tics detected by the operator no. 1 (expert neurologist) and by the WD are compared.

In these dataset motor, facial and vocal tics are included even if borderline with the goal of the study being very probably not detectable with a WD mounted onto the trunk of the subject. In any case we decided to use the raw data under the hypothesis that also facial tics produce a perturbation of the body equilibrium so that an actigraph could be suitable to measure also this kind of events. Instead, these data indicate that the WD approach produces an underestimation of events with respect to the clinical classification given by doctors. The percentage of correspondence for tics observed by the WD and tics observed by Operator no. 1 (expert clinician) was only 44.5%, with an average value of 47,66% ± 16,49% (SD) among the 9 subjects.

Table 1. Tic classification in body positioning and in severity as carried out by both clinical operators for each subject, and tic count for each severity level according to the subjective assessment by Operator no.1.

Subject	Tic typology	Level 1	Level 2	Level 3	Level 4	Level 5
1	Eyes, trunk	6	8			
2	Eyes, facial grimacing	17	19			
3	Trunk	5	15	14	3	
4	Trunk, facial grimacing	2	14	10		
5	Grimace, eyes	8	11	6		
6	Trunk	3	9	8	3	1
7	Eyes	13	13			
8	Eyes, head, trunk	1	4	11	2	
9	Vocal, trunk	4	11	21		

Table 2. Comparison of tics recognized by the Operator no. 1 and the WD.

Subject	Op.1	WD	% Corresp.
1	14	12	85,71
2	36	15	41,67
3	40	12	30,00
4	26	14	53,85
5	25	8	32,00
6	24	12	50,00
7	26	10	38,46
8	18	9	50,00
9	36	17	47,22
Tot.	245	109	44,49

This low value could be also related to the absence of a specific single subject calibration but a simple thresholding approach, but more probably they could be due to a wrong (but mandatory) sensor positioning onto the subject (in fact in case of facial tics it is unacceptable for the subject to wear a sensing sensor onto the face). Therefore, we conducted a more detailed analysis in case of mild episodes or facial tics.

In the performed experiments, the main criticisms arise with low intensity events that occur in anatomical districts far from the sensing system, i.e. the WD that is usually placed onto the trunk, so that it is not able to detect them; from parallel video check, this seems to be the main cause determining underestimation. Excluding the subjects presenting only facial tics (i.e. S2, S5, and S7) and excluding the facial tics by the occurrences detected both by the operator and the WD (null in the analyzed data) the situation significantly improves as reported in the following Table 3.

Table 3. Comparison of tics recognized by the operator 1 and the WD (related to tics only involving the trunk).

Subject	Op.1	WD	%Corresp.
1	13	12	92,31
3	37	12	32,43
4	18	14	77,78
6	24	11	45,83
8	15	9	60,00
9	24	17	70,83
Tot.	129	75	57,25

The total correspondence percentage increases at 57,25% and the average agreement level raises at 63,20% ± 21,80% (SD). This is a good result but still not optimal for introduction into the clinical practice.

A similar analysis is performed between the experienced operator (Op.1) and the non-expert neurologist (Op.2): data are reported in Table 4.

Table 4. Comparison of tics recognized by the two clinical operators.

Subject	Op.1	Op.2	%Corresp.
1	14	4	28,60
2	36	12	33,30
3	40	16	40
4	26	1	3,80
5	25	13	52
6	24	19	79
7	26	15	57,70
8	18	1	6
9	36	21	58,30
Tot.	245	102	41,60

The unexpert operator (Op.2) had a tic recognition percentage of 41.6% compared to the expert operator. It is also noticeable the high variability in not-experienced evaluation: the average correspondence percentage is 39,86% ± 25,56% (SD).

Comparing the results of the expert operator with the results of the inexperienced operator and the WD recognition capability, we can conclude that the WD behaves as an inexperienced operator presenting a small difference and a lower variability in judgements. This makes the developed system a useful tool for preliminary analysis in clinical practice.

For further application in long term and remote monitoring, the algorithm could and should be optimized to recognize severe events that are discarded now, because they are considered as voluntary movements (e.g. walking). This is a limitation of the present method and has to be considered in the future developments. Similarly, but at the opposite, another source of error in the method are other rapid movements but not related to the pathology could happen that can overcome the imposed acceleration threshold so that they are classified as tics by the software. This would have produced an overestimation but the experiments did not elicit this occurrence.

4 Conclusions

Improving the quality of life and social distress are factors that affect TS. The repeated visits, the pharmacological changes, anxiety and depression are entrusted to the treating physician for evaluation of the symptoms that afflicts them and their care. In the absence of an objective quantification of the "tics" associated with the syndrome, it becomes difficult to assess the evolution of the disease, monitor the changes and rate any improvements. The proposed systems aims at offering a novel solution to intervene in these cases and to support clinician in their decisions.

The proposed approach based on an actigraph and simple two-level thresholding in low and high trunk acceleration shows good discriminatory capacity for tic event classification in subjects with high intensity scales (scale 3–4), but it is underperforming in recognizing low severity tics as facial grimacing or vocal tics. The WD approach has a smaller increase in reliability to detect motor tics with respect to an unexperienced operator. The experienced operator, i.e. the skilled neurologist, is the gold standard in our study. Data analysis revealed that the WD is unable to detect the facial or voice tics given its positioning on the body. Considering the inexperienced operator, the difference is due to the separation capacity of the tic events and their scale. For example, the operator 2 recognizes one tic even twenty minutes in duration. This is not realistic and consistent with the clinical significance and interpretation. From a global point of view, the unskilled operator and the WD showed a similar overall evaluation.

The objective measures provided by the WD system can be a valuable addition to the medical evaluation, in order to offer a more detailed up-to-date clinical picture of the patient to neurologists, neurosurgeons and psychiatrists.

Acknowledgments. The authors would like to thank you all the subjects that took part to the study for their patients, commitments and motivated collaboration.

References

1. Shapiro, A.K., Shapiro, E.S., Young, J.G., Feinberg, T.E.: Gilles de la Tourette Syndrome, 2nd edn. Raven Press, New York (1998)
2. Bernabei, M., Preatoni, E., Mendez, M., Piccini, L., Porta, M., Andreoni, G.: A novel automatic method for monitoring Tourette motor tics through a wearable device. Mov. Disord. 25(12), 1967–1972 (2010)
3. Goetz, C.G., Tanner, C.M., Wilson, R.S., Shannon, K.M.: A rating scale for Gilles de la Tourette's Syndrome: description, reliability, and validity data. Neurology 37, 1542–1544 (1987)
4. Goetz, C.G., Pappert, E.J., Louis, E.D., Raman, R., Leurgans, S.: Advantages of a modified scoring method for the rush video-based tic rating scale. Mov. Disord. 14, 502–506 (1999)
5. Sistemi per Telemedicina. http://www.sxt-telemed.it/
6. Laboratorio Sensibilab, Politecnico di Milano. http://www.sensibilab.lecco.polimi.it

7. Aubert, O., Prié, Y.: Advene: active reading through hypervideo. In: Proceedings of ACM Hypertext 2005, pp. 235–244 (2005)
8. Bajwa, R.J., de Lotbinière, A.J., King, R.A., Jabbari, B., Quatrano, S., Kimberly, K., Scahill, L., Leckman, J.F.: Deep brain stimulation in Tourette's Syndrome. Mov. Disord. **22**(9) (2007)

Assessment of Physiological Signals During Happiness, Sadness, Pain or Anger

Nima TaheriNejad[✉] and David Pollreisz

Institute of Computer Technology, TU Wien, Vienna, Austria
nima.taherinejad@tuwien.ac.at

Abstract. With the advancement of technology, non-intrusive monitoring of some physiological signals through smart watches and other wearable devices are made possible. This provides us with new opportunities of exploring newer fields of information technology applied in our everyday lives. One application which can help individuals with difficulty in expressing their emotions, e.g. autistic individuals, is emotion recognition through bio-signal processing. To develop such systems, however, a significant amount of measurement data is necessary to establish proper paradigms, which enable such analyses. Given the sparsity of the available data in the literature, specifically the ones using portable devices, we conducted a set of experiments to help in enriching the literature. In our experiments, we measured physiological signals of various subjects during four different emotional experiences; happiness, sadness, pain, and anger. Measured bio-signals are Electrodermal activity (EDA), Skin Temperature, and Heart rate. In this paper, we share our measurement results and our findings regarding their relation with happiness, sadness, anger, and pain.

Keywords: Physiological signals · Smart watch · Characterization · Emotional experiences · EDA · Skin temperature · Heart rate · Happiness · Sadness · Pain · Anger

1 Introduction

Although expressing emotions is often considered a given ability, many people struggle with them on daily basis. For example, studies have shown that many individuals on autism spectrum suffer speech impairment [1–3]. They may also show atypical facial expressions [3,4]. To make the matters worse, their expressions are more poorly recognized by others, whether autistic or neurotypical individuals [5]. Therefore, trying to understand their feelings using alternative methods -such as physiological signal analyses- can be significantly helpful.

One of the major problems with using bio-signals for such applications has been the complexity of measurement device setups and their cost, which can render them impractical outside laboratories [6,7]. However, with the rise of simple wearable gadgets which are able to measure physiological signals, e.g.

© ICST Institute for Computer Sciences, Social Informatics and Telecommunications Engineering 2017
P. Perego et al. (Eds.): MobiHealth 2016, LNICST 192, pp. 107–114, 2017.
DOI: 10.1007/978-3-319-58877-3_14

[8,9], using this information in everyday applications is more feasible than ever. This motivates us to look into the relation of these signals and emotional experiences.

Although there are some works in the literature regarding the physiological signals and their correlation with emotional experiences, the accuracy of the analysis seems to be dependent on the data set [6,10,11]. Therefore, further body of work seems essential to expand existing knowledge. Moreover, the literature is more sparse when it comes to experiments using portable devices [12] and often the scope of these works are limited to one or two types of signals or emotions [8,13]. Through this work, we hope to contribute to the literature by presenting our measurement results using a smart watch, namely Empatica E4, and regarding three different bio-signals; Electrodermal activity (EDA), Skin Temperature, and Heart rate. We also discuss the observed relations between these signals and four emotions: happiness, sadness, pain, and anger.

The rest of this paper is organized as the following: In the next section, we will cast a brief glance over the literature. In Sect. 3, we explain our data collection setup and present the measurement results. In Sect. 4, we discuss our findings regarding the collected data and put it into further light by comparing it to the existing knowledge in the literature. Finally, Sect. 5 concludes the paper.

2   Literature Overview

In this section, we will have a brief glance into the some of the most recent works in the literature. More specifically, those that are most similar or relevant, which inspired us in parts of our data collection and research procedures.

A common traditional approach for emotion recognition using physiological signals have been using Electrocardiography (ECG) signals. For example, in [7], the authors used an ECG to measure the changes in the heart rate variability. The participants had to sit still for 120 s after the ECG was attached to them, so their baseline could be measured. Afterwards, the participants watched a slide show of pictures and listened to music. Measuring ECG seems to be too complicated for everyday applications, however, their experimental setup was inspiring in designing our setup as well.

In [6,12], the experimental setups were similar too. First, the participants had to sit still fore 60 s so their baseline could be measured. After that, they watched a short clip to experience some emotions. In [6], the participants had to fill out a Self Assessment Manikin (SAM) to show how strongly they felt each emotion. Both groups used an ECG, an EDA and a skin temperature sensor. In addition, the authors of [12] used an EEG sensor too.

Many groups that tried to identify emotions out of bio-signals used more than one device and often bulky devices to recognize emotions [6,14]. Only a few groups tried to measure emotions using portable devices. In [8], the authors used wearable EDA sensor (wore on the wrist) for measurements. The EDA was measured at two positions on each hand, and they used two different devices to measure the EDA signals. The experimental setup was similar to the ones mentioned before. The participant had to sit still so that their baseline could be measured, and after that, they had to do some tasks such as pedaling for five minutes, or watching a short clip.

Last but not least, Ayzenberg and Picard [15] tried to combine a portable device and a long term measurement. The participant had to wear an EDA sensor on their wrist, with which, not only the EDA was measured, but also the skin temperature and the movement too. The participants wore the sensor for 10 days. Every time an event occurred (e.g. getting scared), the subject had do write it down. They analysed the signals for different peaks in a period of ten minutes, and thus characterized the signals. Then, they characterized the emotions using the information of peaks and the changes in the movement. The information about peaks, as it will be described in the next sections, proved to be an important distinguishing character in our collected data-set as well.

3   Data Collection

3.1   Subjects

For this work, ten subjects participated in the data collection. All of the participant were male university students, between 20 to 25 years old. Every subject was in perfect health without any medical condition. None of them reported consumption of any medication. Before the experiments, the procedure was explained to them and they were asked for their consent. They were not compensated for their participation.

3.2   Smart Watch

For the measurements, the E4 Smart Watch from Empatica was used [9]. The watch has four embedded sensors: EDA-sensor to measure the skin conductance, Photoplethysmogram (PPG) to measure heart rate, temperature sensor to measure skin temperature, and a 3-axis accelerometer to measure movements. The latter of which was not used in our experiments since the subjects were seated and had no physical activity or movement. In addition, the watch has a button to tag events, such as the beginning and the end of the application of stimuli.

3.3   Experiments Setup and Stimuli

At the beginning of the experiment, the procedure was explained to the participants. They were then seated in front of a computer and had to put on the Empatica E4 smart watch [9] on their left wrist and a headset. The procedure consisted of watching six stimulating videos between 1.5 to 3.5 min. The videos were chosen to solicit following emotions: happiness (2 videos), sadness (2 videos), anger, and fear. The videos were played in a random order. To solicit pain, the participants were pinched in the arm. Before and after each stimulus, the subjects had to sit still for one minute so that their baseline could be obtained. Beginning and end of each stimulation were tagged (shown by red starts in the figures) by pressing the button embedded in the watch for this purpose. After each stimulus, the participants had to fill a Self-Assessment Manikin (SAM) to state what emotion they experienced and how strongly they felt it.

Table 1. Number of samples marked by the subjects as each of the solicited emotions.

Solicited emotions	Samples marked as such
Happiness	16
Sadness	15
Anger	8
Pain	8
Fear	2

3.4 Computations

After experiments the collected data were downloaded on a computer, then analysed and plotted in Matlab. In the Matlab code of this analysis, a "small" peak has a height between 0.05 to $0.4\,\mu S$, and a "big" peak has a height larger than $0.4\,\mu S$. Accordingly, in the rest of this paper, a "few" peaks means 2–4 peaks, whereas "some" implies 5–7 and "many" means more than 8 peaks. Moreover, for the heart rate, a change between 3 and 9 bpm was considered as a slight change. For skin temperature, on the other hand, the slight change implies a change between 0.06 and $0.2\,°C$. The signals were analysed by the aforementioned Matlab code in the window between the beginning and end of the application of stimuli (tagged during the experiments by the button on the watch and shown by red stars on the figures).

3.5 Results

As found out in other works as well [11,16], the stimuli were not unanimously successful in soliciting the intended emotions. Based on the filled SAM, from the 70 samples of emotional experiences (60 videos and 10 sample of pain), emotions were tagged as shown in Table 1. As we can see in this table, number of samples tagged with "fear" were very low and hence, this emotion was discarded from this study.

Figures 1 and 2 show a sample of the results. In Fig. 1, we see the various changes in the measured physiological signals corresponding to three different emotions. We can see that some signals show no particular change or any significant correlation to some emotion (e.g. the skin temperature during pain as shown in Fig. 1(a)). However, most other signals have some correlation; some demonstrate slow and very monotonic behavior (e.g. the skin temperature during happiness shown in Fig. 1(b)), some have somewhat larger or less monotonic changes (e.g. the heart rate during anger shown in Fig. 1(c)). On the other hand, some other signals show a sizable and faster changes (e.g. the EDA signal corresponding to the pain, Fig. 1(d)), which leads us to the next important feature we observed in some signals.

In Fig. 2, we see two more plots representing a different characteristics that we found distinguishing, namely peaks. This characteristic proved specifically significant in EDA signals, a few examples of which are shown in Fig. 2. The number

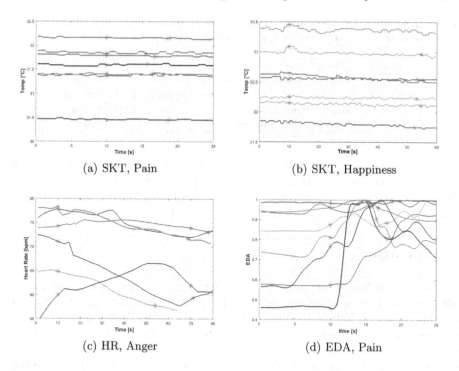

Fig. 1. Measurement results of different bio-signals as a result of various stimuli (a) SKT for Pain, (b) Skin Temperature (SKT) for happiness, (c) Heart Rate (HR) for Anger, and (d) EDA for Pain.

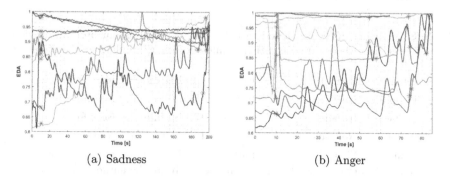

Fig. 2. EDA measurements; number and size of the peaks seems to be the main characterizing factor in EDA signals for different emotions.

and size of these peaks can point to different emotions, as seen in Figs. 1(d) and 2[1]. We often observe one big peak (Fig. 1(d)) during pain, whereas we see more big peaks during anger (Fig. 2(b)). We often notice many small peaks during sadness (Fig. 2(a)), although they occur sometimes during happiness too.

---

[1] For the sake of better presentation and quality of the plots, EDA signals in all figures were normalized to their maximum.

Table 2. Summary of the observed trends in the collected data. The darker the cell color, the bigger the number of samples showing the respective trend.

Emotion	Heart Rate	EDA	EDA Peaks	Skin Temp.
Happiness	slight increase	increase	small & few	slight decrease
Sadness	decrease	increase	small & many	slight decrease
Anger	slight decrease	increase	big & some	slight decrease
Pain	no change	increase	big & one	no change

We have summarized our observations in Table 2, where the intensity of cell color shows the frequency of observing the respective trend in various samples. The darker the cell color, the bigger the number of samples showing the respective behavior.

4   Discussion

To put our findings in perspective, compared to the existing knowledge in the literature, we summarized the characteristics we found in the literature and tabulated them in Table 3. The colored cells in this table, show where our observations differ from what we found in the literature. The lighter the cell color, the more in accordance are the findings; i.e. no cell color shows full accordance of our findings and the ones in the literature. We further remark that since the insets of Table 3 are taken from various works, they do not necessarily follow our definitions in Table 2, Sect. 3.5. As we see in Table 3, the available information is very sparse regarding the changes of the values after experiencing emotions.

Table 3. Summary of the characteristics of emotions based on our literature review. Colored cells show where our observation is different from the findings in the literature.

Emotion	Heart rate	EDA	EDA peaks	Skin temp.
Happiness	No change [17]	Increase [15]	Many [15]	No info.
Sadness	No info.	Increase [17]	No info.	No info.
Anger	No info.	Increase [17]	Many [15]	No info.
Pain	Slight Increase [6]	Increase [6]	Few[a] [6]	No change [6]

[a]This information was obtained by inference. In [6] the authors mention that the number of peaks during pain are lower than surprise, which similar to happiness and anger, stands higher in the arousal scale.

We observe in Table 3, that all of our findings are in complete accordance with the ones in the literature, except for two cases. For the case of heart rate during happiness, only three out of sixteen samples had no change, whereas seven has a slight increase. Hence, the difference in the findings could be due to the dependency on the sample set or accuracy of measurement devices. In the case of the heart rate during pain, the observed 'increase' in [6] is significantly small which makes the discord rather negligible. On the other hand, our observation was not very confident (no cell color in Table 2). The reason being that four out of eight samples showed no change, three showed a slight decrease, and one showed a slight increase. All of which does not give a strong statistical indication as to its "normal" behaviour or tendency.

A similar observation was made for the heart rate during sadness. In this case, we had six slight increases, and one large increase (larger than 9 bpm), whereas four slight decreases and four large decreases (larger than 9 bpm). This and the aforementioned observations confirm the high variation of the results and their high dependency on instances as discussed in Sect. 1. Another example of which is that in [17], in contrast with our work and that of [15], no change was observed in the EDA value during happiness. Furthermore, it is worth mentioning, that our current observation table is different compared to our own previous observation table inserted in [18], which was based on primary measurements on only four subjects.

Last but not least, we notice that in [15], the authors do not associate the number of peaks with specific feelings and rather observe it as a potential sign for arousal, which includes various emotions such as happiness and anger. Moreover, they don't specify what exactly many (or a "large number" as they call it) means, in contrast to what we did in Sect. 3.5. Nevertheless, since they measured the number of peaks during ten minutes, compared to our study in which we observed few peaks in approximately two minutes, observing many peaks in ten minutes is expected as a natural extrapolation.

5   Conclusion

Advancement of the technology has led to wearable devices which can measure physiological signals on-line and without interrupting daily life of the subject. This has opened up new opportunities to study the association of the bio-signals with emotional experiences and consequently to recognized them. Although there have been data collection campaigns in the literature, there is still a need for collecting further data. Especially, considering the high variation of the measured data and their strong dependency on the samples in experiments, as well as the considerable sparsity of data measured by wearable devices.

In this paper, we tried to contribute to the literature by reporting the results of our data collection campaign. In our experiments, we used Empatica E4 watch to measure Heart Rate, EDA, and Skin Temperature of the subjects while experiencing Happiness, Sadness, Anger, and Pain. Through this campaign, we could add new information to the literature, and verify the existing knowledge further. One of the key observations of our work was finding the association between EDA peaks and the four emotions. Number and size of the EDA peaks proved to be one of the most distinguishing characteristics of the four emotions subject to this study. Given the intrinsic high variation of the data, collecting more data in order to increase the confidence of the observed trends seems to be important for further enhancement of the existing knowledge in the literature and consequently applications which are developed based on this knowledge.

References

1. Diehl, J.J., Bennetto, L., Watson, D., Gunlogson, C., McDonough, J.: Resolving ambiguity: a psycholinguistic approach to understanding prosody processing in high-functioning autism. J. Brain Lang. **106**(2), 144–152 (2008)
2. Diehl, J.J., Paul, R.: Acoustic differences in the imitation of prosodic patterns in children with autism spectrum disorders. J. RASD **6**(1), 123–134 (2012)
3. Grossman, R.B., Edelson, L.R., Tager-Flusberg, H.: Emotional facial and vocal expressions during story retelling by children and adolescents with high-functioning autism. JSLHR **56**(3), 1035–1044 (2013)
4. Stagg, S.D., Slavny, R., Hand, C., Cardoso, A., Smith, P.: Does facial expressivity count? how typically developing children respond initially to children with autism. Autism (2013). doi:10.1177/1362361313492392
5. Brewer, R., Biotti, F., Catmur, C., Press, C., Happé, F., Cook, R., Bird, G.: Can neurotypical individuals read autistic facial expressions? Atypical production of emotional facial expressions in autism spectrum disorders. Autism Res. **9**(2), 262–271 (2016)
6. Jang, E.-H., Park, B.-J., Park, M.-S., Kim, S.-H., Sohn, J.-H.: Analysis of physiological signals for recognition of boredom, pain, and surprise emotions. J. Physiol. Anthropol. **34**(1), 25 (2015). London
7. Yu, S.-N., Chen, S.-F.: Emotion state identification based on heart rate variability and genetic algorithm. In: 37th Annual IEEE EMBC, pp. 538–541, August 2015
8. Poh, M.Z., Swenson, N.C., Picard, R.W.: A wearable sensor for unobtrusive, long-term assessment of electrodermal activity. IEEE Trans. Bio-Med. Eng. **57**(5), 1243–1252 (2010)
9. Garbarino, M., Lai, M., Bender, D., Picard, R.W., Tognetti, S.: Empatica E3—a wearable wireless multi-sensor device for real-time computerized biofeedback and data acquisition. In: EAI 4th Mobihealth, pp. 39–42. IEEE (2014)
10. Wagner, J., Kim, J., Andre, E.: From physiological signals to emotions: implementing and comparing selected methods for feature extraction and classification. In: IEEE International Conference on Multimedia and Expo, pp. 940–943 (2005)
11. Jang, E.H., Park, B.J., Kim, S.H., Eum, Y., Sohn, J.H.: Identification of the optimal emotion recognition algorithm using physiological signals. In: ICEI, pp. 1–6, November 2011
12. Dai, Y., Wang, X., Li, X., Zhang, P.: Reputation-driven multimodal emotion recognition in wearable biosensor network. In: IEEE I2MTC, pp. 1747–1752 (2015)
13. Faghih, R., Stokes, P., Marin, M.-F., Zsido, R., Zorowitz, S., Rosenbaum, B., Song, H., Milad, M., Dougherty, D., Eskandar, E., Widge, A., Brown, E., Barbieri, R.: Characterization of fear conditioning and fear extinction by analysis of electrodermal activity. In: 37th IEEE EMBC, pp. 7814–7818, August 2015
14. Park, M.W., Kim, C.J., Whang, M., Lee, E.C.: Individual emotion classification between happiness and sadness by analyzing photoplethysmography and skin temperature. In: Fourth WCSE, pp. 190–194, December 2013
15. Ayzenberg, Y., Picard, R.: Feel: a system for frequent event and electrodermal activity labeling. J-BHI **18**(1), 266–277 (2014)
16. Lee, C., Yoo, S., Park, Y., Kim, N., Jeong, K., Lee, B.: Using neural network to recognize human emotions from heart rate variability and skin resistance. In: 27th IEEE-EMBS 2005, pp. 5523–5525, January 2005
17. Sharma, T., Bhardwaj, S., Maringanti, H.: Emotion estimation using physiological signals. In: TENCON 2008, pp. 1–5 (2008)
18. TaheriNejad, N., Jantsch, N., Pollreisz, D.: Comprehensive observation and its role in self-awareness; an emotion recognition system example. In: FedCSIS, pp. 123–130, September 2016

Customising the Cold Challenge: Pilot Study of an Altered Raynaud's Phenomena Assessment Method for Data Generation

Isobel Taylor[(✉)]

FCT, University of Porto, Porto, Portugal
mail@isobeltaylor.com

Abstract. The objective of the study is to develop a methodology for gathering data on phalanges to be utilised in wearable technology research with the potential to assist Raynaud's Phenomena (RP) sufferers. This paper gives an overview of a pilot study using a method developed from an existing medical practise called 'cold challenge', which is used in the clinical analysis of RP, and amended for data collection. Due to the alterations that differentiate the pilot study from the clinical exam, it is expected that adjustments will be required to the methodology before a full study is undertaken. The paper centres on the pilot study and the developments made through the analysis of the pilot study results for implementation in further research. The pilot study illustrates a method trialled in the early stages of R&D within PhD design research.

Keywords: Pilot study · Raynaud's Phenomenon · Medical technology research

1 Introduction

The focus of the research study is a medical condition called Raynaud's Phenomenon (RP), which 'describes excessive vasoconstriction of the digital microvasculature in response to cold exposure and emotional stress' [1]. The present pilot study aims to develop a methodology for data generation for use in design and research towards mobile technology development. Clinical analysis of RP is conducted in controlled environments and with patient information [2]. There are variations on the thermographic analysis of RP; in this study the 'cold challenge' method developed by Anderson et al. [3] was used as the framework. The cold challenge method states a single subject and includes: an environmentally controlled room to which the subject adjusts before taking the cold challenge, blood tests, an assessment of the subject's medical and family history, and the subject abstaining from smoking or caffeine intake for 4 h prior to the test.

Tests in clinical environments are carefully developed for diagnostic and clinical purposes; the anticipated outcome of this research and pilot study is not a diagnostic tool but the generation of data towards a database that would be beneficial with regard to mobile technology development. Aspects of the cold

© ICST Institute for Computer Sciences, Social Informatics and Telecommunications Engineering 2017
P. Perego et al. (Eds.): MobiHealth 2016, LNICST 192, pp. 115–121, 2017.
DOI: 10.1007/978-3-319-58877-3_15

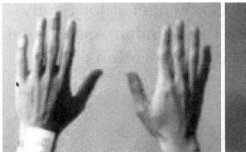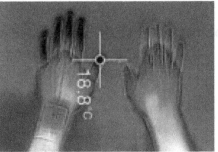

Fig. 1. Images of a participant's hands obtained during the pilot study. (a) Photograph. (b) Thermal image. Images by Isobel Taylor @ 2016

challenge not considered in this pilot study include fixed environments, family history, and medical data. Eliminating these factors allows for a simpler, more time efficient testing method, allowing the assessment of data for fingers from a range of subjects, regardless of their medical and family history, in quotidian situations. In this pilot study, hand submersion was carried out in containers of 15 °C water and ice. The temperature was set to 15 °C to trigger RP and cause vasoconstriction within the clinical examination of RP. Alternatively, ice is known to cause vasodilation and was also used within the pilot as a record of the effect. The research looks towards mobile outputs that create changing environments; therefore, the environment in which the test is conducted was recorded but not fixed for each group tested. Part of the overall study that will follow this pilot will involve testing specific focus groups, such as athletes and particular age groups, which is known as purposive sampling [4]. The subsequent sections of the paper outline the method used in the pilot study, the results, and the amendments to be made to the methodology for the full study. This study also acts as an example of multidisciplinary research, as it spans the fields of medicine, design, and technology.

2   Pilot Study

The participants volunteered from within the University of Porto. The session was conducted in a classroom environment at a temperature of 22 °C with the windows closed and no direct sunlight, heating, or air conditioning for the duration of the study. Participants were given information on RP and the study and an opportunity to ask questions. To the participants' knowledge, none have RP, and none have had RP diagnosed.

A container of ice cubes and a container of 15 °C water were prepared for the hand submersions. Both were stirred and their temperatures regularly checked. Participants each had a number attached to their hands (see Fig. 1), preserving anonymity whilst identifying age bracket and gender, which are known factors in RP. The FLIR ONE 2nd Gen thermal imaging camera and FLIR ONE 2nd

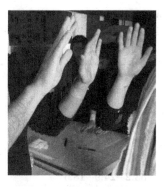

Fig. 2. Photograph hands held at chest height whilst queuing for thermal imaging. Photograph by participant no. 2

Gen iOS software were used for imaging. Participants had their temperatures taken through thermal imaging at regular intervals for 20 to 30 min following submersion. The following instructions were given to the participants. Submerse both hands, one person at a time, and form a queue for thermal imaging, looping until the time frame ends. Hold hands above the table surface for the thermal imaging to eliminate temperature contamination. Hold hands up at chest height whilst queuing and do not let hands touch anything for the duration of the test (see Fig. 2). Following the study, the participants were given a chance to ask questions & fill out a feedback form. The pilot study, gathering data on the nine participants, was completed in 1 h.

Method

1. Participants had a base temperature reading taken.
2. Participants submersed their hands: right hand in 15 °C water, left hand in a container of ice cubes. Group A: duration of 60 s, five participants. Group B: duration of 120 s, four participants (see Table 1).
3. Paper towels were used to dab dry hands.
4. Thermal images were taken at regular intervals for 20 to 30 min.
5. Temperature readings were gathered from the thermal imagery at the nail bed of the index and ring fingers and recorded.

Results. Tables and graphs were created for each participant, and initial data has been generated. The results for four of the nine participants are included in this paper as illustrative examples of the different variables considered in this study: one male and one female for each submersion time of 60 and 120 s. The charts include the first temperature taken before submersion; the gradient shows the drop from the base temperature to that post-submersion and the subsequent climb in temperature over time (see Figs. 3, 4, 5 and 6). The two lines in each graph show temperature taken from the nail beds of the index finger and ring

Table 1. Submersion times and temperature ranges obtained during the pilot study for four participants. All temperature data in table were taken from the index finger. Isobel Taylor @ 2016

Participant no., gender and submersion time in seconds	15 °C (right hand) base−highest−lowest, temperature in °C	Ice (left hand) base−highest−lowest, temperature in °C
No.8 Male 60 s	29.9−23.2−20.5	30.5−20.9−17.4
No.1 Female 60 s	24.2−28.5−7.9	25.1−32.8−10.2
No.6 Male 120 s	33.2−31.6−19.4	33.2−12.2−32.5
No.7 Female 120 s	33.2−24.9−18.6	24.6− 9.9−19.8

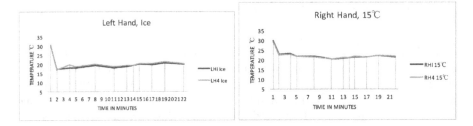

Fig. 3. Charts for participant 8: male, submersion duration of 60 s. The left hand showed a slight temperature increase following submersion in ice over 22 min, and the right showed very little temperature increase following the 15 °C submersion. Isobel Taylor @ 2016

finger of the same hand. The results show that although they can be very close in temperature, fingers on the same hand do not change temperature at exactly the same rate.

3 Amendments

Although the pilot study yielded useful temperature data results, the method requires some alterations before being conducted on a larger scale. The core changes are as follows.

3.1 Gloves

Within the pilot, the participants were asked to dab their hands dry with paper towels; however, this is problematic, as any leftover dampness alters skin temperature readings. In the Raynaud's cold challenge method, thin latex gloves are worn during the submersion and removed prior to the thermography to avoid this problem.

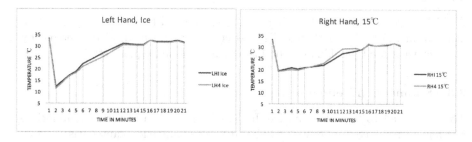

Fig. 4. Charts for participant 6: male, submersion duration of 120 s. The left hand showed a slightly faster temperature rise over time than the right hand, as expected from the vasodilation effect of the ice, and the right hand showed rewarming following the 15 °C submersion. Isobel Taylor @ 2016

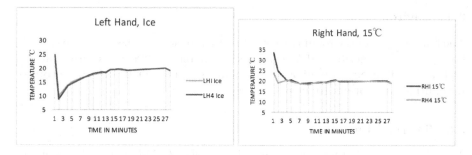

Fig. 5. Charts for participant 7: female, submersion duration of 120 s. The right hand showed very little temperature rise over time, and the base temperature of the ring finger was higher than that of the index finger. Isobel Taylor @ 2016

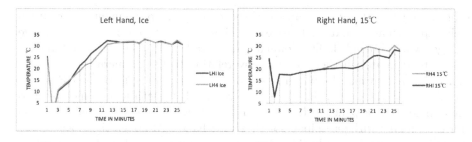

Fig. 6. Charts for participant 1: female, submersion duration of 60 s. This not only showed the faster rewarming following ice submersion but also a final finger temperature that was higher than the base temperature in the same hand. Isobel Taylor @ 2016

3.2 Back Drop

A thick piece of white matte paper was used to avoid the reflection of temperature from the table. In Raynaud's cold challenge and medical thermography, black cloth is used [5]. This will be incorporated in subsequent studies.

3.3 Submersion Temperature

The pilot used 15 °C water and ice. Ice has been used in historic examinations but has been rejected more recently because ice submersion causes vasodilation rather than triggering a Raynaud's attack. Ice submersion was included in the pilot to obtain a record of the effect of vasodilation. The problem with conducting two tests on one person is that their body is likely to be effected by both hands; therefore, within the pilot, neither measurement is a reading of the response to 15 °C water or ice but a measurement of the effect of one hand in each temperature.

3.4 Environment

The temperature of the room the participants were acclimatised to was recorded; however, a more accurate device is needed for reliable results. Considerations such as wind speed, time of year, temperature, and climate will be recorded when using outdoor environments.

3.5 Thermal Imaging

The battery on the thermal imaging device (FLIR ONE 2nd Gen) is short. Because of this, the data contains a gap from when the device required charging. For future studies the FLIR will remain connected to a power supply during the study to keep it charged [6].

3.6 Target Group and Participants

For the pilot test, the age ranges of the pilot study participants were 21–30 (eight participants) and 31–40 (one participant). In future work, a larger range of ages will be included. The dominant hand and hand strength should also be noted to evaluate whether this has any relation to the temperature readings. This information may be useful based on advice currently given to RP sufferers that exercise is beneficial [7]. Therefore, hand strength will be measured to determine if participants with stronger hands show any unique temperature patterns compared with participants with weaker hands. Although the labels on the participants' hands were legible, they were not easy to read. In future studies, participant labelling should be clearer. Amendments to the explanation of the exam given to the volunteers identified from the pilot study include the following addition to the information sheet based on the question most commonly asked by the participants: 'What happens if it turns out I have or may have RP?' From this, a section will restate that this test is not a diagnosis but is aimed at data collection and that if the condition has not previously affected the participants, this study will not change that.

4   Conclusion

The pilot study was successful in recording temperature ranges when exposing hands to specific stimuli and the identification of improvements for the full study. The data collected is clear and usable, and additional information, such as hand strength information, has been identified for inclusion in further studies. As a designer working across disciplines, I have found creating this pilot study to be highly beneficial as a crash course in obtaining a more in-depth understanding of RP not just from papers and discussions but from live testing and observation. As this pilot is the early stages and research is ongoing, the results of how this pilot and the method of study it informs are inconclusive, as they cannot be fully evaluated until the study is further developed. The test and results will also be discussed with medical experts for feedback and further alterations.

Acknowledgements. This work is ongoing and funded by Fundação para a Ciência e a Tecnologia, Foundation of Science and Technology (FCT), Porto, Portugal. The pilot study was conducted by myself, Isobel Taylor, PhD student in Design, with assistance from the volunteers who participated in the study. Special thanks to the participants, Prof Heitor Alvelos, Dr. John Pauling, and Dr. Kevin Howell.

References

1. Pauling, J.D.: Evaluating Digital Vascular Perfusion and Platelet Dysfunction in Raynaud's Phenomenon and Systemic Sclerosis. Doctoral dissertation, University of Bath (2013)
2. Murray, A., Pauling, J.D.: Non-invasive methods of assessing Raynaud's phenomenon. In: Wigley, F.M., Herrick, A.L., Flavahan, N.A. (eds.) Raynaud's Phenomenon: A Guide to Pathogenesis and Treatment. Springer, New York (2015)
3. Anderson, M.E., et al.: The 'distal-dorsal difference': a thermographic parameter by which to differentiate between primary and secondary Raynaud's phenomenon. Rheumatology **46**(3), 533–538 (2006)
4. Devers, K.J., Frankel, R.M.: Study design in qualitative research - 2: sampling and data collection strategies. Educ. Health **13**(2), 263–271 (2000)
5. Hildebrandt, C., Raschner, C., Ammer, K.: An overview of recent application of medical infrared thermography in sports medicine in Austria. Sensors **10**, 4700–4715 (2010)
6. FLIR ONE 2nd Gen user guide. http://www.flir.com/flirone/press/FLIR-One-ios-android-user-guide.pdf
7. SRUK: Managing Raynaud's. https://www.sruk.co.uk/raynauds/managing-raynauds/

IOT - Internet of Things

A Context-Aware, Capability-Based, Role-Centric Access Control Model for IoMT

Flora Malamateniou[✉], Marinos Themistocleous, Andriana Prentza,
Despina Papakonstantinou, and George Vassilacopoulos

Department of Digital Systems, University of Piraeus, 80 Karaoli and Dimitriou street,
Piraeus, Greece
{flora,mthemist,aprentza,dpap,gvass}@unipi.gr

Abstract. The Internet of Medical Things (IoMT) can be described as connecting everyday devices and wearables to the Internet in order to intelligently link them together, thus enabling new forms of communication between things (medical devices) and people (patients) and between things themselves. This paper describes a context-aware access control model that hinges on the role-based and attribute-based access control (RABAC) and the capability-based access control (CapBAC) models. A prototype access control mechanism based on the model is intended to be incorporated into a personal health record (PHR) platform.

Keywords: IoMT · Access control · Role-centric model · Capabilities-based model

1 Introduction

Recently, there has been a noted shift in the healthcare sector from episodic-care to continuous-care and from traditional hospital care to connected care when and where possible [2, 9]. As a result, there is growing interest for home care services in order to support better health management and independent living, especially for the elderly [1, 9, 10].

Basically, home care services aim at providing continuous patient monitoring and immediate response by healthcare professionals in case of either emergency situations, indicated by abnormal physiological data and medical measurements, or risk situations, indicated by patient abnormal behavior (e.g. less movement, lack of personal care). Moreover, it has been suggested that continuous, connected healthcare, based on the "Internet of Medical Things (IoMT)" is an important component of smart cities of the present and of the future, since, increasingly, patients want to heal at home and connected care at home allows this to happen [1, 9, 10]. Hence, connected healthcare is an alternative to institution-based healthcare that has not been designed to keep up with demand or the desire for patients to heal and age at home.

Along with growth, healthcare organizations have been developing a whole new digital health strategy. Instead of using systems that push information from one hospital and physician to the other, they employ personal health records (PHRSs) and patient portal technology that encourage patient engagement and patient-centered care [2–4]. For the

© ICST Institute for Computer Sciences, Social Informatics and Telecommunications Engineering 2017
P. Perego et al. (Eds.): MobiHealth 2016, LNICST 192, pp. 125–131, 2017.
DOI: 10.1007/978-3-319-58877-3_16

patient, the PHR stores all of the patient data in one place and is easy to use providing access to patient data and more online, round the clock and at their convenience, which is fulfilling their needs and demands. However, when IoMT are integrated around a PHR platform, various security challenges have to be confronted, such as patient privacy, end-to-end security, user authentication, access control and resilience to attacks [3, 6].

This paper presents a context-aware capability role and attribute-based access control (CapRABAC) model that has been developed for connected medical devices that have been integrated around a PHR platform and hinges on the role and attribute-based access control (RABAC) and the capability-based access control (CapBAC) models [3, 5–8]. Thus, through a capability transfer the model allows to delegate to certain role holders both contextually constrained permissions and roles.

2   Motivation

The basic motivation of this research stems from our involvement in a recent project concerned with development of an authorization mechanism for connected medical things. Table 1 shows an extract of authorization policies regarding PHR and medical device-produced data accesses by physicians.

Table 1.   Extract of **authorization** policies

No	Authorization policy
1	A physician assigned to treat a patient (patient's attending physician) is allowed to access the PHR and to read data produced by connected medical devices that have been assigned to the patient and are related to his/her specialty
2	A physician assigned to do a night or holiday duty (duty physician) is allowed to access the PHR and to read data produced by connected medical devices that have been assigned to the patients and are related to his/her specialty
3	A physician requested to provide consultation on a patient (patient's consulting physician) is allowed to access the PHR and to read data produced by connected medical devices that have been assigned to the patient and are related to his/her specialty, on delegation by the patient's attending physician

The authorization policies of Table 1 surface certain permission delegation and propagation requirements with regard to the three physician (functional) roles involved: attending physician, duty physician and consulting physician. In fact, the role "attending physician" corresponds to a relationship (physician, patient), the role "duty physician" corresponds to a relationship (physician, healthcare unit) and the role "consulting physician" corresponds to a relationship (attending physician, physician). These roles are revoked when the relationship occurrences cease to exist.

Since PHRs empower patients with data ownership, it is the patients themselves who are entitled to grant permissions on accessing their own data to others. However, this may be proved infeasible in the stressful medical environment (e.g. in emergency cases or, even, in ordinary cases). Hence, there is a need to somehow automatically allow physicians receive the least possible authorizations (just-in-time and at the suitable level of granularity) for performing their healthcare activities.

A realistic scenario of the need for automatic delegation of authority (the data access permissions that have been assigned to the role) is as follows: Upon assignment to a patient, a physician takes up the role of the "attending physician" for the patient automatically; upon request to provide consultation for a patient, the requested physician takes up the role of the "consulting physician" for the patient automatically; and, upon assignment to a night or holiday duty, a physician takes up the role of the "duty physician" automatically.

3   Capability-Based RABAC Model Overview

On the above premises, a context-aware capability role and attribute-based access control (CapRABAC) model has been developed for controlling access to data objects from connected IoMTs which are integrated around a PHR platform [4, 11]. Basically, CapRABAC is an extension of the RABAC model obtained by integrating a CapBAC mechanism into a context-aware RABAC model (that dynamically adjusts role and permission assignments based on contextual information so that users are provided with tight, just-in-time permissions). Moreover, the model addresses the issue of flexible delegation of capabilities subject to capability propagation constraints [5, 6, 8]. To reduce the complexity of the model only positive authorizations are considered.

Figure 1 shows the context-aware CapRABAC model that includes the following main components:

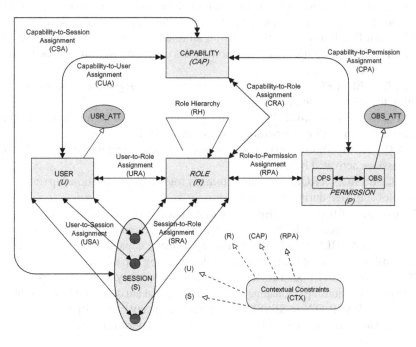

Fig. 1. The context-aware CapRABAC model.

- *USER:* A user is an entity whose access is being controlled. Patients are super-users as the owners of their PHR data.
- *ROLE:* A role may be assumed as a named collection of capabilities or permissions which define the division of work and the lines of authority based on job functions and seniority. Thus, roles encapsulate sets of permissions, they are assigned to users through a many-to-many relationship and they may be activated at run time, possibly with regard to contextual constraints. Thus, roles encapsulate the minimum sets of permissions which are tailored to run time access needs of users by taking into account the context (i.e. are constrained by context rules) so that users are provided with tight, just-in-time permissions.
- *PERMISSION:* A permission is an approval to access one or more protected objects in certain modes.
- *CAPABILITY:* A capability is a communicable, unforgeable token consisting of an object identifier and a list of permitted operations for that object. Hence, a capability represents a self-authenticating permission to access a specific object in permitted operations, whereby owners of the capability can access the object without any authentication. Moreover, it is used for delegation of authority, usually achieved in three steps performed by the delegator (i.e. a user who wishes to delegate authority to another user): (1) capability creation, (2) assignment of some permissions and/or roles to the capability, and (3) transfer of the capability to the intended delegate (i.e. receiver of the capability). Thus, a user can delegate both permissions and roles by a capability transfer.
- *SESSION:* A session is a set of user interactions with the system during which a user is assigned a set of roles. One of these roles will be active for each interaction. Role activation and deactivation may be performed dynamically during a session.
- $RH \subseteq ROLE \times ROLE$, a partial order on all roles, called the role dominance relationship (also, indicating which functional roles can be derived from which organizational roles).
- $URA \subseteq USER \times ROLE$, a many-to-many user to role assignment relationship (indicating the roles assigned to users).
- $RPA \subseteq ROLE \times PERMISSION$ is a many-to-many role to permission assignment relationship (indicating the permissions assigned to roles).
- $USA \subseteq USER \times SESSION$ is a one-to-many user to session relationship (indicating the sessions activated by a user).
- $SRA \subseteq SESSION \times ROLE$ is a many-to-many role to session relationship (indication the roles activated during a session).
- $CUA \subseteq CAPABILITY \times USER$ is a many-to-many capability to user to assignment relationship (indicating both the delegators and the delegates of capabilities).
- $CRA \subseteq CAPABILITY \times ROLE$ is a many-to-many capability to role assignment relationship (indicating the roles that are delegated by capabilities).
- $CPA \subseteq CAPABILITY \times PERMISSION$ is a many-to-many capability to permission assignment relationship (indicating the permissions that are delegated by capabilities).
- $CSA \subseteq CAPABILITY \times SESSION$ is a many-to-many capability to session relationship (indicating the capabilities that are activated during a session).

The model of Fig. 1 indicates that some additional components have been introduced to the original RABAC model, namely, a set of capabilities, a mapping to determine the owners of the capabilities and the assignment of roles and permissions to capabilities. Note that in terms of these assignments both roles and permissions are treated as delegation units.

3.1 Contextual Rules

Context is a set of context types evaluated during a session (at run time) which constrains the available set of access permissions. Context types may correspond to domain-dependent or domain-independent concepts. For example, with regard to medical device data accesses, domain-dependent context types may be user (userCtx) and object (objCtx) and domain-independent context types may be time (timeCtx) and location (locCtx).

Based on the context types, three kinds of context components may be defined: (a) contextual attributes (corresponding to user and object attributes of the RABAC model), (b) contextual sets (corresponding to set valued attributes of the RABAC model), and (c) contextual functions (corresponding to the filter functions that are boolean expressions based on user and object attributes of the RABAC model) [7]. These are expressed in the syntax <context type>.<component>.<name>.

For example, in a medical situation, the context type *userCtx* may include the contextual attribute *(userCtx.Att.user_id)*, representing user identity, and may be related to the contextual set (userCtx.Set.physician), representing that the user is actually a physician, and to the contextual function (userCtx.Fn.attending(pat_id)), specifying that the user is an attending physician to the patient with the particular pat-id. Hence, a role defined by a relationship between a physician and a patient (e.g. attending physician, consulting physician) may be represented by a contextual function.

Contextual rules relate contextual information, considered relevant to a particular situation, in logical expressions that constrain an access control policy with regard to protected objects. Essentially, they are parameterized expressions whose arguments are evaluated at run time to determine whether an attempted access should be permitted (if they evaluate to *"True"*) or denied (if they evaluate to *"False"*). For example, the rule *homecare(pat-id) {pat-id in pat.Ctx.Set.home_care_patients}*, where *"in"* checks whether *pat-id* belongs to the set of home_care_patients of a hospital or a health district, yields *"True"* if the patients identified by *pat-id* is a homecare patient.

3.2 Authorization Rules and Capabilities

On the above considerations, the authorization rules *AUTH* and the capabilities *CAP* of the context-aware CapRABAC model for IoMT are of the form

$$AUTH = \{R, (M, O/P/MD), CON, \delta\} \quad /Authorization\ rule$$
$$CAP = \{R, (M, O/P/MD), CON, \delta\} \quad /Permission\ capability$$

The authorization rule *AUTH* indicates that a user holding the role R may exert permission (M, O/P/MD), (for performing operation M on the object O/P/MD of medical device MD connected to patient P), under a set of contextual constraints (expressed as contextual rules) CON that must be fulfilled (evaluated to *"True"*) and that this permission may or may not be passed on by the role holder as denoted by flag δ. Similar interpretations hold for the corresponding capability *CAP*.

This definition presumes that users holding specific roles may be granted sets of permissions by a role holder who holds all the permissions (in the case of a PHR platform, the latter user holds the *"patient"* role who owns his/her data). Subsets of these permissions may then be passed on by the grantees to other role holders.

4 Concluding Remarks

Success of connected care largely depends on protecting patient information security and privacy. This paper presents CapRABAC, an access control model for healthcare information stored into a PHR and connected medical devices. The model is an attempt to provide a flexible approach for managing information security with regard to medical devices used by patients and connected to a PHR platform. Hence, the use of ontologies has been adopted that results into suitable context-aware authorizations for users. Model implementation into a mechanism, which is intended to be incorporated into an experimental PHR platform, is still in progress focusing, among the rest, on intelligent, ontology-based approaches for automatic delegation of roles and of context-aware permissions and for enabling such devices, agents and services interact securely and with the least user intervention.

References

1. Bhide, V.: A survey on the smart homes using Internet of Things (IoT). Int. J. Adv. Res. Comput. Manage. **2**(12), 243–246 (2014)
2. Calvillo, J., Roman, I., Roa, L.M.: Empowering citizens with authorization mechanisms to their personal health resources. Int. J. Med. Inform. **82**, 58–72 (2013)
3. Carrion, I., Aleman, J., Toval, A.: Accessing the HIPAA standard in practice: PHR privacy policies. In: Proceedings of the 33rd Annual International Conference of the IEEE EMBS, Boston, Massachusetts, USA (2011)
4. Chen, T.S., Liu, C.H., Chen, T.L., Chen, C.S., Bau, J.G., Lin, T.C.: Secure dynamic authorization scheme of PHR in cloud computing. J. Med. Syst. **36**(6), 4005–4020 (2012)
5. Gusmeroli, S., Piccione, S., Rotondi, D.: A capability-based security approach to manage access control in the Internet of Things. Math. Comput. Model. **58**(5–6), 1189–1205 (2013)
6. Hernandez Ramos, J., Jara, A., Marın, L., Skarmeta, A.: Distributed capability-based access control for the Internet of Things. J. Internet Serv. Inf. Secur. (JISIS) **3**(3/4), 1–16 (2013)
7. Jin, X., Sandhu, R., Krishnan, R.: RABAC: role-centric attribute-based access control. In: Kotenko, I., Skormin, V. (eds.) MMM-ACNS 2012. LNCS, vol. 7531, pp. 84–96. Springer, Heidelberg (2012). doi:10.1007/978-3-642-33704-8_8
8. Li, F., Rahulamathavan, Y., Conti, M., Rajarajan, M.: LSD-ABAC: lightweight static and dynamic attributes based access control scheme for secure data access in mobile environment. In: Proceedings IEEE Local Computer Networks (IEEE LCN 2014), Edmonton, Canada (2014)

9. Pang, Z., Zheng, L., Tian, J., Kao-Walter, S., Dubrova, E., Chen, Q.: Design of a terminal solution for integration of in-home health care devices and services towards the Internet-of-Things. Enterp. Inf. Syst. **9**(1), 86–116 (2015)
10. Uckelman, D., Harrison, M., Michahelles, F. (eds.): Architecting the Internet of Things. Springer, Heidelberg (2011)
11. Weber, R.: Internet of Things – new security and privacy challenges. Comput. Law Secur. Rev. **26**, 23–30 (2010)

Modular IoT Platform for AAL and Home Care Using Bluetooth Low Energy

Johannes Kropf$^{(\boxtimes)}$, Samat Kadyrov, and Lukas Roedl

AIT Austrian Institute of Technology, Vienna, Austria
johannes.kropf@ait.ac.at
http://www.ait.ac.at

Abstract. This work describes a standard conform Java based modular IoT framework for context-aware applications for AAL and home care. An extensive support of Bluetooth Low Energy personal health devices as well as various home sensor networks is provided.

Keywords: IoT · Java framework · AAL middleware · Home care support · ehealth · Bluetooth low energy · Personal health devices

1 Introduction

During the past decades, consumer driven health care in conjunction with web-based platforms and electronic health records have led to an array of improved health-care solutions. In recent years, also a big amount of smart phone apps for physiological status monitoring became available. However, despite being an important step towards personalized medicine, these solutions often suffer from scalability, security, interoperability and privacy issues. Furthermore, such solutions are only able to provide a snapshot of physiological conditions rather than a continuous view of the overall health status over the course of many years [1].

Despite the increasing number of mobile phones, their supported wireless PAN or WAN technologies are limited, i.e. not all devices support all the available types of wireless PAN or WAN. Therefore interoperability between the sensor devices and mobile phones becomes very restricted. Another common issue when using mobile phones for transmission of data from personal health devices or other sensors is that the application that is receiving the sensor data has to be initiated and cannot always be available for receiving sensor data.

Internet of Things and pervasive computing is becoming more and more important, not only in home care. Furthermore the number of data acquiring devices in households is increasing dramatically. Current systems for the home care and Ambient Assisted Living (AAL) domain available on the market are very often isolated solutions without interfaces for third party applications. In this project, the authors aim to create an inter-operable, standard conform and flexible framework for collecting and analyzing data in the user's home on low-cost hardware. Furthermore, smart home and health related data will be combined and analyzed, to get a continuous and deeper insight into the patient's

© ICST Institute for Computer Sciences, Social Informatics and Telecommunications Engineering 2017
P. Perego et al. (Eds.): MobiHealth 2016, LNICST 192, pp. 132–137, 2017.
DOI: 10.1007/978-3-319-58877-3_17

health status, by e.g. comparing smart home activity data with vital parameters. This paper describes the main features and the architecture of the system and how it is integrated in real world scenarios using low-cost hardware.

2 Related Work

In the moduLAAr project [2,3], an NFC-based (near field communication) system was used to monitor vital parameters of older adults in their homes remotely. The system makes use of NFC for both identification via an NFC card and data acquisition via NFC-enabled personal health devices using a smart phone [4]. During the long time field trial a few problems appeared concerning usability (two step approach) as well as robustness of the NFC technology. The users asked for a less obtrusive and simpler solution whereby the system was successfully used in other settings with a different target group. However, the project has shown that there is a demand for cheap, simple to use and non-obtrusive solutions for supporting home care and health care in the AAL domain. Further more, real world use of mobile phone based systems has shown the difficulty to maintain multi-purpose devices.

From the platform perspective, there are existing various AAL middleware solutions as outcome of research projects. The most prominent one is the universAAL open platform and reference specification for building AAL systems [5]. The universAAL project created a reference architecture or an ontology based AAL middleware platform, whereby its core consists of three buses for context, services and user interaction. The reference implementation was done in Java using an OSGi framework.

Beside commercial smart home systems, there exists a number of open source smart home platforms, focusing on the remote control of devices and some AAL platforms providing some more functionality like reminders etc., but a ready-to-use, sustainable, flexible, extensible and modular middleware for AAL providing the whole spectrum of required features like sensing the smart home environment plus the inhabitant, integrated data analysis and context aware multi-modal user interaction which could be used on a large scale is not available so far, even though many research projects attempted to provide certain aspects. The authors aim to close this gap with the provided solution described in this paper.

3 Platform Overview

Our group has developed the HOMER (HOMe Event Recognition) [6] system, a modular software platform, for integration of many kind of devices (smart home environment, body worn and health related devices), data acquisition and analysis of multi-modal data. The platform itself, written in Java, is open source with its core functionalities and makes use of OSGi technology to facilitate modularity and to reduce complexity. Moreover, HOMER runs inside the Apache Karaf framework [7], which is a modern and polymorphic container and supports features like hot deployment, console advanced logging and dynamic configuration.

Besides that OSGi also offers advantages regarding versioning, runtime-flexibility and maintenance. To realize important aspects of such a platform (such as security, modularity, extendibility or interoperability), standards for medical device communication and home automation networks are also integrated. The platform enables integration of other transport types (transport abstraction) as well as device abstraction, that uses a standardized abstraction model (ISO 11073-10471 [8]) in order to enforce interoperability [9]. Based on that hardware abstraction layer deterministic rules, respectively finite-state-machines are configured to trigger various actions. Within the scope of the current work the platform was extended in terms of management and handling of health related data. The implementation is based on the ISO 11073-20601 and accompanying standards for specific health device profiles.

Based on the modular architecture HOMER supports the full signal chain from raw sensor data to abstracted data fusion, connection to remote players and multi-modal intelligent user interaction. This makes HOMER a ready-to-use platform for AAL and home care applications. Even initially designed as a research platform, HOMER can be used for real world applications which require functionalities on top of a smart home like intelligent multi-modal user interaction or human behaviour recognition.

4   Bluetooth Low Energy Integration

Bluetooth Low Energy (BLE) is an emerging wireless technology developed by the Bluetooth Special Interest Group (SIG) for short-range communication. In contrast with previous Bluetooth flavors, BLE has been designed as a low-power solution for control and monitoring applications [10]. Since the BLE communication protocol is well documented and closely related to the ISO 11073 [11] standard and the Continua Health Alliance design guidelines, the creation of standard-conform devices would be quite straight forward, however, the number of standard conform BLE devices on the market is poor. Instead, manufacturers tend to create custom profiles with a custom data encryption even if a device profile exists for their device class.

Within this work a flexible Java framework for integration of BLE enabled devices, both standard-conform and proprietary, was developed and integrated in the platform described above. Due to the aim to create low-cost unmaintained systems for the health care domain the focus was on the Linux operating system using the BlueZ stack. The framework makes use of the Java D-Bus API to connect to the BlueZ daemon and provides generic BLE profiles, services etc. as well as certain proprietary devices. A template class makes the definition of new profiles fast and easy and the integration into the HOMER system provides the connection to an IoT enabled gateway as well as a generic multi-modal data analysis. Moreover, due to the modular architecture the generic BLE library, represented by the Common bundle in the stack of OSGi bundles, is designed to be reused within other applications and operating systems, e.g. Android or Windows. The interconnection of the modules and the data flow from a BLE device up to the application is depicted in Fig. 1.

Even though a small number of open BLE libraries for Java exist, so far none of them is complete in terms of providing all services, characteristics and profiles, and flexible enough to add additional standardized and proprietary devices. The provided solution aims to help to close this gap.

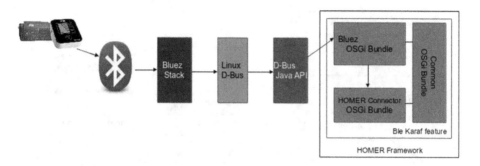

Fig. 1. Bluetooth integration in Karaf feature and OSGi bundle hierarchy

5   Integrated Raspberry Pi Prototype

The whole framework runs on a Raspberry Pi (RPi) which was enhanced with a small LCD display as well as a finger print sensor for user identification in a multi-user setting. Using the newest version 3 of the RPi with on-board Bluetooth and wireless LAN, no additional hardware (in form of USB dongles) is necessary. This allows the construction of a low-cost and stand-alone and non-obtrusive device acting in the background and able to get integrated in the home environment.

6   Applications

The HOMER platform was tested in a few research projects involving extensive user trials. On a larger scale it was used in the moduLAAr project to monitor vital parameters and to detect unusual situations in 50 households e.g. no activity due to a fall [9]. Moreover, a tablet based user interface, which was especially designed for elder users, was provided with functionalities like smart home control. reminders or shared pictures.

In the RelaxedCare project [12] HOMER was used for audio and smart home based activity recognition, and in the Doremi project [13] it was used to design, configure and provide sensor configuration for 40 test flats.

These examples show that our platform is flexible enough and ready-to-use for research projects in the AAL and home care domain on the one hand, and ready for deployment on a larger scale on the other hand.

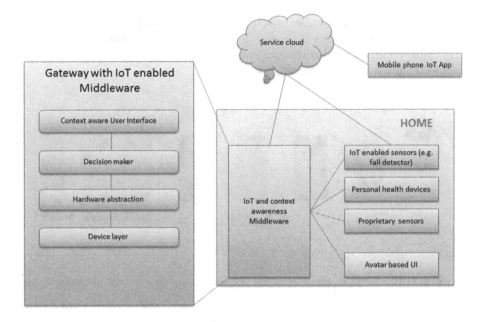

Fig. 2. Overall architecture of the solution

7   Conclusion and Future Work

The solution described in this work forms a flexible and scalable framework for various applications in the AAL and home care domain and is able to run on low-cost hardware. In addition to the original aim to collect data from the home environment, Bluetooth Low Energy based personal health devices were integrated in a modular, non-obtrusive and flexible way. With the ability to collect data from arbitrary sensors and devices, it can and will be used as a context aware middleware platform interacting with the end-user following the ubiquitous computing paradigm. Currently, HOMER platform is being further improved by integrating avatar based user interfaces and a context aware decision making module combing data from the home environment and personal health devices. A detailed architecture of the framework and how it is embedded into a home care setup is depicted in Fig. 2. A service cloud and a mobile app enables the connection to remote players like service provider and informal care givers. Furthermore, unlike mobile phones and tablets, this solution makes it easy to integrate interfaces for different transport types and communicate with sensor devices without having to worry about the underlying transport type and is always available for collecting sensor data.

References

1. Acampora, G., Cook, D.J., Rashidi, P., Vasilakos, A.V.: A Survey on ambient intelligence in health care. Proc IEEE Inst. Electr. Electron. Eng. **101**(12), 2470–2494 (2013)

2. Siegel, C., Prazak-Aram, B., Kropf, J., Kundi, M., Dorner, T.: Evaluation of a modular scalable system for silver-ager located in assisted living homes in Austria-study protocol of the modulaar ambient assisted living project. BMC Public Health **14**(1), 736 (2014)

3. Kropf, J.: Modulaar project (2016).http://www.modulaar.at. Accessed 11 May 2016

4. Morak, J., Kumpusch, H., Hayn, D., Modre-Osprian, R., Schreier, G.: Design and evaluation of a telemonitoring concept based on nfc-enabled mobile phones and sensor devices. IEEE Trans. Inf Technol. Biomed. **16**(1), 17–23 (2012)

5. Hanke, S., Mayer, C., Hoeftberger, O., Boos, H., Wichert, R., Tazari, M.R., Wolf, P., Furfari, F.: In: UniversAAL - An Open and Consolidated AAL Platform. Springer, Heidelberg (2011)

6. AIT: Home Event Recognition System (2016). http://homer.aaloa.org. Accessed 25 May 2016

7. Apache Software Foundation: Apache Karaf Framework (2016). http://karaf.apache.org. Accessed 9 Nov 2016

8. ISO, IEEE: ISO/IEEE 11073–10471: Health Informatics - Point-of-care medical device communication - Part 10471: Device specialization - Independant living activity hub (2010)

9. Kropf, J., Roedl, L., Hochgatterer, A.: A modular and flexible system for activity recognition and smart home control based on nonobtrusive sensors. In: 2012 6th International Conference on Pervasive Computing Technologies for Healthcare (PervasiveHealth), pp. 245–251. IEEE (2012)

10. Gomez, C., Oller, J., Paradells, J.: Overview and evaluation of bluetooth low energy: an emerging low-power wireless technology. Sens **12**(9), 11734–11753 (2012)

11. ISO, IEEE: ISO/IEEE 11073–20601: Health informatics - Point-of-care medical device communication - Part 20601: Application profile - Optimized exchange protocol (2010)

12. Morandell, M., Steinhart, J., Sandner, E., Dittenberger, S., Koscher, A., Biallas, M.: Relaxedcare: A quiet assistant for informal caregivers. In: Proceedings of the ACM CSCW Workshop on Collaboration and Coordination in the Context of Informal Care, pp. 11–21 (2014)

13. Bacciu, D., et al.: Smart environments and context-awareness for lifestyle management in a healthy active ageing framework. In: Pereira, F., Machado, P., Costa, E., Cardoso, A. (eds.) EPIA 2015. LNCS, vol. 9273, pp. 54–66. Springer, Cham (2015). doi:10.1007/978-3-319-23485-4_6

Non-conventional Use of Smartphones: Remote Monitoring Powered Wheelchairs in MARINER Project

Paolo Meriggi[1(✉)], Ivana Olivieri[1], Cristina Fedeli[1], Diana Scurati[1],
Giovanni Ludovico Montagnani[2], Elena Brazzoli[1], Marina Rodocanachi[1],
and Lucia Angelini[1]

[1] Fondazione Don Carlo Gnocchi Onlus, Centro S.M. Nascente,
Via Capecelatro 66, 20148 Milan, Italy
{pmeriggi,iolivieri,cfedeli,
dscurati,ebrazzoli,mrodocanachi,langelini}@dongnocchi.it
[2] Politecnico di Milano and Istituto Nazionale di Fisica Nucleare, Sezione di Milano, Milan, Italy
giovanniludovico.montagnani@polimi.it

Abstract. In this paper we will present the prototype of a system meant to quantitatively and continuously monitor the information measured during the daily use of powered wheelchairs, early adopted by severely impaired children. The system is based on a non-conventional use of a common smartphone, and it may represent an interesting application for long-term remote monitoring of health-related information.

Keywords: Quantitative remote monitoring · Powered wheelchair · Smartphones · Cloud

1 Introduction

Powered Wheelchairs (PWs) represent a fundamental aid to severely impaired people, especially children [1]. Because of their key role, there should be a careful pre-provision assessment and accurate follow-ups to verify the subjects' capabilities, as well as to adapt these devices to the users' changes. However, despite the high costs of these aids and their increasing demand, the assessments are usually limited to some pre-provision ones (not always performed by skilled professionals), and the follow-ups are seldom done, usually by means of phone calls to caregivers [2]. According to a recent review these assessments are, moreover, generally of qualitative nature [3]. The lack of post-provision quantitative evaluations, regarding "how long" and "how well" PWs are actually used, becomes particularly relevant when dealing with children, whose needs and capabilities are evolving with subjects' growth. Of course, without a continuous monitoring of the actual PW's use, such an important and sophisticated aid might turn into a less relevant support, or even useless and then abandoned, if it becomes difficult to be controlled or even dangerous to be operated by the user.

In 2014 we started a study (funded by Italian Lombardy Region), with the aim to assess the effects of early adoption (4–5 years old) of PWs in children with Cerebral Palsy, by evaluating changes in quality of life and in development of cognitive functions.

© ICST Institute for Computer Sciences, Social Informatics and Telecommunications Engineering 2017
P. Perego et al. (Eds.): MobiHealth 2016, LNICST 192, pp. 138–143, 2017.
DOI: 10.1007/978-3-319-58877-3_18

Within this framework, we specifically designed a subproject (named Project MARINER – MonitorAggio Remoto carrozzIne ElettRoniche), to gather quantitative information about the real use of PWs in a non-invasive manner, without the need for parents or caregivers to fill in daily questionnaires or reports. The goal for this monitoring subproject was to remotely and automatically collect data, allowing the operators to have an insight in terms of the number of hours of actual motion with the PW, as well as other parameters that might result useful to better understand their daily use by the child.

We initially considered the control module already shipped with each PW, but such device is usually meant to operate the connected actuators only (i.e. motors, etc.), and it is designed to export raw data about PW's motion only for rare fine-tuning of the PW's parameters, performed by skilled technicians.

We then analyzed possible alternative solutions already on the market, without finding anything completely suitable for the purpose. In the growing areas of wearable devices and the Internet of Things, many products are able to continuously capture inertial data up to a few hours, but they have limited capacity to store and transmit this information to the Internet and to be connected with other electronic devices. Furthermore, among the industrial and fleet tracking solutions, despite the abundance of devices, these have very limited capacity of continuously recording inertial data. Since no available solution fully met the desired requirements, we finally opted to develop and integrate a custom designed system on the PW, to gather information from the motion, without interfering with the PW's controls.

In the following paragraphs we will briefly describe the system designed and integrated for the MARINER project, and we will highlight some possible future developments.

2   Materials and Methods

Nine children, 4 to 6 years old, were recruited, for an observation period of one year. Each of them was given a PW Skippy (Otto Bock Mobility Solutions GmbH, Germany), bundled with *seat modules*, to extend the low-level I/O capabilities. Every PW was then equipped with the custom developed remote monitoring system.

We wanted to collect three types of information: the actual number of hours each PW was actually used per day, quantitative data about "how well" the PW was operated, and finally issue some alerts in case of major problems (in particular empty battery and system overheating). While the first and the last types of information are rather straight-forward to manage, respectively by monitoring the number of hours the motors are powered on and the presence of certain conditions (i.e. battery voltage drop under 20% of full charge, temperature raising above 50 °C), there is not a single way to assess the "how well the wheelchair is used" issue. For this preliminary study, we hence decided to simply collect all the available kinematic information (acceleration and angular speed), to be further analyzed in order to derive meaningful indexes, also by comparing these quantitative data with the qualitative impressions and considerations from the caregivers, by means of periodic phone calls.

Given these goals, we wanted the monitoring system to be energetically autonomous and rechargeable, equipped with inertial sensors (an accelerometer and a gyroscope) to measure the PW's use and an I/O interface to detect PW conditions. The monitoring system also needed to be firmly attached to the PW, and capable to autonomously transfer the acquired data to the Internet.

The final prototype of the monitoring system was thus built around a commercial smartphone (Galaxy S4, Samsung, Seoul, South Korea). The external information provided by each PW as pulse-width modulation signals (activation status of the electric brake) are low-pass filtered by a custom made RC filter (10 ms time constant) and acquired by a multi I/O board (Maxi I/O, Yoctopuce Sarl, Cartigny, Switzerland) connected to the smartphone through an USB cable (see Fig. 1).

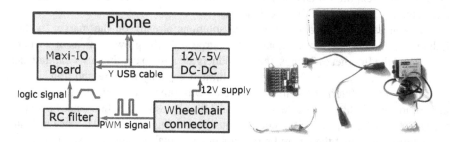

Fig. 1. Acquisition system scheme (left) and a photo of the actual elements (right).

During the PW's activity, the whole system is powered from the main PW's battery (12 V) through a common 12 V to 5 V DC-DC converter, which may provide up to 3A @ 5 V. This converter provides the required power supply either to the smartphone and the I/O board, thanks to a dedicated Y-cable (VAlarm, California, USA).

The smartphone is placed into a rugged plastic box, right above another enclosure hosting the DC-DC converter, the multi-IO board and the cables, as in Fig. 2.

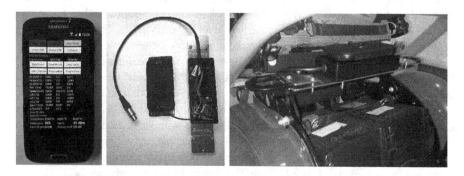

Fig. 2. The Galaxy S4 smartphone running the app (left), a view of the devices placed in the plastic box and rugged enclosure (center). Final setup in the back side of the wheelchair (right) with the custom metal plate.

These boxes are set very close to the wheels' center of rotation, through a 3 mm thick metal plate designed and realized on purpose.

The overall cost of the hardware components is around €500.

The smartphone runs a custom Android app we developed to acquire, store and transmit data to the back-end architecture. The inertial measures are sampled @ 50 Hz from the smartphone's triaxial accelerometer and gyroscope, only during the movements of the PW, while the smartphone's temperature is continuously sampled, ten times per minute (@ 0.167 Hz). All of these data are stored as timestamped values in separate files on the smartphone (*tracings*).

Each single change in PW conditions (Power ON/OFF, Motor ON/OFF, battery level change, etc.) is timestamped and stored at the time of its occurrence, and considered an *asynchronous event*. The sequence of asynchronous events, as well as the tracings, are locally processed on the smartphone to extract some basic indexes. These basic indexes describing the PW's condition (percentage of activity, temperature of the smartphone, battery level, GSM/UMTS/4G signal level, etc.) are sent to the back-end architecture according two different timings: once every hour, the *Hourly Events,* to give a fast and synthetic view of the conditions, and once a day the *Daily Events*, which consist of a more thorough insight (including the number of hours of activity, number of daily power ON/OFF, number of daily motor ON/OFF and other data regarding the use of the wheel-chair for that day). These latter data are sent every day, at 2:00 am, when the PW is not in use. At 2:0 am, furthermore, all the *tracings* acquired during that day are transferred to the appropriate back-end part (the blob repository).

In case a major problem or in case a major threat is detected (i.e. the temperature of the smartphone goes above a certain threshold – namely 50 °C, or battery below a certain threshold – namely 20% of full charge), this information is sent to the back-end architecture as an *Asynchronous Event*, the acquired data are saved locally on the phone, and a text message is directly sent from the smartphone to an operator.

The back-end side for collecting *Events* (simple set of few bytes of information) and *Tracings* (the files containing the signals acquired during the motion of the wheelchair) is briefly depicted in the scheme in Fig. 3. It has been developed using Microsoft Azure Cloud (Microsoft Corp., Redmond, USA), by using some of the key elements that have been specifically developed for the Internet of Things, like the Event Hub and the Stream Analytics, and using also a blob repository for the tracings and an SQL database for the final storage of the valuable information (indexes).

Once the tracings are transferred to the blob repository, they are further processed by the so called *workers* (custom developed algorithms coded in C#), to provide other indexes (min/max, mean, standard deviation, etc.) to the database. More sophisticated indexes (i.e. describing the distribution of accelerations and angular velocities and their asymmetries, etc.), which could be derived from the acquired tracings, will be further investigated and evaluated in the future.

The ultimate goal of this architecture is to provide both a simple lively overview of the current PWs' use by subjects, by accessing the SQL database, while allowing further detailed analysis and post-processing, once the tracings are available in the blob repository.

We have estimated to store up to 20 MB for tracings in the blob repository and some KB of data stored in the SQL database per day per wheelchair.

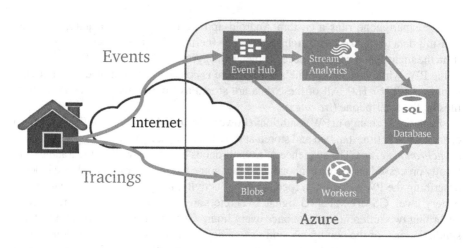

Fig. 3. Simple scheme of the dual data flow from the Power Wheelchair to Event Hub (events) and the blob repository (tracings), and after some processing steps, to the SQL database.

3   Conclusions and Future Perspectives

The prototype system described in the present paper is aimed at evaluating the feasibility and the clinical relevance in long-term quantitative monitoring of PWs' daily use, even going from some months up to various years.

To our knowledge, after the provision, there are no efforts in this direction regarding PWs, not only used by children, but also by adults and elderlies, unless (in some cases) diaries filled in by caregivers or phone/email contacts from operators.

Once this information and the related indexes will be thoroughly assessed and validated, this quantitative approach could give a significant contribution in the field of PW's use. Due to the high costs of the PWs (easily above €5000), and the increasing need of cost-effectiveness in the public healthcare systems, it is reasonable that such an approach, based on a minimally invasive and relatively low-cost "black box", could be used to derive more robust and useful measures of outcome in the provision of PWs.

Finally, since the project is based on a mobile Android app, it is foreseeable that almost the same backend architecture and a part of the front-end one could be easily adapted to gather quantitative information in a non-obtrusive manner on a broad spectrum of biomedical measures, valuable for the health conditions of patients (children, adult and elderly), directly from the smartphone or from other wearable devices (watches, etc.). This will allow a variety of novel forms of daily quantitative remote monitoring in a long-term perspective, not only limited to the use of PWs.

Further and larger studies will be of course required to foster the subject, because of the number of psychological, social and economic implications.

Acknowledgments. Authors would like to thank Microsoft Corp. for the provision of their Azure Cloud solutions to Fondazione Don Gnocchi, as a part of their support program for non-profit organizations. Authors would also like to thank Samsung Electronics Italia SpA for their support in the early stage of the project, by providing some mobile solutions to be tested and integrated.

Finally, authors would like to acknowledge Amper S.r.l. (Milano, Italy) who manufactured and provided all the mechanical components required for the proper system placement on the PWs.

References

1. Bray, N., et al.: Wheelchair interventions, services and provision for disabled children: a mixed-method systematic review and conceptual framework. BMC Health Serv Res. **14**, 309 (2014)
2. Salatino, C., et al.: An observational study of powered wheelchair provision in Italy. Assistive Technol. **28**(1), 41–52 (2016)
3. Livingstone, R., Field, D.: Systematic review of power mobility outcomes for infants, children and adolescents with mobility limitations. Clin. Rehabil. **28**(10), 954–964 (2014)

Intelligent Automated EEG Artifacts Handling Using Wavelet Transform, Independent Component Analysis and Hierarchal Clustering

Shaibal Barua[✉], Shahina Begum, and Mobyen Uddin Ahmed

School of Innovation, Design and Engineering, Mälardalen University,
72123 Västerås, Sweden
{shaibal.barua,shahina.begum,mobyen.ahmed}@mdh.se

Abstract. Billions of interconnected neurons are the building block of the human brain. For each brain activity these neurons produce electrical signals or brain waves that can be obtained by the Electroencephalogram (EEG) recording. Due to the characteristics of EEG signals, recorded signals often contaminate with undesired physiological signals other than the cerebral signal that is referred to as the EEG artifacts such as the ocular or the muscle artifacts. Therefore, identification and handling of artifacts in the EEG signals in a proper way is becoming an important research area. This paper presents an automated EEG artifacts handling approach, combining Wavelet transform, Independent Component Analysis (ICA), and Hierarchical clustering. The effectiveness of the proposed approach has been examined and observed on real EEG recording. According to the result, the proposed approach identified artifacts in the EEG signals effectively and after handling artifacts EEG signals showed acceptable considering visual inspection.

Keywords: Electroencephalogram (EEG) · Ocular artifacts · Muscle artifacts · Hierarchical clustering

1 Introduction

The Electroencephalogram (EEG) signal represents the electrical activity of the brain that is recorded along the scalp. EEG signal analysis has become an important research area in the clinical research and Brain Computer Interfaces (BCI) applications. It has also become useful physiological measurement for sleep study, epilepsy, and cognitive science research. However, the problem with the EEG signal is that, it is non-stationary and non-linear, and contaminates with other biological signals e.g., Electrooculogram (EOG), Electromyography (EMG), Electrocardiogram (ECG) [1, 2]. EEG artifacts are referred to any undesired signals or potential differences due to extra-cerebral source that interfere with the recorded signal [3, 4]. Artifacts make EEG signals uninterruptable and in the EEG signal analysis these can lead to a serious misinterpretation. Moreover, in the EEG signal processing such as power spectral analysis or topographic displays, artifacts can cause false conclusion unless artifactual data are handled or excluded from the EEG data.

© ICST Institute for Computer Sciences, Social Informatics and Telecommunications Engineering 2017
P. Perego et al. (Eds.): MobiHealth 2016, LNICST 192, pp. 144–148, 2017.
DOI: 10.1007/978-3-319-58877-3_19

The sources of the EEG artifacts are the ocular and the muscle activities; and both kind of artifacts overlap with the neural brain activity, which increase the difficulty to correctly interpret the EEG signals. The hypothesis on the artifacts is that, they are independent from the brain activity, either collected from normal or pathologic subjects [5]. Over the years, several methods have been proposed for artifacts removal from EEG signal. Daly and his colleagues [6] have developed the FORCe: Fully Online and automated artifact Removal tool for BCI application that combines wavelet transform, ICA and thresholding. Thresholding was applied on the independent components (ICs) to identify artifactual components, and resulting signals were obtained by removing the ICs that are identified as artifacts. LAMIC [7] is a clustering algorithm that has been developed to remove artifacts automatically from EEG signal. Blind source separation algorithm called the Temporal Decorrelation Source Separation (TDSEP) has been applied to decompose EEG signals. Later, clustering has been done on the components, based on the similarity of their lagged Auto-Mutual Information (AMI). ICA and clustering algorithms have been used to classify artifacts in EEG signals in [8, 7].

This paper proposed an approach, combining wavelet transform, Independent component analysis (ICA), and Hierarchical clustering methods to handle artifacts in the EEG signals. Here, recorded EEG signals are decomposed to approximation and details coefficients using wavelet transforms. Then ICA has been applied on the set of approximation coefficients to separate coefficients into ICs. Thereafter, features are extracted from each IC and all the ICs are grouped through Hierarchical clustering to identify clusters containing artifactual ICs, which are used to remove artifacts.

2   Materials and Methods

EEG signals are recorded at 2048 Hz sample rate following the international 10–20-electrode placement system with 19 channels EEG settings. A controlled data collection scenario was used during the data collection and participants were asked to perform different ocular and muscle movement activities to generate artifacts in the recorded EEG data.

A step-by-step process of the proposed system for artifacts handling is presented in Fig. 1. In the pre-processing, 50 Hz channel noise is removed from the recorded EEG signals using notch filter and signals are divided into 1 s segments. After pre-processing, recorded EEG signals are decomposed using wavelet transform that provides a set of approximation and details coefficients. Then approximations coefficients are further decomposed applying ICA to obtain ICs [6, 9].

In order to identify artifactual components i.e., the ocular and the muscle artifacts, several features are extracted from each IC (Hurst exponent, Kutosis, 1/frequency distribution, gamma power spectral density, spectral ratio i.e. the power spectral ratio of two frequency ranges (ratio of 30–60 Hz and 4–30 Hz), energy ratio i.e., $E(55 \text{ Hz} \leq f \leq 100 \text{ Hz})/E(f < 20 \text{ Hz})$, spectral edge frequency (SEF)) [10].

To identify artifactual components the Hierarchical Clustering algorithm is applied. The Hierarchical algorithm clusters data over a variety of scales by creating a hierarchical structure (tree) or 'dendrogram'. The tree is not a single set of clusters, but rather a

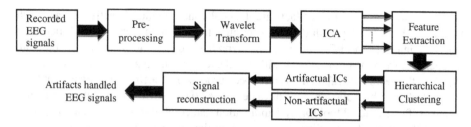

Fig. 1. Steps of the proposed approach in order to handle artifacts in EEG signals

multilevel hierarchy, where clusters at one level are joined as clusters at the next level [11]. In Hierarchical clustering, the distance between pairs of objects is calculated using Euclidean distance as a 'correlation' parameter of the MATLAB function 'pdist'. The linkage function applies 'complete' (i.e. Furthest distance) as a parameter, which determines the objects in the data set that should be grouped into clusters. Finally, cluster function with 'cutoff' value 1.1 is applied to group the data into random number of clusters. In addition, to label each cluster a 1-D feature vector is estimated that consists of 8 features (topography histogram, spectrum fit 1 and 2, frontal and peripheral location scores, average auto-correlation, Lorentz threshold, and Symlets wavelet (sym3) repeatability). Then a distance measure is applied to identify clusters containing artifactual components based Chauvenet's Criterion threshold value of 0.75 [12].

3   Evaluation and Results

EEG recording with artifacts during saccades and body movement activity are shown in Figs. 2(a) and 3(a) respectively. The resulting signals after artifacts handling are depicted in Figs. 2(b) and 3(b). By comparing two signals (the recorded EEG signals and the signals after handling artifacts), it is visible from the visual inspection that the artifacts are handled in the recorded signals.

Saccades movement EEG Recoding

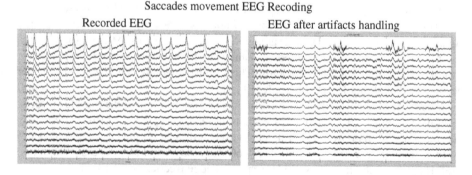

Fig. 2. (a) EEG signal with artifacts (b) EEG signal after artifacts handling

Body movement EEG Recoding

Recorded EEG   EEG after artifacts handling

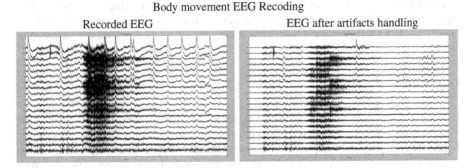

Fig. 3. (a) EEG signal with artifacts (b) EEG signal after artifacts handling

However, the ratio between the recorded signal and the artifacts handled signals is also important issue to observe. Thus, an experiment has performed to observe the difference considering Signal Quality Index (SQI) in different artifacts activities.

Here, SQI in terms of standard deviation of the amplitude values (StdAmp), maximum amplitude values (MaxAmp) and Kurtosis are calculated for saccades, body movement. The calculated values for EEG with and without artifacts are presented in Table 1.

Table 1. Signal quality index of EEG signals with and without artifacts

Activity	Parameter	With artifacts	Without artifacts	Difference in percentage
Saccades	StdAmp	21.03	11.75	44.09%
	MaxAmp	88.9	59.79	32.74%
	Kurtosis	4.3	5.03	15.42%
Body movement	StdAmp	23.54	10.28	56.33%
	MaxAmp	156.82	84.04	46.41%
	Kurtosis	7.4	8.0	08.01%

4 Conclusion

EEG signal measures the electrical activity of the brain and is a valuable physiological measurement in clinical application and research. In the EEG signal processing, it is important to handle artifacts i.e., the interference of physiological signals other than brain activity. This paper proposed an automatic approach for handling ocular and muscle artifacts in the EEG signals. Here, the proposed approach combines wavelet transform, ICA, and Hierarchical clustering. In addition, a distance measure has been applied using Chauvenet's Criterion threshold value of 0.75 to label the artifactual clusters. From the results it is noticeable that for the ocular artifacts handling it can improve signal quality index in the range of 15% to 44% and for the body movement signal quality index the improvement is 8% to 56%. In addition, the proposed approach does not require any reference signal to identify artifactual components from the independent components of ICA.

Acknowledgement. This research work is supported by the Vehicle Driving Monitoring (VDM) project funded by Swedish Governmental Agency for Innovation Systems (VINNOVA) and partially by the ESS-H profile and SafeDriver project funded by the Knowledge Foundation of Sweden.

References

1. Klonowski, W.: Everything you wanted to ask about EEG but were afraid to get the right answer. Nonlinear Biomed. Phys. **3**, 1–5 (2009)
2. Migotina, D., Calapez, A., Rosa, A.: Automatic artifacts detection and classification in sleep EEG signals using descriptive statistics and histogram analysis: comparison of two detectors. In: Spring Congress on Engineering and Technology (S-CET), pp. 1–6 (2012)
3. Chadwick, N.A., McMeekin, D.A., Tan, T.: Classifying eye and head movement artifacts in EEG signals. In: 2011 Proceedings of the 5th IEEE International Conference on Digital Ecosystems and Technologies Conference (DEST), pp. 285–291 (2011)
4. Klass, D.W.: The continuing challenge of artifacts in the EEG. Am. J. EEG Technol. **35**, 239–269 (1995)
5. Romo-Vazquez, R., Ranta, R., Louis-Dorr, V., Maquin, D.: EEG ocular artefacts and noise removal. In: 29th Annual International Conference of the IEEE Engineering in Medicine and Biology Society, EMBS 2007, pp. 5445–5448 (2007)
6. Daly, I., Scherer, R., Billinger, M., Muller-Putz, G.: FORCe: fully online and automated artifact removal for brain-computer interfacing. IEEE Trans. Neural Syst. Rehab. Eng. **23**(5), 725–736 (2014)
7. Nicolaou, N., Nasuto, S.J.: Automatic artefact removal from event-related potentials via clustering. J VLSI Sign Process. Syst. Sign **48**, 173–183 (2007)
8. Barua, S., Begum, S., Ahmed, M.U., Funk, P.: Classification of ocular artifacts in EEG signals using hierarchical clustering and case-based reasoning. In: Workshop on Synergies Between CBR and Data Mining at 22nd International Conference on Case-Based Reasoning, Cork, Ireland (2014)
9. Ghandeharion, H., Erfanian, A.: A fully automatic ocular artifact suppression from EEG data using higher order statistics: improved performance by wavelet analysis. Med. Eng. Phys. **32**, 720–729 (2010)
10. Barua, S., Begum, S., Ahmed, M.U.: Clustering based approach for automated EEG artifacts handling. In: 13th Scandinavian Conference on Artificial Intelligence (SCAI 15), Halmstad, Sweden (2015)
11. Chen, G., Jaradat, S.A., Banerjee, N., Tanaka, T.S., Ko, M.S.H., Zhang, M.Q.: Evaluation and comparison of clustering algorithms in anglyzing ES cell gene expression data. Statistica Sinica **12**, 241–262 (2002)
12. Hames, E.C.: EEG Artifact Removal and Detection via Clustering. Electrical and Computer Engineering, Ph.D. Texas Tech University (2014)

Mobile Application for Health

Crowdsourced Data Collection of Physical Activity and Health Status: An App Solution

Daniel Kelly[1]([⊠]), Brian Caulfield[2], and Kevin Curran[1]

[1] Computer Science Research Institute,
Ulster University, Coleraine, Northern Ireland
d.kelly@ulster.ac.uk
[2] INSIGHT Center, University College Dublin, Dublin, Ireland

Abstract. Health status measurements are vital in understanding a patient's health. However, current means of measuring health status, such as questionnaires, are limited. Research has shown that there is a need for more objective and accurate methods of measuring health status. We postulate that novel sensor solutions could be used to make observations about a patients' behaviour and make predictions relating to their health status. In order to achieve this overall goal, the problem of building a dataset comprising behaviour observations, from sensors, and health status measure must be addressed. In this work, we propose a crowd-sourced solution to this dataset problem where a Smartphone App is developed in order to facilitate in the collection of behaviour data, via sensors, and health status information. Results show that, after just 4 months, 1311 people have downloaded the App and 541 participants have completed a health status questionnaire (SF-36). Preliminary analysis of the data also shows a statistically significant correlation between the amount of time a participant is active and the health status of the participant.

1 Introduction

Chronic diseases are the most common causes of death and disability throughout the world [1]. In the UK, for example, 70% of all healthcare costs are chronic disease related [2]. Health Status measurements, such as Health Related Quality of Life (HRQOL), are used as a means of quantifying the impact of chronic disease on a patients' daily life [3]. These measures are vital in understanding a patients health and their response to particular treatments and have become a central feature in many chronic disease studies [4]. Questionnaires are used to evaluate health status. However, evidence suggests questionnaire results are only useful in large groups and should not be relied upon on an individual basis [5]. It is only worth continuing to prescribe symptomatic treatments if the patient can report benefit, but due to the limited reliability of health status questionnaires for individual patients there is currently no way of accurately accessing that benefit.

There is therefore a need for accurate and individualized methods for clinicians to assess functional aspects of a patient's life. An innovative solution to

© ICST Institute for Computer Sciences, Social Informatics and Telecommunications Engineering 2017
P. Perego et al. (Eds.): MobiHealth 2016, LNICST 192, pp. 151–159, 2017.
DOI: 10.1007/978-3-319-58877-3_20

this need is to utilize remote sensing technologies in the community, rather than questionnaires, to compute accurate, objective and individualized QOL measurements.

Our overall research goal is therefore to develop an unobtrusive sensing system which can objectively measure a persons' longitudinal behaviour and make accurate predictions about their health status based on their behaviour. However, there exists an initial problem which must be solved prior to solving this overall problem health status prediction. This initial problem relates the collection of appropriate data. In order to accurately model the mapping between sensor data and health status, a data-set comprising mobile sensor data and corresponding health status information must be acquired. The data-set must include participants with a broad spectrum of health measurements. Recording patient data alone would represent only a small window in the health status spectrum.

Modern smartphones are equipped with multiple sensors. The combination of these sensors, built within the common and non-invasive form factor of a mobile phone, have the potential of tracing human activities at scales that were previously unattainable. Smartphones can therefore enable a new type of data collection by harnessing the power of the crowd. Crowdsourced data collection, using smart-phones, presents a major opportunity to collect sensor data from a large, and varied, set of participants. The aim of this work is therefore to develop a smartphone App to facilitate the crowdsourced based data collection of motion sensor data and health status information. Additionally, we will discuss preliminary observations made from data which have been collected.

2   Methods

In this section, we will describe the development of an Android App aimed at recording motion sensor and health status information.

2.1   Motion Sensors

The Accelerometer, built into a participants' Smartphone, is used by the App to measure physical activity. Sensor data capture and recording is performed in the background, and data is recorded constantly while the App is enabled.

We postulate that features, extracted from motion signals, relating to the duration a person was stationary and active could potentially be used as a health status indicator. For example, using the total time a person was active as a feature. In order to investigate this, we propose two duration based measures: (1) Total Movement Duration (TMD) and (2) Average Stationary Period (ASP). TMD specifies the total amount of time in which the phone was detected as moving during a given day. The phone was deemed to be moving if the variance of the accelerometer magnitude was greater than a predefined threshold. For each 2 s window where the phone was deemed to be moving, 2 s were added to the overall TMD measure for that day. ASP was calculated as the average of a set of stationary period durations for a given day. The set of stationary period durations store the set of times between when the phone stopped moving and when the phone started to move again (i.e. the amount of time the phone was stationary). ASP therefore stores the average period of time a participant's phone was stationary during a given day.

In order to reduce the size of data being uploaded by a participant, we implement a system whereby each hour of motion sensor data is processed on the Smartphone, and extracted features for each hour are then uploaded to the server. These features include TMD and ASP features, as well as additional Accelerometer and Gyroscope statistical feature to be utilized in future works. Additional data processing and feature extraction can then be performed on the server using the hourly data.

2.2   User Interface

The App features two main User Interface (UI) sections. The first provides users with activity feedback and the second provides a means for users to take a health status questionnaire.

Activity Feedback. A study carried out in 2012 showed that 1 in 5 smartphone users had a health tracking App installed on their phone [6]. Health tracking is therefore a genre of App which the general public actively install on their smartphone. In order to get potential participants interested in and contributing to our data collection, we postulated that the App should be designed and marketed as a Health tracking App. Based on a review of the top health tracking Apps on the Google Play store, we found that a common feature of all health tracking Apps was that some level of quantitative feedback was provided to the user on their activity levels.

To increase App downloads, and improve user retention within the experiment, the App was therefore designed to provide users with visual feedback on the duration and intensity of their activities over time using graphs and statistics calculated from motion sensors (see Fig. 1). The App has received 14 reviews on Google Play, with an average rating of 4.6/5.

Health Status Interface. A key aim of this study is to record health status for a set of participants with a broad spectrum of health measurements. We utilize the Short-Form 36 (SF-36) survey in order to measure participant health status. The SF-36 is a non-illness specific health status measure which has been validated in a general adult population [7] and in a chronic illness patient population [8,9].

The SF-36 is a general health instrument that measures eight health related concepts: physical functioning (PF-10 items), role limitations due to physical problems (RP-4 items), bodily pain (BP-2 items), general health perceptions (GH-5 items), vitality (VT-4 items), social functioning (SF-2 items), role limitations due to emotional problems (RE-3 items), and perceived mental health

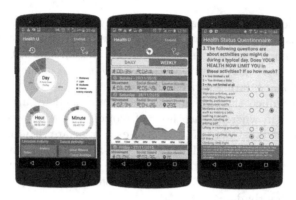

Fig. 1. "Health-U" App - (Left) Visual feedback showing current activity, (Middle) Activity history showing daily activity, (Right) Health status questionnaire.

(MH-5 items). These eight scales can be aggregated into two summary component measures: the Physical (PCS) and Mental (MCS) Component Summary Scores [10]. A questionnaire UI screen was integrated into the App to allow users to answer the SF-36 questions (See Fig. 1 (Right)). Questions are multiple choice and radio buttons are used to select answers to individual questions.

3   Results

The key aims of this study is to (1) develop an App based crowdsourced data collection platform which can record motion sensor and health status information and (2) investigate the feasibility of using such an App to build a dataset which can be later used to develop models linking activity to health status.

The App, named "Health-U", was published on Google Play and anyone with an Android phone could download and install the App and participate in the study. Upon launching the App for the first time, participants are shown a participant consent screen where details about the study, and data collected during the study, are explained. Participants are then given the choice to consent via a button labelled "I Consent" or to reject via a button labelled "Do not participate". Ethical approval for this study was granted by Ulster University Ethics committee and the contents of the participant consent screen was reviewed by the Ethics Committee.

The App was downloaded by a total of 1311 users in the first four months that the App was live. Of the 1311 downloads, 541 participants completed the SF-36 questionnaire. An average of 114 h of sensor data was uploaded by each participant. Of the 541 participants who completed the questionnaire, 263 participants (48.6%) uploaded at least 1 h of sensor data. This statistic shows approximately half of all users which downloaded the App and completed the questionnaire, disabled the sensing, or uninstalled the App, within an hour of installing the App. Figure 2 details the number of participants that uploaded a minimum number of hours. For example, it can be seen that 115 participants uploaded at least 72 h of data.

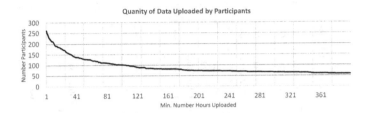

Fig. 2. Quantity of data uploaded by participants

Based on the SF-36 data uploaded by the 541 participants, Table 1 details the mean and standard deviation SF-36 scores, for the 8 different concepts and the 2 summary measures, of participants based on categories of gender, age and country. It can be seen, for example, that PF is generally higher in younger participants. Conversely, MH is generally higher for older participants.

It can be seen that the majority of the average scores are lower when compared to the study conducted in 2007 by Burholt et al. [11]. A possible explanation for this is that it has been shown that lower SF-36 scores are obtained when the questionnaire is self-administered when compared with scores which were obtained when the questionnaire was interviewer-administration [12].

3.1 Activity Duration

An initial statistical analysis of sensor information was carried out by computing the overall mean and standard deviation (SD) for the TMD and ASP measures. Results showed that, on average, a participants' phone moves for an average of 1 h and 33 min per day (SD = 4 min 50 s). Additionally, a participants' phone stays stationary for an average period of 22 min (SD = 14 min).

A qualitative analysis of movement data was performed in order to investigate potential links between movement and health status. Figure 3 shows movement duration data (TMD), and individual SF-36 scores, for two female participants (both aged 40–50). As detailed in the Fig. 3, Participant A has significantly lower SF-36 measures than Participant B. Interestingly, it can be seen that a large portion of Participant A's time is stationary, while data for Participant B shows that movement occurs regularly between 10 am and 11 pm. This does give an indication of the potential merit of using activity duration as an indicator of health status.

Further to the qualitative analysis above, we perform a quantitative evaluation to further investigate potential links between SF-36 scores and movement durations. Table 2 details correlations between the 10 SF-36 scores (8 SF-36 concepts and 2 summary measures) and the two duration measures TMD and ASP.

Table 1. SF-36 scores for participant demographics (Gender, Age, Country).

	N	PCS Mean (SD)	MCS Mean (SD)	PF Mean (SD)	RP Mean (SD)	BP Mean (SD)	GH Mean (SD)	VT Mean (SD)	SF Mean (SD)	RE Mean (SD)	MH Mean (SD)
Gender											
Female	306	49.0 (9.0)	48.6 (9.5)	71.8 (26.6)	75.1 (30.7)	66.3 (28.3)	52.5 (23.3)	45.3 (21.5)	61.9 (28.5)	60.8 (33.3)	53.7 (23.8)
Male	234	51.2 (7.8)	51.7 (7.6)	75.2 (27.2)	78.2 (30.0)	72.9 (23.9)	58.0 (20.9)	52.2 (17.8)	67.4 (28.4)	67.0 (31.6)	61.2 (21.2)
Age											
18–21	105	50.5 (8.0)	49.4 (9.0)	77.0 (25.3)	76.8 (30.1)	72.0 (26.5)	55.5 (21.2)	47.5 (19.0)	63.0 (29.0)	61.5 (34.0)	55.1 (23.6)
22–25	77	51.2 (7.6)	49.3 (9.2)	79.2 (22.8)	82.3 (23.8)	73.1 (21.1)	53.3 (21.8)	46.9 (19.9)	65.1 (27.9)	61.2 (31.8)	54.5 (23.0)
26–30	62	49.0 (8.0)	48.7 (9.7)	72.2 (25.9)	73.0 (32.2)	70.1 (26.2)	52.2 (21.6)	44.9 (21.0)	59.5 (26.8)	59.3 (33.3)	55.6 (25.1)
31–35	61	49.2 (8.0)	48.6 (8.3)	72.3 (25.3)	75.9 (26.0)	67.8 (25.9)	52.0 (21.0)	48.3 (21.4)	57.9 (28.7)	60.1 (33.3)	52.6 (20.6)
36–40	55	50.0 (8.8)	50.9 (8.4)	68.9 (27.5)	73.4 (31.6)	72.4 (28.2)	57.9 (22.5)	50.7 (19.4)	65.0 (29.2)	60.5 (32.4)	60.7 (22.3)
41–50	90	48.8 (10.4)	50.1 (8.9)	70.1 (32.7)	74.0 (36.9)	65.7 (28.8)	52.5 (25.2)	46.8 (21.7)	63.1 (29.4)	69.0 (30.7)	58.5 (22.9)
51–60	49	49.9 (8.9)	51.9 (9.0)	68.3 (26.9)	75.5 (31.4)	62.8 (30.8)	59.5 (23.5)	50.8 (20.5)	73.0 (28.1)	69.6 (33.3)	61.5 (21.5)
60+	38	51.1 (8.1)	52.5 (6.9)	73.1 (23.9)	80.3 (24.8)	65.4 (24.1)	59.6 (20.0)	55.0 (16.0)	72.8 (24.4)	69.0 (28.8)	61.8 (21.8)
Country											
UK	145	50.1 (9.3)	49.7 (9.4)	75.1 (29.0)	79.1 (31.2)	69.4 (28.1)	52.5 (23.0)	46.8 (20.6)	63.3 (29.6)	65.6 (34.1)	56.4 (24.4)
USA	82	49.5 (8.6)	51.0 (9.2)	70.2 (28.2)	73.0 (32.1)	65.6 (25.0)	57.1 (23.6)	48.6 (22.1)	69.7 (29.3)	67.8 (33.3)	60.1 (24.7)
Ireland	75	50.6 (9.0)	49.7 (9.1)	76.0 (25.9)	78.7 (30.2)	71.9 (29.0)	55.7 (23.8)	47.2 (20.4)	64.0 (28.9)	64.7 (32.3)	55.9 (24.1)
Canada	57	49.6 (7.3)	48.4 (8.5)	77.5 (22.4)	79.6 (26.1)	68.0 (23.9)	50.2 (20.2)	43.4 (20.8)	60.9 (29.1)	61.1 (32.4)	55.0 (20.7)
Spain	27	52.7 (7.1)	53.3 (8.3)	78.1 (20.9)	80.4 (26.1)	76.5 (28.2)	61.5 (16.7)	57.0 (19.1)	69.4 (28.3)	70.7 (32.6)	63.7 (20.6)
Australia	48	48.4 (8.6)	49.1 (7.8)	67.4 (27.8)	72.2 (30.6)	64.0 (24.4)	53.6 (22.0)	48.7 (17.8)	63.8 (23.7)	55.1 (31.5)	55.4 (20.4)
New Zealand	33	50.9 (6.7)	49.4 (8.2)	78.0 (23.2)	82.2 (27.2)	69.6 (24.4)	55.9 (19.7)	46.0 (17.7)	62.2 (29.3)	63.9 (28.4)	55.5 (20.6)
Other	74	49.3 (8.3)	50.2 (8.3)	67.4 (26.4)	68.7 (30.6)	71.4 (26.0)	56.9 (23.0)	53.2 (17.9)	62.0 (26.7)	58.5 (30.9)	56.3 (21.1)
Overall	541	49.9 (8.6)	49.9 (8.9)	73.3 (26.9)	76.4 (30.4)	69.2 (26.7)	54.7 (22.5)	48.3 (20.2)	64.2 (28.6)	63.6 (32.7)	56.9 (23.0)
Burholt [11]	*13917*	*N/A*	*N/A*	*77.8 (30.0)*	*78.3 (32.3)*	*70.1 (28.9)*	*66.2 (24.0)*	*57.3 (22.3)*	*80.2 (28.1)*	*87.0 (26.0)*	*74.0 (19.9)*

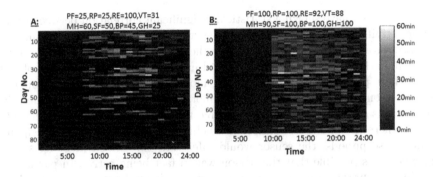

Fig. 3. Sample movement durations (TMD) for each day and hour, for 2 participants. Blank (black) areas of the graph denote no motion recorded for that hour. This can be due to the sensor being turned off, or because the phone remained stationary for the entire hour

Results showed that correlations between ASP and the SF-36 measures were not significant. However, results do show that the was a statistically significant correlation between TMD and the PCS, MCS, PF, RP, RE and SF concepts of the SF-36 scale. In particular, a correlation of $r = 0.221$ was shown between TMD and the RP component. The largest correlation between SF-36 and ASP was for the BP component, with $r = 0.042$. Table 2 also details the average TMD and ASP for 5 different ranges of scores for the different SF-36 concepts.

Table 2. Correlation between duration measures and SF-36 scores ($*$ = Statistically significant correlation, where p-value < 0.05, calculated using two-tailed test)

Measure SF-36 Activity	Correlation	SF-36 Bands				
		0-20 Mean (SD)	21-40 Mean (SD)	41-60 Mean (SD)	61-80 Mean (SD)	81-100 Mean (SD)
		$N=0$	$N=76$	$N=419$	$N=46$	$N=0$
PCS *(TMD)*	0.195*		54m (2m:23s)	100m (4m:54s)	101m (5m:39s)	
(ASP)	0.017		30m (12m:44s)	21m (13m:10s)	17m (16m:35s)	
		$N=0$	$N=77$	$N=393$	$N=71$	$N=0$
MCS *(TMD)*	0.150*		63m (3m:3s)	100m (5m:3s)	96m (4m:51s)	
(ASP)	0.038		30m (13m:10s)	21m (13m:8s)	18m (15m:18s)	
		$N=28$	$N=47$	$N=102$	$N=86$	$N=278$
PF *(TMD)*	0.206*	66m (2m:56s)	68m (3m:19s)	70m (4m:32s)	99m (5m:31s)	105m (4m:48s)
(ASP)	-0.021	32m (12m:53s)	20m (13m:15s)	28m (13m:53s)	21m (13m:47s)	20m (13m:47s)
		$N=34$	$N=53$	$N=55$	$N=86$	$N=312$
RP *(TMD)*	0.221*	75m (3m:2s)	66m (5m:19s)	64m (3m:21s)	74m (3m:23s)	109m (5m:9s)
(ASP)	-0.043	23m (13m:46s)	27m (14m:19s)	24m (13m:5s)	25m (10m:52s)	20m (13m:54s)
		$N=61$	$N=57$	$N=131$	$N=77$	$N=211$
RE *(TMD)*	0.182*	56m (2m:36s)	89m (4m:20s)	77m (3m:44s)	127m (6m:56s)	104m (4m:45s)
(ASP)	0.051	37m (12m:17s)	16m (14m:34s)	19m (14m:23s)	21m (12m:47s)	22m (13m:15s)
		$N=66$	$N=98$	$N=230$	$N=110$	$N=37$
VT *(TMD)*	0.114	69m (4m:22s)	99m (3m:45s)	89m (4m:55s)	119m (5m:32s)	83m (4m:12s)
(ASP)	0.031	24m (12m:42s)	21m (11m:36s)	23m (14m:9s)	19m (12m:56s)	20m (14m:30s)
		$N=41$	$N=95$	$N=206$	$N=111$	$N=88$
MH *(TMD)*	0.105	55m (2m:51s)	95m (4m:34s)	92m (5m:3s)	116m (5m:1s)	90m (4m:36s)
(ASP)	0.022	33m (14m:15s)	17m (11m:5s)	21m (14m:20s)	20m (12m:43s)	20m (13m:54s)
		$N=27$	$N=100$	$N=79$	$N=143$	$N=186$
SF *(TMD)*	0.138*	46m (2m:10s)	89m (4m:20s)	77m (4m:59s)	115m (5m:7s)	96m (4m:47s)
(ASP)	0.068	24m (11m:43s)	23m (13m:13s)	20m (13m:55s)	20m (11m:44s)	22m (14m:27s)
		$N=24$	$N=56$	$N=111$	$N=111$	$N=201$
BP *(TMD)*	0.057	102m (3m:34s)	80m (3m:36s)	83m (4m:11s)	115m (6m:1s)	89m (4m:35s)
(ASP)	0.096	20m (11m:29s)	24m (11m:9s)	24m (12m:27s)	17m (14m:30s)	22m (14m:6s)
		$N=48$	$N=105$	$N=174$	$N=152$	$N=60$
GH *(TMD)*	0.062	72m (4m:50s)	92m (5m:17s)	97m (4m:49s)	95m (3m:54s)	100m (5m:52s)
(ASP)	-0.019	25m (10m:46s)	27m (14m:2s)	21m (12m:52s)	20m (12m:27s)	22m (16m:46s)

While results have shown a statistically significant correlation between duration of activity and health status, these correlations are not strong enough to make accurate predictions about a persons' health status. Based on these results, we conclude that due to the real world and inherent uncontrolled nature of this study, where participants use the sensing modality without researcher supervision, duration of activity on its own cannot be used to consistently infer the health status of a participant. It is possible that periods of inactivity relate to periods where the phone was simply not being used/carried by the participant. During these periods, the sensor would infer that the person in being sedentary when it is possible that the person was in fact being active. In particular, the ASP measures showed no correlation with the health status measures. However, results did show that while correlation between TMD and different SF-36 components were negligible, the correlations were statistically significant.

The preliminary investigates discussed in this work have therefore indicated that additional features should be investigated to compliment the duration based features. Additional features could relate to activity intensity, type and frequency computed from accelerometer and gyroscope sensor data.

4   Conclusion

We postulate that smartphone sensors could be used to make automatic predictions about patient health status. In order to move towards this overall goal, we must first propose solutions to the problem of recording a large dataset of behaviour observations and health status information from a broad spectrum of participants. In this work, we propose a crowd-sourced solution to this problem, where a smartphone App is developed to record behaviour observations, via the recording of sensor data, and health status information, via a built-in SF-36 questionnaire.

Preliminary analysis of data obtained from our proposed crowd-sourced system demonstrates the feasibility of our solution. In just 4 months, 1311 people downloaded the App and, of these downloads, 541 participants completed the SF-36 questionnaire. Initial examination of the sensor data showed a correlation between the total amount of movement performed per day, by a participant, and the health status of the participant. While this correlation was statistically significant, the correlation was not strong. We therefore conclude that while these results demonstrate the potential of our proposed solution, further work is needed in terms of developing more discriminant features and evaluating regression models to make health status predictions.

References

1. Viswanathan, M., Golin, C.E., Jones, C.D., Ashok, M., Blalock, S.J., Wines, R.C.M., Coker-Schwimmer, E.J.L., Rosen, D.L., Sista, P., Lohr, K.N.: Interventions to improve adherence to self-administered medications for chronic diseases in the United States: a systematic review, pp. 785–795, December 2012

2. UK Department of Health: Long Term Conditions Compendium of Information, 3rd edn. (2012)
3. Kocks, J.W.H., Tuinenga, M.G., Uil, S.M., van den Berg, J.W.K., Ståhl, E., van der Molen, T.: Health status measurement in COPD: the minimal clinically important difference of the clinical COPD questionnaire. Respir. Res. **7**(i), 62 (2006)
4. Jones, P.W.: Health status measurement in chronic obstructive pulmonary disease. Thorax **56**(11), 880–887 (2001)
5. Pitta, F., Troosters, T., Probst, V.S., Spruit, M.A., Decramer, M., Gosselink, R.: Quantifying physical activity in daily life with questionnaires and motion sensors in COPD. Eur. Respir. J.: Official J. Eur. Soc. Clin. Respir. Physiol. **27**(5), 1040–1055 (2006)
6. Fox, S., Duggan, M.: Mobile Health 2012, Pew Research Center. Technical report (2012)
7. Bize, R., Johnson, J.A., Plotnikoff, R.C.: Physical activity level and health-related quality of life in the general adult population: a systematic review, pp. 401–415 (2007)
8. Boueri, F.M., Bucher-Bartelson, B.L., Glenn, K.A., Make, B.J.: Quality of life measured with a generic instrument (Short Form-36) improves following pulmonary rehabilitation in patients with COPD. Chest **119**(1), 77–84 (2001). http://www.ncbi.nlm.nih.gov/pubmed/11157587
9. Ståhl, E., Lindberg, A., Jansson, S.-A., Rönmark, E., Svensson, K., Andersson, F., Löfdahl, C.-G., Lundbäck, B.: Health-related quality of life is related to COPD disease severity. Health Qual. Outcomes **3**, 56 (2005)
10. Farivar, S.S., Cunningham, W.E., Hays, R.D.: Correlated physical and mental health summary scores for the SF-36 and SF-12 Health Survey, V. 1. Health Qual. Life Outcomes **5**(1), 54 (2007)
11. Burholt, V., Nash, P.: Short Form 36 (SF-36) health survey questionnaire: normative data for wales. J. Publ. Health (Oxf. Engl.) **33**(4), 587–603 (2011)
12. Lyons, R.A., Wareham, K., Lucas, M., Price, D., Williams, J., Hutchings, H.A.: SF-36 scores vary by method of administration: implications for study design. J. Publ. Health Med. **21**(1), 41–45 (1999)

Skinhealth, A Mobile Application for Supporting Teledermatology: A Case Study in a Rural Area in Colombia

Juan Pablo Sáenz[1]([✉]), Mónica Paola Novoa[2], Darío Correal[1],
and Bell Raj Eapen[3]

[1] Systems and Computing Engineering Department,
Universidad de los Andes, Bogotá, Colombia
{jp.saenz79,dcorreal}@uniandes.edu.co
[2] Fundación Universitaria de Ciencias de la Salud,
Hospital San José, Bogotá, Colombia
mopanoca@hotmail.com
[3] Kaya Skin Clinic, Dubai, United Arab Emirates
bell.eapen@gmail.com

Abstract. Background: The use of mobile applications in dermatology to support remote diagnosis is becoming more important each day, particularly in rural areas where dermatology services are commonly managed by healthcare personnel with no speciality training.
Objective: The aim of this study is to assess the reliability of mobile applications to support remote dermatological diagnosis, when used together with a dermatological ontology in underprivileged areas.
Methods: A mobile application that allows characterization of skin lesions was developed. The experiment was conducted in a remote area without access to a dermatologist. A total of 64 dermatological queries were recorded in the mobile application.
Results: The results showed that the probability of obtaining a correct diagnosis was between 64.4% and 85.6% and a confidence interval of 95%.
Conclusions: This study demonstrates the implementation of a Teledermatology strategy based on mobile applications and domain ontology-driven knowledge base to provide timely assistance to healthcare professionals. This approach was found to be pertinent in the Colombian rural context, particularly in forest regions where dermatology specialists are not available.

Keywords: mHealth · Teledermatology · Remote consultation · ONTODerm · Colombia · Latin America

1 Introduction

According to the Colombian Association of Dermatology, there were 1.25 dermatologists per 100,000 inhabitants in 2011, with a large number of them in

© ICST Institute for Computer Sciences, Social Informatics and Telecommunications Engineering 2017
P. Perego et al. (Eds.): MobiHealth 2016, LNICST 192, pp. 160–163, 2017.
DOI: 10.1007/978-3-319-58877-3_21

larger and more densely populated cities (3 per 100,000 inhabitants), thus leaving rural areas without specialized dermatological care options. There, some complex queries are sent to specialists through means such as email, and the answers may take several days to arrive.

Against this backdrop, mobile teledermatology is established as a technically feasible [1–5] and diagnostically reliable method of increasing access to dermatologic expertise in poorer regions of the world where access to computers with Internet is unreliable or insufficient.

In this paper, we present Skinhealth, a system that supports the diagnostic process of skin lesions by using ontology and knowledge base along with its integration with a mobile application. ONTODerm [6] is an ontology for dermatology that was originally designed for collaborative development by domain experts to analyse, modify and visualize the ontology in a convenient and accurate manner without the need of technical instructions.

Likewise, this paper reports the results of the first-time use of Skinhealth in a rural area in Colombia. The use of the application was made within the context of a program called Health Brigades in Colombia. Health brigades have been carried out since 2003 and are organized by the foundation "Alas Para la Gente" (Wings for the People) [7].

2   Skinhealth Overview

To illustrate Skinhealth application, let us consider the process presented in Fig. 1. In step one, the health care professional in a remote area uses Skinhealth to capture the information that corresponds to the parameters that describe the lesion. Skinhealth then connects to an application server located in the Systems and Computing Department (DSIC) of the Universidad de los Andes, in Bogotá, and transfers the information. In step two, the application server transfers the query to ONTODerm by using a web service hosted in an external server (gulfdoctor.net/dermbase). Once the external web service receives the request, it formulates a query that is sent to ONTODerm. In step three, the web service

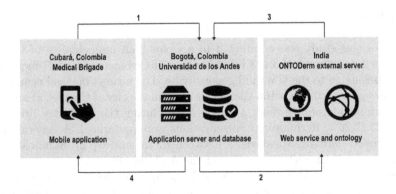

Fig. 1. Skinhealth overall perspective

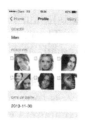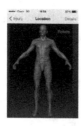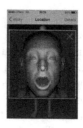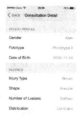

Fig. 2. Screenshots of the Skinhealth mobile application

returns eight differentials to the application server in Bogotá. In step four, the application server records the differentials for the query and sends them to the mobile application in the rural area. This information is used by the health care professional during the diagnosis process. Figure 2 presents the mobile application used by doctors.

3   Methods

To analyse the ability of Skinhealth and ONTODerm in supporting remote diagnosis of dermatological lesions, a health brigade conducted in a rural area in Colombia without immediate access to a dermatologist was selected as the scenario. The study population included all patients who attended the brigade without any exclusion criteria. The study was conducted in two stages. The first stage involved a general physician of the health brigade with no special training in dermatology and an assistant in charge of Skinhealth. The second stage is performed once the health brigade concludes. A dermatologist with broad experience in skin diseases examines the characterization of each query and compares this information with the diagnosis made by the general practitioner. The physician's diagnosis is marked accurate if it corresponded with the dermatologist's diagnosis.

4   Results

Phase 1 of this study was conducted in a Colombian municipality of Cubará, which has a population of 3,118 inhabitants; 1,551 women and 1,567 men, most of them belonging to the U'wa indigenous tribe. The nearest medical center with a dermatologist available is 166 kilometres away in the city of Cúcuta, at an eight-hour overland journey through a jungle area. During the three-day brigade, a total of 65 (7.26%) dermatology consultations were performed. A general physician attended dermatological visits between 8 a.m. and 5 p.m. Skinhealth was installed on a tablet with version 4.2 of the Android OS.

Phase 2 of the study took place in Bogotá, two weeks after the brigade. Coincidentally, the point estimate of the proportion of correct diagnoses in men and women was the same. It should be noted that the sample size for men is not large enough; thus, confidence intervals are very broad and do not provide accurate information. In contrast, confidence intervals for women are smaller and allow the formulation of more precise observations. Most skin lesions were identified in the face and hair, comprising 60% of total observations. Since the volume of pooled data was high, it was possible to separately analyse the queries of lesions on the face and the queries of lesions on the hair in order to determine the degree of accuracy in each case. The percentage of accurate queries in which the face was identified as the affected area was 96%.

5 Discussion

In the present study we proposed the integration of a mobile application and its respective connectivity and portability features with the ability of inference and learning of a dermatological ontology. We tried to ascertain the potential of this solution in dermatological diagnostic work carried out by general practitioners in rural and geographically marginalized municipalities where there are no specialists.

Besides assessing the accuracy of results, this study demonstrated the implementation of a different strategy of teledermatology that relies on mobile applications and domain ontology to immediately assist a general practitioner who answers dermatological consultations. This approach was found relevant in the Colombian context, particularly in geographically and economically marginalized regions. However, since the sample size is small, more studies would be necessary to validate the findings. The conclusions drawn in this paper do not represent a final validation of Skinhealth but a preliminary evaluation in order to determine its potential as a tool that can support medical staff in regions where there are not dermatology specialists.

References

1. Brewer, A., Endly, D.C., Henley, J., et al.: Mobile applications in dermatology. JAMA Dermatol. **149**(11), 1300–1304 (2013)
2. Kanthraj, G.R.: Classification and design of teledermatology practice: what dermatoses? Which technology to apply? J. Eur. Acad. Dermatol. Venereology **23**(8), 865–875 (2009)
3. Wurm, E.M.T., Peter Soyer, H.: Mobile teledermatology. In: Peter Soyer, H., Binder, M., Smith, A.C., Wurm, E.M.T. (eds.) Telemedicine in Dermatology, pp. 79–85. Springer, Heidelberg (2012)
4. Kaliyadan, F., Amin, T.T., Kuruvilla, J., Ali, W.H.A.B.: Mobile teledermatology - patient satisfaction, diagnostic and management concordance, and factors affecting patient refusal to participate in saudi arabia. J. Telemedicine Telecare **19**(6), 315–319 (2013)
5. Brewer, A., Sampson, B., Endly, D., Henley, J., Amir, M., Dellavalle, R.: There's an app for that: the emergence of mobile applications in dermatology. J. Am. Acad. Dermatol. **68**(4), AB90 (2013)
6. Eapen, B.R.: ONTODerm-a domain ontology for dermatology. Dermatol. Online J. **14**, 16 (2008)
7. Alas para la gente. http://alasparalagente.com

Smartphone-Based Detection of Location Changes Using WiFi Data

Anja Exler$^{(\boxtimes)}$, Matthias Urschel, Andrea Schankin, and Michael Beigl

Karlsruhe Institute of Technology (KIT), TECO, Karlsruhe, Germany
{exler,urschel,schankin,michael}@teco.edu
https://www.teco.edu

Abstract. Context information, in particular location changes as indicator for motoric activity, are indicators for state changes of patients suffering from affective disorders. Traditionally, such information is assessed via self-report questionnaires. However, this approach is obtrusive and requires direct involvement of the patient. Related work already started to rely on unobtrusively gathered smartphone data. Despite its ubiquitousness, WiFi data was barely considered yet. Due to the increasing availability of public hot spots we want to focus on this data source. We investigate the usefulness of WiFi data in two use cases: detect location changes and estimate the number of nearby persons. In a two-week study we captured MAC addresses, WiFi SSIDs and timestamps to identify current location and location changes of ten subjects in a five minute interval. We achieved a recall of 98% for location changes which proves the usability of WiFi data for this purpose. We confirm a basic feasibility of using WiFi data for unobtrusive, opportune and energy-efficient detection of location changes.

Keywords: Mobile sensing · WiFi · Location changes

1 Introduction

In clinical psychology the assessment of states and state changes of patients suffering from affective disorders – e.g. depression, bipolar or borderline personality disorder – is important to perform an appropriate treatment [1,2]. Location changes are relevant as they can provide insights about motoric activity (lethargically staying at home vs. moving from one place to another) or avoidance of other people (staying at home vs. changing location) which are symptoms of depression [3].

Traditionally, experience sampling questionnaires are used for the assessment. However, they cause a disruption in the patients' daily routines. Smartphones are personal wearables and simultaneously a powerful sensor system. Related work already suggests to rely on automatically gathered smartphone data in psychology [4]. A wide range of contexts and sensors is already covered. Though, until now, WiFi information was barely considered. The increasing number of

© ICST Institute for Computer Sciences, Social Informatics and Telecommunications Engineering 2017
P. Perego et al. (Eds.): MobiHealth 2016, LNICST 192, pp. 164–167, 2017.
DOI: 10.1007/978-3-319-58877-3_22

public hot spots and access points suggest to investigate this data. But is it possible to infer location changes only based on smartphone WiFi data? We present results of a first feasibility study to answer this question.

2   Related Work

Smartphones offer different sensors to assess location and location changes. The most common example is GPS (Global Positioning System). However, this is delicate in terms of data protection as it reveals the actual position in fine granularity. In addition, it is fairly expensive in terms of energy consumption. Therefore, we neglect this option. Low-cost alternatives for location detection are GSM, Bluetooth or WiFi [5,6].

GSM (Global System for Mobile Communications) is a standard for mobile communication and digital cellular networks. Via GSM it is possible to identify the cell tower a mobile device is connected to or to create a fingerprint of nearby cell towers. This allows location detection with coarse granularity. It was already used in related work, e.g. [7]. However, location tracking via GSM is too inaccurate for our setting as a person can be connected to two different towers while being at the same location (urban areas) or be connected to the same tower but changing location significantly (rural areas).

An alternative is *Bluetooth* which was used in [8]. Bluetooth is a wireless technology that allows data exchange over short distances. It is possible to create location fingerprints based on nearby devices, even though this is not always accurate. Alternatively, it is possible to equip locations with Bluetooth beacons and identify locations by their unique beacons. However, the process of labeling locations with Beacons is inefficient and not suitable for real-world scenarios in which we do not know where a user will go. In addition, smartphone manufacturers restrict the visibility of devices via Bluetooth: it is only visible while the Bluetooth menu is the foreground app[1].

WiFi is a technology that allows devices to connect to wireless LAN (WLAN). Nowadays, WiFi is often used as a synonym for WLAN as most WLAN rely on this standard. Within the last years, WiFi access became omnipresent[2], especially in urban environments. Some researches already used WiFi for location detection [9,10]. They relied on WiFi fingerprints which were labeled in advance. Again, the pre-labeling is expensive and not suitable for real-world assessment.

In summary, relying on WiFi data is a promising approach. It is suitable for real-world scenarios if no pre-labeling is required. We present an approach to detect location patterns based on unlabeled WiFi fingerprints. This allows identification of location changes or duration of a stay at a location, for example.

---

[1] https://support.google.com/nexus/answer/2819579?hl=en-GB.

[2] http://www.statista.com/statistics/218596/global-number-of-public%2dhotspots-since-2009/.

3   Detecting Location Changes via Smartphone WiFi Data

We build an Android app to collect WiFi information using the 2.4 GHz and the 5 GHz frequency band. We decided to assess MAC addresses instead of SSIDs, because networks may use the same SSID or broadcast their SSID from multiple access points. We only want to consider long-term stays at locations and location changes between them. This shall avoid counting passing a location as a location change during a transit of the user. We decided to log the currently available WiFi networks every five minutes. This is also a very energy-efficient sampling rate. Location changes can be detected by comparing the available WiFi networks detected by the smartphone at two or three consecutive points in time. In this context a location change occurs when none of the set of access points recorded in measurement M_1 is present in the set of access points recorded in measurement M_2 (five minutes later) or M_3 (ten minutes later).

4   Evaluation

Study Design. The study lasted ten days and was taken by ten subjects (70% male, 30% female), aged between 21 and 68 (mean: 28.8). All subjects were informed about the objective of the study and the data that is captured by the app. Afterwards, we asked them to sign a consent form. In the study, subjects used their own smartphones. We asked them to use the smartphones as usual. As ground truth subjects recorded their location changes in a chart, providing start and end times for stays at every location they visited. We asked them to provide the type of location from which they were coming and going to in the format "P→B". We differentiated between *private* ("P"), *business* ("B"), and *public* ("Ö", in German "öffentlich") locations, analog to location labels in [8].

Results. Location change data of only nine subjects were included in the data analysis. One subjects missed to restart the app after a smartphone restart. During the study 17,406 different access points were detected overall and between 458 and 3426 per subject. We counted 1,065 location changes in total and between 33 and 208 per subject.

The collected data was compared to the manually recorded ground truth to determine the recall (a.k.a. sensitivity) of our detection. This metric specifies how many location changes were detected by our approach. We noticed that when only considering the last two measurements, the recall is rather low, e.g. 0.76 for Subject 1. The high number of errors is caused by fluctuations in the WiFi data, e.g. due to loss of WiFi connection during the measurements or caused by subjects moving to another room within the same but large building. Hence, we decided to take the last three measurements into account, i.e. all measurements within the last 10 min. We achieve an average recall of 98% (95% confidence interval [CI] = 97.1–99.6). The remaining errors are caused by location changes that were logged by the subject but were shorter than the five or ten minute minimum that our app requires.

5   Conclusion

Movement and location changes are interesting measurements in clinical psychology to identify states and state changes in subjects suffering from affective disorders such as depression. However, assessing these metrics requires automatic, privacy-aware and energy-efficient approaches.

We presented results of a study conducted to investigate the feasibility of purely WiFi-based detection of location changes using smartphones. A recall of 98% proves a successful detection of location changes by our approach. We see a high potential of these findings for context recognition in clinical psychology. Apart from the mere number of location changes, WiFi information can reveal regularity, duration, and frequency of location visits. These aspects can give a deeper insight into affective disorder symptoms such as loss of interest to perform usual activities, decreasing motoric activity, or avoidance of other people.

We intend to design and conduct further studies with patients suffering from affective disorders as subjects. Thereby, we want to gain insights about their location change behavior and evaluate the usefulness of our location detection for phase change detection.

References

1. Trull, T.J., Ebner-Priemer, U.: Ambulatory assessment. Ann. Rev. Clin. Psychol. **9**, 151 (2013)
2. Trull, T.J., Ebner-Priemer, U.W.: Using experience sampling methods/ecological momentary assessment (ESM/EMA) in clinical assessment and clinical research: introduction to the special section (2009)
3. Davidson, G.C., Neale, J.M.: Abnormal Psychology. Wiley Publishing Co., New York (1996)
4. Miller, G.: The smartphone psychology manifesto. Perspect. Psychol. Sci. **7**(3), 221–237 (2012)
5. Gaonkar, S., Li, J., Choudhury, R.R., Cox, L., Schmidt, A.: Micro-blog: sharing and querying content through mobile phones and social participation. In: Proceedings of the 6th International Conference on Mobile Systems, Applications, and Services, pp. 174–186. ACM (2008)
6. Paek, J., Kim, J., Govindan, R.: Energy-efficient rate-adaptive GPS-based positioning for smartphones. In: Proceedings of the 8th International Conference on Mobile systems, Applications, and Services, pp. 299–314. ACM (2010)
7. Eagle, N., Pentland, A.S.: Reality mining: sensing complex social systems. Pers. Ubiquit. Comput. **10**(4), 255–268 (2006)
8. Pejovic, V., Musolesi, M.: InterruptMe: designing intelligent prompting mechanisms for pervasive applications. In: UbiComp 2014 (2014)
9. Chen, Y., Kobayashi, H.: Signal strength based indoor geolocation, 1 (2002)
10. Mok, E., Retscher, G.: Location determination using WiFi fingerprinting versus WiFi trilateration. J. Location Based Serv. **1**(2), 145–159 (2007)

Adaptive Motif-Based Alerts for Mobile Health Monitoring

Ekanath Rangan[1] and Rahul Krishnan Pathinarupothi[2(✉)]

[1] School of Medicine, Amrita Vishwa Vidyapeetham (University), Kochi, India
[2] Center for Wireless Networks and Applications,
Amrita Vishwa Vidyapeetham (University), Kollam, India
rahulkrishnan@am.amrita.edu

Abstract. We have developed a rapid remote health monitoring architecture called RASPRO using wearable sensors and smartphones. RASPRO's novelty comes from its techniques to efficiently compute compact alerts from sensor data. The alerts are computationally fast to run on patients' smartphones, are effective to accurately communicate patients' severity to physicians, take into consideration inter-sensor dependencies, and are adaptive based on recently observed parametric trends. Preliminary implementation with practicing physicians and testing on patient data from our collaborating multi-specialty hospital has yielded encouraging results.

Keywords: Mobile healthcare · Severity detection

1 Introduction

Remote health monitoring through the use of clinically approved wearable sensors, integrated with the smartphones, are emerging as a promising technological intervention to overcome the lack of affordable access to quality healthcare and timely delivery of critical care. Sensors are now available for monitoring as many as 30 vital cardio-metabolic health indicators, including blood pressure (BP), blood glucose, electrocardiogram (ECG), and oxygen saturation (SpO2) to alert any impending cardiac conditions such as ischemic events or syncope. Perego et al. [1] propose that wearable sensing can be employed even as early as in newborn babies. Frederix et al. [2] present a mobile smartphone based application for monitoring coronary artery disease. Such systems enable physicians, who are located in specialty hospitals far from the patients, to assess the patient's physiological condition based on received sensor values, viewed in the context of patients' historical electronic health records (EHR). The physicians can then initiate delivery of timely treatment through proximally located healthcare service providers.

Extensive survey of remote health monitoring devices is presented in [3]. However, in an experimental deployment of such systems of sensors and smartphones, we observed the following limitations:

© ICST Institute for Computer Sciences, Social Informatics and Telecommunications Engineering 2017
P. Perego et al. (Eds.): MobiHealth 2016, LNICST 192, pp. 168–176, 2017.
DOI: 10.1007/978-3-319-58877-3_23

- **At the physician end:** Physicians started to receive voluminous data from the sensors attached to their patients. The data volume is amplified by the increased number of patients, multiplicity of sensors on each patient, and frequent sensing of vital parameters. Physicians, overwhelmed by this data volume, practically started to ignore, let alone even attempt to interpret, and there was diminished chance of making a suitable treatment decision in real-time.
- **At the patient end:** The use of popular smartphones to receive, multiplex, and transmit sensor data continuously causes rapid power draining. As a result, there is a good chance of inadequate power just when all sensors are required to fire in the event of an unforeseen health condition.

A solution to overcome these challenges is to summarize the data on the patients' smartphones prior to transmission. Recent hardware advances in both sensors and mobile wireless devices have led to increasing quantum of interest and research in this area. Banaee et al. [4] recognize that, recently, research in health monitoring systems has shifted from simple reasoning of wearable sensors readings to the advanced level of data processing.

Much of the recent research in summarization has focused on complex machine learning techniques to aid in disease diagnosis [5]. Whereas this is a promising direction for the future, our interactions and observations with our medical collaborators in our inter-disciplinary research team is that, physicians are not yet ready to accord an influential role for automated diagnosis in their patient care. We have chosen a practical compromise: Summarization whose outcome is alerts with following attributes:

- Alerts have to accurately communicate the severity of the patient's condition to the physician. Alerts are computed from the sensor measurements and can take multiple levels.
- Alerts should take into consideration observed trends in intra-sensor measurements, and also inter-sensor severity dependencies.
- Alerts should have a feedback influence on adapting the frequency of both the sensor measurements and summarization. By dynamically reducing the frequency during low severity conditions, significant savings in the power can be achieved, without compromising on the accuracy. Conversely, during high alert conditions, rapidity of measurements and related summarization can be accelerated since delays can be life threatening. So, in this paper, we set forth to address the challenge of accurate and timely processing of alerts.
- Alerts should be dynamically adjustable based on the physicians' perception of the patients' vulnerability to health conditions.
- Alerts should be computationally inexpensive to run efficiently on edge devices such as smartphones.

To our best knowledge, the alert mechanisms already proposed in literature, like the one proposed by Bai et al. [6] are targeted towards generating alarms in an ICU, and could not satisfy all of the above requirements that we set out with.

In this paper, we propose a novel interventional time-inverted adaptive feedback alert mechanism, which we call as RASPRO (Rapid Alerts Summarization for Effective Prognosis) to analyze the data at the edge devices (e.g., smartphones), followed by transmission of alerts to the remote physician. We have based this mechanism on our previous work [7], where we have used a motif-based representation for multi-sensor medical data.

The remainder of this paper is organized as follows: Sect. 2 presents the overall architecture of the RASPRO remote health monitoring system. Section 3 presents the adaptive feedback based alert computation techniques. Section 4 presents implementation and preliminary results, and Sect. 5 concludes the paper.

2   RASPRO Architecture

The patient side architecture (see Fig. 1) begins with sensors attached to human body for measuring and monitoring a variety of physiological parameters such as, pulse rate, blood pressure, blood oxygen, ECG, respiratory rate, blood sugar, temperature, etc., together constituting the sensing subsystem. Each of the sensors output analog signals that are then digitized into a raw data sequence. In general, let us consider N vital sensors, $s_1, s_2 ..., s_N$, each with a sampling frequency, F. The sampling proceeds continuously for an interval of I time units, following which there may be a gap of Γ time units, and then the sampling resumes for the next interval I, etc. Many such intervals constitute the total observation window Φ. For instance, sampling may occur for $I = 1$ h every day in a week, in which case, $\Gamma = 23$ h and $\Phi = 7$. The relative durations I, Γ, and Φ are patient and disease specific and are set by the physician.

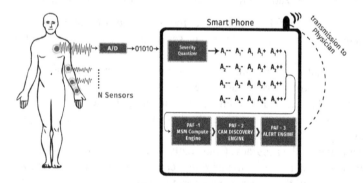

Fig. 1. RASPRO remote health monitoring patient-side architecture, with three physician assist filters (PAFs) running on patient's smartphone. Matrices (MSM) and Motifs (CAM) are introduced later in this section.

Then a sensor data specific comparator quantizes the digital sequence into one of Q possible severity symbols. For instance, if Q is taken to be five, the levels are labeled A−−, A−, A, A+ , and A++ with the symbol A indicating normality, and subscripts "−" and "+" indicating sub-normal and above normal levels of increasing severity. More complex parameters could be derived from sensor data and can employ domain specific reference patterns corresponding to various severity levels. The different severity levels are selected from the medical interpretation as well as physician's input based on the patient profile. For instance the normal range of BP is 120/80 to 140/90 and there are different severity levels of hypertension and hypotension above and below this normal range.

The severity symbol sequences, all assumed to be of same frequency, are multiplexed at the granularity of one symbol per sensor. Its output is a sequence of timed vectors, with each vector consisting of N values, one from each sensor sampled at that particular instant. Any missing sensor values (for whatever reason), are filled in by duplicating the most recent value of that particular sensor.

These vectors become the elements of a three dimensional Multi-Sensor Matrix (MSM), with F * I columns, and Φ rows, and each element depth equal to N. The MSM can be thought of as consisting of N two dimensional Single Sensor Matrices (SSM [1], SSM [2],..., SSM[n],... SSM[N]), each of F * I columns and Φ rows. In the next stage of RASPRO, the MSM is used for discovering frequent trends in sensor values that is called consensus abnormality motifs (CAM). This is dealt with in detail in our previous work [7].

The above modules are implemented as Physician Assist Filters (PAFs), and are named MUX-MSM Compute Engine, CAM Discovery Engine, and Alert Delivery Engine and they run on the patient smart phone. The computed alerts and its semantic interpretation are promptly transmitted to the physician by the Alert Delivery Engine via popular messaging platforms such as SMS and Whatsapp, based on the network bandwidth availability, power constraints and severity of the alerts.

3 Alert Computation Techniques

Building on our previous works on developing a rapid severity detection and summarization algorithm, we propose the use of consensus abnormality motifs as a representation of frequent abnormality in a large time series data.

3.1 Motifs

Candidate Motif, $\mu_{CAN}[n]$ is a temporally ordered sequence of quantized values, A^*_t, A^*_{t+1}, A^*_{t+2}, ..., A^*_{t+L} of length L that is selected from SSM [n]. So, the first row of an SSM can be selected as a μ_{CAN} by selecting $L = F * I$ and starting symbol as element $(1,1)$ in SSM.

Normal Motif, $\mu_{NOR}[n]$ is a candidate motif in which all values represent the normal severity level, which means each and every value is equal to A.

Consensus Motif, $\mu_{CON}[n]$ is a candidate motif satisfying the following two conditions: its hamming distance from $\mu_{NOR}[n]$ does *not* exceed a physician prescribed sensor-specific near normality bound, $d_{NOR}[n]$ and, its total hamming distance from all other $\mu_{CAN}[n]$ is the minimum. μ_{CON} represents the observed patient-specific near normal trend.

Consensus Abnormality Motif, $\mu_{CAM}[n]$, is a candidate motif satisfying the following two conditions: its hamming distance from $\mu_{NOR}[n]$ exceeds a physician prescribed sensor-specific near normality bound, $d_{NOR}[n]$ and, its total hamming distance from all other $\mu_{CAN}[n]$ is the minimum (Fig. 2).

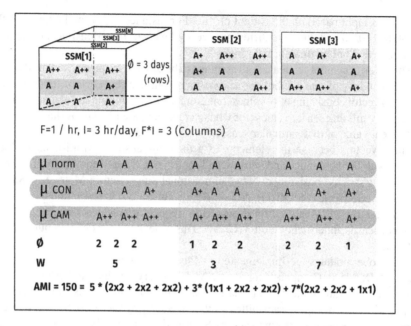

Fig. 2. Computation of the Motifs and Alerts from sensor matrices

It should be noted that, whereas an isolated abnormal sensor reading is indicated by A++, A+ , A–, A––, etc., μ_{CAM} represents the most frequently occurring abnormality trend over the entire observation period. The parameter d_{NOR} can be set specific both to the patient and to the vital parameter, by the attending physician. The discovery of the motifs is dealt with in detail in our previous work [7]. In this paper, we now present novel techniques for computing alerts from these motifs.

3.2   Alert Measure Index

At the end of each observation window Φ_r, for every patient, we define an aggregate alert score, called the **Alert Measure Index (AMI)**. This is calculated as

$$AMI[\Phi_r] = \sum_{i=1}^{N} W[i] * \sum_{j=1}^{F*I} \mathbf{num}(\mu_{cam}[i][j]) * \Theta[j] \tag{1}$$

Wherein, the inner summation takes each severity value in the μ_{CAM} of the ith sensor, converts it into a numerical value (e.g., A± is assigned 1, A++/–– is assigned 2), scales it up by a severity specific factor $\Theta[j]$, and the outer summation scales it up by a sensor specific weightage $W[i]$, both of which are derived from medical domain expertise. We call these two factors W and Θ as severity factors, and the resulting AMI is indicative of the immediacy of patient priority for physician's consultative attention.

3.3   Interventional Time-Inverted Alerts

We propose a goal directed approach to determining the severity factors W and Θ. The goal of delivering the alerts to the physician is to indicate the upper bound on the time that can elapse before which the physician's intervention is imperative to pull the patient out of danger. In order to capture this, we define the severity factors W and Θ as follows:

$$\Theta[\alpha] = \frac{K1}{\Delta[\alpha]}, \quad W[n] = \frac{K2}{\Delta[n]} \tag{2}$$

where, $\Delta[\alpha]$ is the upper bound on the time for intervention for severity level α (which can take on values A++, A+ , etc.), $\Delta[n]$ is the upper bound on the time for intervention for sensor n. In (2), constants K_1 and K_2 can be set by the physician considering the context of patient's health condition (including historical medical records and specific sensitivities and vulnerabilities documented therein). The inverse linear equation relating the severity factor to interventional time may be substituted by more complex equations for progressively complicated disease conditions. For instance, cardiologists prefer an exponential increase in alert levels if the monitored patients' ECG shows significant ST level depression: a direct indicator of myocardial infarction.

$$\Theta(\alpha) = e^{\left(\frac{K1}{\Delta(\alpha)}\right)} \tag{3}$$

We are currently engaged in active dialog with collaborating physicians from our medical school to determine the severity level - interventional time relationships for different specialties.

AMIs also serve as a feedback mechanism to modulate sensing frequency and alert computation instants. A low AMI is used to effect three adjustments: (1) Reduce the frequency F of future sensor measurements to a medically allowed minimum bound, (2) Increase the gap Γ between successive monitoring intervals, and (3) Increase the subsequent inter-alert window Φ, thereby saving power and bandwidth of transmission. By the same token, a high AMI causes F to increase, Γ to decrease, and Φ to increase. We have used a linear model to relate each of these factors:

$$F_{r+1} = F_r[1 + C_1 * (AMI(\Phi_r) - AMI(\Phi_{r-1}))]$$
$$\Gamma_{r+1} = \Gamma_r[1 - C_2 * (AMI(\Phi_r) - AMI(\Phi_{r-1}))] \tag{4}$$
$$\Phi_{r+1} = \Phi_r[1 - C_3 * (AMI(\Phi_r) - AMI(\Phi_{r-1}))]$$

where, C_1, C_2, C_3 are positive feedback constants adaptively set by physician's preferences. A very high frequency causes redundancy in summarization while a lower frequency may result in missing sudden short duration spikes in parameters. An optimum frequency for SDS has to be specific to the patient, sensor and severity. A detailed discussion on setting of these constants is outside the scope of this paper.

4   Implementation and Preliminary Results

We have built an initial implementation of the RASPRO architecture (see Fig. 3), and carried out preliminary testing of the alerting techniques on anonymized patient data at our 1500-bed super-specialty hospital, namely, the Amrita Institute of Medical Sciences. Secure network protocols are used to transmit alerts (AMIs) over mobile networks, and standard encryption techniques are used to ensure privacy. Upon viewing the received AMI pertaining to a patient, the doctor may initiate a data pull mechanism called Detail Data on Demand, abbreviated as "*DDoD*", originating from the doctor's device to the cloud. The DDoD may further propagate to the patient's smartphone if part or whole of the data requested is still remnant on the patient's smartphone.

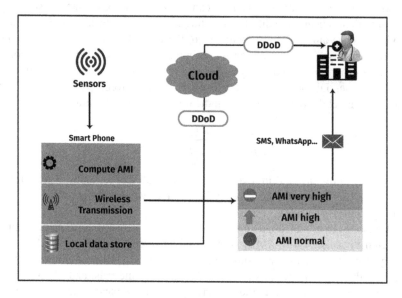

Fig. 3. Implementation of the alert delivery mechanism on Mobile networks with Detail Data on Demand (DDoD) feature

We have seen very encouraging results during the early trials of the system at the hospital, both among the physician community as well as the patients. As early adopters of the RASPRO system, the physicians identified the following target patient groups. Cardiac patients with history of ischemia, diabetes, syncope and hypertension have been using our wearable monitoring and alerting devices [8] and integration of RASRPO alerting technique is slated to be a key enabler in identifying patients who need immediate help. Another target group are patients who need to be identified with sleep apnea and given warnings when their heart rate and respiratory rate variability is asynchronous in nature.

Figure 4 shows blood glucose levels measured using interstitial chips from two patients as a representative of this group. The continuously collected 24 h raw values are analyzed for severity and summarized at a fixed frequency and then using the adaptive feedback technique of (4), where $\Phi = 3$ h in the beginning and then decreased to 2 h, 1 h, and then finally to 20 min, corresponding to increasing severities.

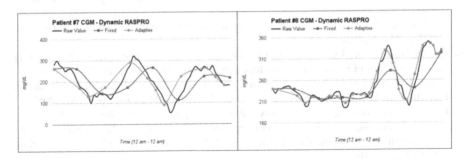

Fig. 4. Performance of adaptive feedback based alerts for blood glucose level variations, as compared to fixed frequency alerts, for multiple patients

We have very interesting observations from these data: (a) fixed frequency alerts might lead to missing spikes of high severity, which might lead to even life-threatening scenarios, (b) since feedback-based alerts adapt the frequency according to rising or falling trends, they are able to pick higher severities with much better accuracy, and (c) both adaptive and fixed alerts are similar in performance during normal times. Similar observations were made in other patient data as well, all though due to space constraints we have omitted from reporting here.

5 Conclusion

We have developed a novel adaptive feedback technique for timely computation of healthcare criticality alerts and a system architecture called RASPRO for their delivery over mobile remote health monitoring networks. The alerts are computed from severity trends represented as motifs, and capture the inter-sensor dependencies. Alerts have great advantages of reducing the bandwidth and energy on smartphones, as well as, avoiding the significant data overload on already very busy doctors saving them from the need to go through voluminous patient reports. Results from our initial pilot implementation carried out jointly with practicing physicians are highly encouraging.

Acknowledgments. We express our deep gratitude to our Chancellor and world renowned humanitarian leader Sri Mata Amritanandamayi Devi (Amma) for her inspiration and support towards working on inter-disciplinary research that has direct societal benefit.

References

1. Perego, P., Andreoni, G., Zanini, R., Bellù, R.: Wearable biosignal monitoring system for newborns. In: EAI 4th International Conference on Wireless Mobile Communication and Healthcare (Mobihealth), pp. 271–274. IEEE (2014)

2. Frederix, I., Sankaran, S., Coninx, K., Dendale, P.: MobileHeart, a mobile smartphone-based application that supports and monitors coronary artery disease patients during rehabilitation. In: IEEE Annual Conference on Engineering in Medicine and Biology, pp. 513–516. IEEE (2016)
3. Mukhopadhyay, S.C.: Wearable sensors for human activity monitoring: a review. IEEE Sens. J. **15**(3), 1321–1330. IEEE (2015)
4. Banaee, H., Ahmed, M.U., Loutfi, A.: Data mining for wearable sensors in health monitoring systems: a review of recent trends and challenges. Sensors **13**(12), 17472–17500 (2013)
5. Keogh, E., Lin, J., Fu, A.: Hot sax: efficiently finding the most unusual time series subsequence. In: Fifth IEEE International Conference on Data Mining (ICDM 2005), 8 p. IEEE (2005)
6. Bai, Y., Do, D., Ding, Q., Palacios, J.A., Shahriari, Y., Pelter, M.M., Boyle, N., Fidler, R., Hu, X.: Is the sequence of super alarm triggers more predictive than sequence of the currently utilized patient monitor alarms. In: IEEE Transactions on Biomedical Engineering, vol. 99. IEEE (2016)
7. Pathinarupothi, R.K., Rangan, E.: Discovering vital trends for personalized healthcare delivery. In: Proceedings of the 2016 ACM International Joint Conference on Pervasive and Ubiquitous Computing: Adjunct, pp. 1106–1109. ACM (2016)
8. Dilraj, N., Rakesh, K., Krishnan, R., Ramesh, M.: A low cost remote cardiac monitoring framework for rural regions. In: Proceedings of the 5th EAI International Conference on Wireless Mobile Communication and Healthcare, pp. 231–236. ICST (2015)

A Portable Real Time ECG Device
for Arrhythmia Detection Using Raspberry Pi

C.A. Valliappan$^{(\boxtimes)}$, Advait Balaji, Sai Ruthvik Thandayam, Piyush Dhingra,
and Veeky Baths

BITS Pilani K.K.Birla Goa Campus, Goa, India
{f2013478,f2013656,f2013489,f2013710,veeky}@goa.bits-pilani.ac.in

Abstract. Arrhythmia related disorders are one of the leading causes
of cardiac deaths in the world. Previous studies have shown that
Arrhythmia can further lead to major cardiac diseases like the Sudden
Cardiac Death (SCD) syndrome. The difficulty in detecting Arrhythmia
in the early stages often results in poor prognosis and presents the need
for a costefficient diagnostic device. To this end, we propose a realtime
portable ECG device with special emphasis on Arrhythmia detection
and classification. The device is centered on a Raspberry Pi 3 (RasPi)
module. RasPi with its signal processing and wireless transfer capabilities acts like an adapter between the sensors and a personalized mobile
device application that is used for tracking the ECG. A highly sensitive
peak detection algorithm was used by RasPi to detect and extract features from the ECG signals at real time. The peak detection algorithm
was tested on the standard MITBIH arrhythmia database and reported
an accuracy of greater than 95%. Hence, we propose a novel low cost
approach towards arrhythmia monitoring and detection with wide applications in mobile health systems.

Keywords: Arrhythmia · Portable · Costeffective · Wireless communication · Mobile health

1 Introduction

Abnormal heart rhythms clinically manifest themselves in the form of arrhythmias. Arrhythmias are relatively quiescent during the initial stages but may provide significant information about the health of an individual and help detect
underlying cardiac anomalies [1]. Cardiovascular diseases like atrial fibrillation
and ventricular fibrillation represent the more severe cases of arrhythmia. One
such disease linked to ventricular fibrillation is the Sudden Cardiac Death (SCD)
syndrome which claims 6 million lives worldwide with a low survival rate of 1%–
5% [2]. As the disease shows very little symptoms early on, it becomes imperative
to come up with diagnostic devices for early detection.

The electrocardiogram (ECG) has been the leading tool for arrhythmia detection and classification, though the bulky 12 lead instrument makes it inconve-
nient for frequent monitoring while data retrieval and interpretation often needs

© ICST Institute for Computer Sciences, Social Informatics and Telecommunications Engineering 2017
P. Perego et al. (Eds.): MobiHealth 2016, LNICST 192, pp. 177–184, 2017.
DOI: 10.1007/978-3-319-58877-3_24

clinical expertise and is expensive in places with limited access to health care [3]. Recently, novel methods have been proposed to use mobile computing for signal processing and data analysis [4]. Previously, use of android based devices for arrhythmia detection using Pan-Tompkins algorithm and feature extraction from mobile devices have been demonstrated [5]. Most of the current algorithms make use of the QRS complex for arrhythmia detection at real time [5,6]. Though these algorithms are quite sensitive to detect the R-R peak intervals, they could fail to abstract other essential features that could detect the presence of other kinds of arrhythmias. The Long QT syndrome characterized by elongation of Q-T interval in ventricular arrhythmias and Premature Atrial Contractions (PACs) associated with Supraventricular arrhythmias are potentially deadly syndromes where characterization of the P and T wave are essential for detection [7]. In our study we present another alternative for ECG tracking with special emphasis on arrhythmia detection. Our approach to this is threefold, (1) Design and development of a portable low cost ECG monitoring device centered on RasPi (2) Developing a highly sensitive algorithm that is capable of detecting P, QRS and T peaks accurately. (3) Developing a mobile application for easy user interface that uses patients medical history for a personalized monitoring of tachycardia or bradycardia. To test the sensitivity and accuracy of our algorithm we tested it on the MIT-BIH arrhythmia and supraventricular arrhythmia database.

2   Design

Raspberry Pi 3 B+. The Raspberry Pi is a portable minicomputer. The Raspberry Pi model B+ has inbuilt wireless LAN 802.11n and Bluetooth 4.1. It has a RAM of 1 GB which makes it ideal for faster calculations and real time implementation. The RasPi model B+ has 40 GPIO pins at its disposal, which allows for greater flexibility to extend the deice for more sensors. The RasPi was booted with Raspbian OS operating system, which is stable open source. Scripting can be carried out using Python 2.7 supported by the Raspbian platform [9]. ECG monitoring system is hardware dependent work, hence Serial Peripheral Interface bus and GPIO pins in RasPi are very useful. The RasPi is powered by 5 V micro USB supply, to make the device portable we have used a standard power bank.

AD8232. AD8232 is a dedicated IC for signal conditioning of ECG signal. In order to achieve the best possible output we are using the AD8232 SparkFun Single Lead Heart Rate Monitor [10]. The evaluation board is mounted with AD8232 and resistors and capacitor. It is designed to filter, amplify ECG signals in the presence of noisy conditions, created by movement or electrode positioning. The board has 3.5 mm jack for connecting sensor pad connection as shown in Fig. 1(C). The usage of 3.5 mm jack reduces the interference of noise. The power supply to the evaluation board is 3.3 V which is provided from the RasPi pinout. The output of the AD8232 is analog, whereas the RasPi read only digital signal. Hence we use MCP3008 for analog to digital convertion.

MCP3008. MCP3008 is capable of taking 8 channel of input and converts it to 10-bit digital value. MCP3008 uses serial peripheral interface (SPI) bus to establish a synchronous serial communication between the master and slave [11]. Here the RasPi is the master and MCP3008 is slave as the clock is being generated by the RasPi. The ADC/MCP3008 is capable of sending 75 Ksps to 200 Ksps based on the supply voltage. The rate at which these samples are read decides the sampling rate. The sampling rate is software programmed by reading after every sampling interval. The ADC is single supply operated and the voltage can be between 2.7 V to 5.5 V. The RasPi has a standard 3.3 V supply, hence we use it to power the MCP3008 which is also used for AD8232 and Vref.

Interface of Components. In order to get a clear ECG signal, 3-electrode method is followed. The sensor pad were placed close to heart forming a right triangle [Fig. 1]. The sensor pads were connected to the tri-conductor sensor cable with the 3.5 mm jack output connected to AD8232. We have developed our device with a three electrode system to have the optimum accuracy as well as make it more user friendly compared to the 12-lead ECG. The analog output of the AD8232 is given to input of the Analog to Digital Converter (MCP3008). The SPI bus was used for serial communication between the MCP3008 and RasPi. The output of the AD8232 varies between 0–3.3 V as per the data sheet, hence the reference voltage of ADC is set as 3.3 V. The ECG output ploted on the Raspi after Digitalisation using MCP3008 is shown in Fig. 1(a)

3 Methodology

In this work, RasPi acts as a central device which analyses the ECG signal and transmits the essential data along with signal to mobile application.

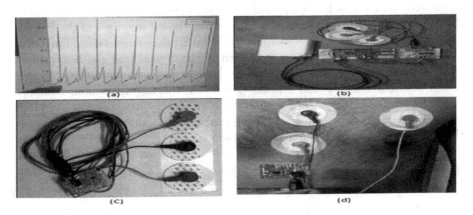

Fig. 1. (a) ECG signals as observed real-time on the RasPi monitor (b) Portable ECG Device powered by a mobile power bank (c) AD8232 with patches (d) Placement of three patches in a right angled triangle

The connectivity between RasPi and the mobile is established by creating a WiFi access point in RasPi. To create hotspot from RasPi, the procedures followed were as given in [9]. The sampling rate is set as 100 samples per second. Every 100th of the second a 10-bit digital value is read by RasPi. The 10-bit value corresponds to a value between 0 to 1024 which is scaled between 0 to 3.3 V. The sampled ECG signal is stored in variable of fixed length of 1000 samples, and updated every 10 s and given as an input signal to the peak detecting algorithm. On the other hand the ECG signal is continuosly transmitter to mobile. This is achieved by using multiple threads. So two variables one stores the current ECG signal incoming and other has the previous 10 s ECG signal for analysis. Time taken for a single run of the algorithm on 1000 samples is on an average 0.080644 s. Every 10 s the stored variable containing the ECG samples is given as input to the peak detecting algorithm. The position of the peaks is being outputed. With these peaks we find the RR interval, PR interval, QT interval and QRS duration (width) which is used to classify the types of pathological condition. This classification is done by mobile application.

Peak Detection Algorithm. An Input signal of 1000 samples was given to the peak detection algorithm. Baseline wandering from the input signal was removed using a moving average filter and the power line noise removal was done by a notch filter designed at 60 Hz. A padding of 100 zeros was then introduced in the start and end of the input signal [12].

To accurately detect R peaks a threshold value was set based on the analysis of all normal ECG signal and all values above the threshold were selected. Threshold value was set as follows:

$$ThresholdValue \geq Mean(Mean(samples) + Max(samples)) \qquad (1)$$

Peaks above the threshold value were further filtered into peaks having less than 10 samples between each of them and the maximum value in this set represents the R- peak. A window of length 20 was chosen to the left and right of the R peak and the minimum values were assigned to Q and S peaks respectively. Further a window of 30 samples was taken to the left of the Q peak and another window of 50 samples was taken to the right of the S peak. The maximum values in this region were assigned to P and T peaks (Fig. 2). At this step the sample numbers of all the peaks are stored. These windows were decided based on the sampling rate. To get the absolute position of the peaks, the padding of 100 zeros from the start is removed from the detected position to get the absolute position. As a check for the abnormal cases, any value below zero or greater than 1000 means that the peak didnt exist. To test the accuracy of the algorithm, samples from the MIT-BIH arrhythmia were taken.

Classification Based on the ECG Wave Characteristics Using Peak Detection Algorithm. In this section, we provide the basis for arrhythmia classification using previously reported classifiers [12], all of which are

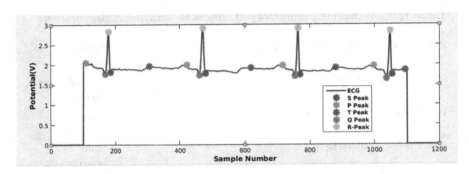

Fig. 2. The P(Yellow), Q(Green), R(Cyan), S(Red), T(Violet) peaks detected by the Peak Detection Algorithm (Color figure online)

incorporated in our algorithm. We are using the peaks detected by using the algorithm and calculating the RR, PR, QRS and QT intervals. Using the R-R interval(samples between R-R peaks) we calculate the heartbeats per minute. Here Fs = Sampling frequency

$$HeartRate = \frac{60 * Fs}{R - Rinterval} \tag{2}$$

Classification based on rhythmic, intervals we also include the conventional heart rate approaches to accurately classify arrhythmia into its specific subclasses as shown in Table 1.

Long QT Syndrome. From the peak position we find the QT interval using (Formula-3). Using Bazetts formula to calculate QTc Values for detecting QT Prolongation [8,13] Where QT and RR are the represent the peak durations respectively.

$$QTc = \frac{QT}{\sqrt{RR}} \tag{3}$$

Mobile Application. The application lets the user create their own account. As soon as RasPi is switched on, it turns on WiFi access point. The user needs to connect the phone to the WiFi hotspot, user can login and start the ECG recording. The transfer of data to mobile from RasPi is achieved using the socket library. The socket library transfers data using UDP protocol. The RasPi does the analysis on the ECG signal and every 10 s data (1000 samples) and updates the information about the peaks during that 10 s interval. The mobile application plots the ECG signal, heart beat.per minute, and RR intervals. Concurrently, it also receives data on the PR, QT and QRS intervals from the RasPi, which are used classification of the signal, which are then displayed in the session log window after recording. The mobile app also helps in heart beat range for the user. Based on the personal information collected from the user for nonsmoking people the lower limit is set to $0.7 * 75$ and the upper limit is set to $220 - 0.48 * Age$.

Table 1. Table showing parameters and criteria for arrhythmia classification.

Parameter	Criteria for detection	Type of disorder
Heart rate	60–100 Bpm	Normal sinus rhythm
Heart rate	100–150 Bpm	Sinus tachycardia
Heart rate	40–60 Bpm	Sinus bradycardia
Rhythm and Heart rate	Irregular rhythm and 40–60 Bpm or 60–100 Bpm	Sinus arrhythmia
QRS width	Width > 0.13 s	Bundle branch block
QRS width	Width < 0.045 s	Premature ventricular contractions
PR interval	Interval > 0.2 s, consistent with every beat	First Degree AV Block
RR interval	Interval > Avg. R-R interval	Escape/AV Block
QTc values	Male > 0.45 Female > 0.47 1–15years: > 0.46	QT syndrome

Studies have shown that people who smoke, their heartrate changes by 11 as compared to people who don't smoke. Hence for smokers, the lower limit increased by 11 and upper limit decreased by 11. A separate thread is created, which keeps track of all the heart-rate measured. The thread keeps running in parallel to check whether the heart-rate falls in the above mentioned range else a message alert is passed to the contacts (Fig. 3).

4   Results

Performance of the Peak Detection Algorithm. In this paper we randomly selected data 100, 101, 109, 113 & 115 from MIT-BIH Arrhythmia Database [14]. Table 2 shows the predicted and the actual heart rate along with the number of peaks in the ECG signal pedicted by our algorithm as compared to MIT-BIH database results.

From Table 3 for data 100, the RR interval, PR interval, are well within the bound whereas the QRS interval wanders around 0.045 s which has a possibility of Premature ventricular contraction & QTc value slightly goes beyond the 0.45. This ECG data corresponds to adult male, so the subject may have prolonged QT syndrome. Similarly for data 101 the all interval (Mean ± std) as shown in are within the bound hence the subject has a normal heart beat. Data 109

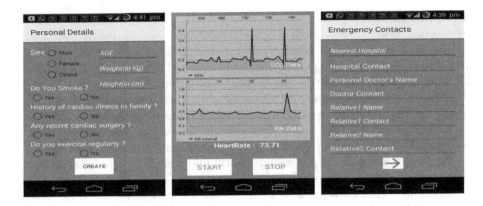

Fig. 3. Screenshot of the personalised mobile application

Table 2. Performance of the peak detecting algorithm.

Data	Predicted HBP	Actual HBP	Predicted R peaks	Actual R peaks
100	75 ± 1	70–89	2268	2273
101	61 ± 3	55–79	1855	1865
109	83 ± 4	77–101	2495	2532
113	62 ± 5	48–87	1865	1795
115	64 ± 5	50–84	1945	1953

Table 3. Results of our analysis on MIT-BIH arrhythmia database

Data	RR	PR	QTc	QRS	HeartRate
100	0.793 ± 0.019	0.152 ± 0.005	0.443 ± 0.013	0.04 ± 0.006	75.62 ± 1.91
101	0.973 ± 0.046	0.152 ± 0.003	0.360 ± 0.083	0.065 ± 0.001	61.78 ± 3.27
109	0.722 ± 0.044	0.196 ± 0.029	0.448 ± 0.078	0.081 ± 0.001	83.28 ± 4.50
113	0.966 ± 0.776	0.131 ± 0.008	0.360 ± 0.029	0.043 ± 0.002	62.52 ± 5.41
115	0.930 ± 0.050	0.184 ± 0.003	0.389 ± 0.018	0.060 ± 0.001	64.70 ± 5.45

has PR interval as 0.1969 ± 0.0290 s hence the subject may suffer from First Degree AV Block. Towards detecting more than one kind of arrhythmia. Further, we also analyzed data 113 and 115. Samples 113 and 115 showed signs of sinus arrhythmia and PVC. Data 115 may have a condition of a AV block, thus the results confirm a strong correlation between the Peak Detection Algorithm and MIT-BIH arrhythmia database. Thus, we were able to predict occurrences of arrhythmia in these sample with high accuracy. In addition to this, our algorithm also picked up instances of the long QT syndrome in Data 100, which werent reported by the database. This may potentially be a case of Ventricular Fibrillation that was detected by our algorithm.

5   Conclusion

In this work, we present a novel device capable of detecting different types of arrhythmia. We have synchronized the RasPi centered device through a wireless LAN, to a mobile app that is user friendly and generate log files, that can be shared with a personal doctor. We also present a highly accurate Peak Detection Algorithm that is sensitive at detecting various types of arrhythmias. Though we have intended to make this device portable, issues like power supply, noise reduction and reducing the overall hardware complexity without compromising on the quality of the signal processing are still major challenges in building real-time tracking devices. In our model, we have tried to reduce these variants to a minimum by introduce a portable USB charger and two peripheral chips along with a RasPi module, to make it a viable prototype for a wearable device.

References

1. Krasteva, V., Jekova, I.: QRS template matching for recognition of ventricular ectopic beats. Ann. Biomed. Eng. **5**(12), 2065–2076 (2007)
2. Mehra, R.: Global public health problem of sudden cardiac death. J. Electrocardiol. **40**(6), S118–S122 (2007)
3. Silva, I., Moody, G.B., Celi, L.: Improving the quality of ECGs collected using mobile phones: the physionet/computing in cardiology challenge 2011. In: 2011 Computing in Cardiology. IEEE (2011)
4. Eskofier, B., Hoenig, F., Kuehner, P.: Classification of perceived running fatigue in digital sports. In: ICPR (2008)
5. Gradl, S., et al.: Realtime ECG monitoring and arrhythmia detection using Android based mobile devices. In: 2012 Annual International Conference of the IEEE Engineering in Medicine and Biology Society. IEEE (2012)
6. Hamilton, P.S., Tompkins, W.J.: Quantitative investigation of QRS detection rules using the MIT/BIH arrhythmia database. IEEE Trans. Biomed. Eng. **12**, 1157–1165 (1986)
7. Gothwal, H., Kedawat, S., Kumar, R.: Cardiac arrhythmias detection in an ECG beat signal using fast fourier transform and artificial neural network. J. Biomed. Sci. Eng. 4(04), 289 (2011)
8. Goldenberg, I., Zareba, W., Moss, A.J.: Long QT syndrome. Curr. Probl. Cardiol. **33**(11), 629–694 (2008)
9. Zhao, C.W., Jegatheesan, J., Loon, S.C.: Exploring IOT application using Raspberry Pi. Int. J. Comput. Netw. Appl. **2**(1), 27–34 (2015)
10. http://www.analog.com/media/en/technical-documentation/data-sheets/AD8232.pdf
11. https://cdn-shop.adafruit.com/datasheets/MCP3008.pdf
12. Naaz, A., Singh, S.: QRS complex detection and ST segmentation of ECG signal using wavelet transform. Int. J. Res. Advent Technol. **3**(6), June 2015
13. Schwartz, P.J., Periti, M., Malliani, A.: The long QT syndrome. Am. Heart J. **89**(3), 378–390 (1975)
14. Moody, G.B., Mark, R.G.: The impact of the MIT-BIH Arrhythmia database. IEEE Eng. Med. Biol. **20**(3), 45–50 (2001)

Design Approach for mHealth Solutions

A Didactic Experience in Designing Smart Systems for mHealth Services

Carlo Emilio Standoli[✉], Maria Renata Guarneri, Marinella Ferrara, and Giuseppe Andreoni

Politecnico di Milano - Dip. di Design, via G. Durando 38/A, 20158 Milan, Italy
{carloemilio.standoli,mariarenata.guarneri,marinella.ferrara,
giuseppe.andreoni}@polimi.it

Abstract. The aim of this paper is to present a didactic experience in designing mobile health systems during a Bachelor Degree class in Industrial Design. The scope is to prove the role of Design in the innovation process and how its approach and methodologies connect research, innovation and technology. As case studies, two projects are presented. In the first one, the students have developed a training suite for figure skating; the second one is related to the development of a system that detects and counts instruments and sterile dressings in the operating suites.

Keywords: Design · Wearable technologies · Mobile technologies · Students' projects

1 Introduction

The aim of this paper is to present the work done during the one-semester class of the second year of the Bachelor Degree in Industrial Design at Politecnico di Milano. The course aimed to design products and systems addressed to sport activities. Moreover, the course focused on the relationship among human healthcare and wellbeing; sports' practice represents a driving force to prevent diseases and to maintain a good health status. One of the goals of Politecnico di Milano and of the class itself is to promote the integration of skills and collaboration different fields, such as social and medical disciplines, to design and develop innovative products, materials, technologies, methodologies and services thanks to a human-centered approach.

The course was coordinated by the prof. Giuseppe Andreoni with the collaboration of the prof. Marinella Ferrara, and the support of TeDH research group (*Technology and Design for Healthcare*). TeDH is a knowledge center specialized in the production and application of research and design (User Centered Design, Participatory Design, Co-design methodology, User research, Ethnographic observation) for product, interior and services development in the health care field. TeDH is an interdisciplinary team including designers, architects and engineers working in permanent connection with people coming from different research field and diverse specializations, such as doctors and nurses belonging to local medical institutions. TeDH's projects range from the design of biomedical wearable devices for remote monitoring of biological signals to the development of health care service scenarios supported by mobile communication technologies.

© ICST Institute for Computer Sciences, Social Informatics and Telecommunications Engineering 2017
P. Perego et al. (Eds.): MobiHealth 2016, LNICST 192, pp. 187–194, 2017.
DOI: 10.1007/978-3-319-58877-3_25

Nowadays Design has a crucial role in the development of technologies and in how the users interact with them. Such interaction could determine the product market success or its failure. In fact, as the International Council of Societies of Industrial Design has stated, *"Design is the central factor of innovative humanization of technologies and the crucial factor of cultural and economic exchange"* [1]. For these reasons, design students have to deal with technologies to solve users' needs. They have to develop products and systems that make technology usable from everyone. Designers involve final users in the product's development since its beginning, to answer properly to their needs. Designers have to understand and to define how products really works and how they are made. They have to develop formal languages and expression, and shapes that reduce the "inside complexity" (Law of conservation of complexity - Larry Poser) [2].

Moreover, healthcare products often show their technological features instead of showing their usability characteristics. Products have to become simpler and understandable without losing their technological features. Human well-being is not only represented by the absence of disease but on the state of satisfaction on the surrounding environment and products. Interacting with objects, we can talk about physiological, psychological, ideological and social pleasure [3, 4]. Healthcare products need a more specific design focus, with regard to their features, such as materials, colors, shapes, textures and visual communication. In this process, Design and Human Factors and their multi-disciplinary approaches are strategic to analyze, define and understand the users' needs and desires, and in which way these needs can be satisfied [5, 6].

2   Materials and Methods

The course dealt with the topic of Sports and Human healthcare and wellbeing. This topic was chosen because of TeDH research group background and its involvement in a Lab named E4Sport [7]. This Lab focuses its research in the measurement and assessment of the athletes' performance and to the design of their equipment. Moreover, in 2016 there were the Olympic and Para-Olympic Games in Rio de Janeiro, and ADI (*Associazione per il Disegno Industriale - Italian Association for the Industrial Design*) established an award for sport and well-being.

Measuring human functions and physiological parameters is also related to healthcare and for this reason the course added also this focus among its objectives. Sports' practice represents a driving force to prevent diseases and to maintain a good health status.

Developing products and systems for healthcare and sports' practice involves different areas of interest: comfort and discomfort, personal and social dimension, emotions and feelings, amusement and training, sports' practice for impaired people. Students were asked to deep investigate these topics before developing a product.

During the course, several experts presented their research and projects, to show students their point of view; doctors, engineers, designers told their experiences.

The course will follow five main phases:

- Theory lessons;
- Supervised analysis and concept generation;
- System design and development;

- Ex-tempore (prototyping/physical computing);
- Presentation and reporting.

The Teachers' team was composed by expert in different disciplines: one expert in biomedical and communication technologies applied to medicine and rehabilitation; one expert in design and materials supporting product and social innovation; one expert in Design for healthcare, ergonomics and Interaction design; one expert in Computer Science and Control Systems; one expert in technologies (hardware and software), wearable devices and Human-Computer Interaction. The Teachers' team expertise are complementary and functional to the topic of the course and the synergy among research and didactic activities allows students to face real case studies and to develop systems and products that answer real needs [8]. This approach is also useful for researchers, that can explain and discuss their research and find different points of view, strengths and weaknesses.

Students were asked to organize into groups of 2 or 3 people and to define a product concept to develop during the course. First of all, they were asked to define a research topic and to characterize the users and their needs. Students were asked to conduct a market and a patent research, to identify what is already produced and patented. At the end of this analysis phase, they were ready to define the general requirements of their concept and to start designing it. Table 1 below shows the groups' features and their topics.

Table 1. Students' groups and corresponding projects

Students' groups	Projects' topic
Group 1 (1 M, 2 F)	Stress monitoring and respiration training tools
Group 2 (2 F)	Swim cap with MP3
Group 3 (2 M)	Wearable monitoring tools for hiking
Group 4 (2 M)	Headphones with heart rate monitoring
Group 5 (3 M)	Martial art chest protector
Group 6 (2 M)	Smart wristband for tennis
Group 7 (2 M, 1F)	Postural shirt
Group 8 (2 M)	Interactive carpet for kids
Group 9 (2 F)	Swim headphones
Group 10 (3 F)	Baby sling
Group 11 (3 F)	Smart helmet for horse-riding
Group 12 (1 M, 1 F)	Smart tools for scuba diving
Group 13 (2 M)	Smart belt for weight-lifting
Group 14 (2 M)	Nutrition tracking system
Group 15 (2 F)	Gloves for people afflicted with the Raynaud Syndrome
Group 16 (2 M)	Mountain bike chest protector
Group 17 (2 F)	Smart garments for ice skating
Group 18 (1 M, 2 F)	Ankle brace
Group 19 (2 M)	Smart swim cap for blind people
Group 20 (2 M)	Rewarding system for gym clients
Group 21 (1 M, 1 F)	Swim vest for kids
Group 22 (1 M, 1 F)	Roller derby protectors
Group 23 (2 M, 1 F)	Smart rescue buoy
Group 24 (1 M, 1 F)	Smart system for detecting surgery instruments
Group 25 (1 M, 1 F)	Smart gym gloves
Group 26 (3 M)	Motocross chest protector
Group 27 (2 M)	Running shoes for preventing ankle twists
Group 28 (1 M)	Swim-board

3   Results and Discussion

In this section, two case studies are presented to prove the good interdisciplinarity achieved and the didactic experience. The first case study is a training suite for Figure Skating. Two students developed this project, both of them with experience in ice skating and artistic gymnastic. The aim was to create a wearable tool that can be used by expert to measure their performance and to prevent injuries or fatigue during their training session. Moreover, this device could give feedback related to their gesture performing an exercise. Their research process started with a deep analysis of the sport activity, using interviews and online form, to understand the critical issues of figure skating and the users' needs. At the same time, they analyzed the Figure Skating from the biomechanics point of view.

After this research phase, they defined their project brief: they would design a wearable monitoring system that could detect the muscular activity during the training session and give real time to inform the user of the muscular stress and avoid injuries. Moreover, the device had to register the training session and send it to a smartphone or a tablet.

They started analyzing the existing technologies, to identify the ones useful for their scope, that answers to their requirements. For measuring the muscular activities, they found interesting dry electrodes for electromyography; for transmitting the data acquired to the control unit, they choose smart textiles. They designed the dimension corresponding to a flexible PCB control unit that can be worn. To give a real time feedback, they identified the Lumigram, an optical fiber that can be sewed. When illuminated, the optical fiber can display which muscle group is activated during the exercise (e.g., an axel jump). Figure 1 below shows the elements and fabrics chosen to answer that needs.

They designed a product named "Electropants", that can be worn during the Figure Skating practice. These "lit pants" and their lighting effects can be seen both by the athlete itself and the coach and the spectators, increasing the involvement during the performance and its magnificent. The students answered the users' needs developing this interactive training suite, investing and cultivating *"the imagination with regard to physical and psychological human needs, and link them to positive experiences such as stimulation, relatedness, and competence"* [9].

According to Sheldon, competence is one of the top-ten psychological human needs based on a review of theories about the content of motives. Others are autonomy, relatedness, influence, pleasure, security, physical thriving, self-actualizing, self-esteem, and money [10].

Moreover, the students developed the UI of an App, that can be used to track the training session. Figure 2 below shows their prototype.

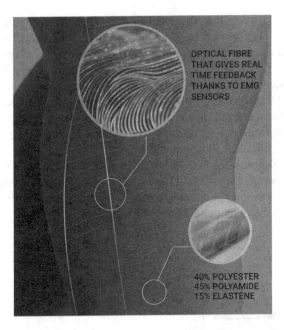

OPTICAL FIBRE
THAT GIVES REAL
TIME FEEDBACK
THANKS TO EMG
SENSORS

40% POLYESTER
45% POLYAMIDE
15% ELASTENE

Fig. 1. Project requirements and related items.

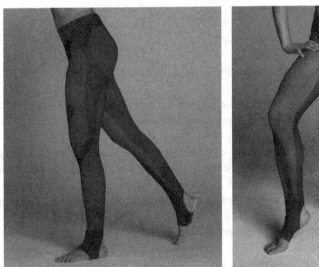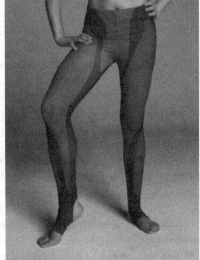

Fig. 2. The concept prototype.

The second project is a system that detects and counts instruments and sterile dressings in the operating suites. Sometimes during or after a surgery, some items disappear or can be left inside the body and it represents a very high risk for both the patient and the medical team. To avoid that, these students developed a system that automatically count the items and in case of items' loss, can detect where it is thanks to a RFID sensor.

They started their research attending a surgery and interviewing the person devoted to the items count. This count is made more times during the surgery: before the beginning, during the surgery and at the end. Sometimes happens that an items could disappear. In that case, all the medical team has to look for the loss item; sometimes the patient must to undergo to other examinations, to detect the loss item. To avoid such problem, the students focused their project on the detection of the instruments, excluding needles and their similar due to their little dimensions.

At the end of this research phase, the students started searching for technologies that can be used to solve the loss of instruments and sterile dressings. They found that the RFID technology is already in use in several UK hospitals, to solve that problem.

Figure 3 shows the functioning of the identified technology.

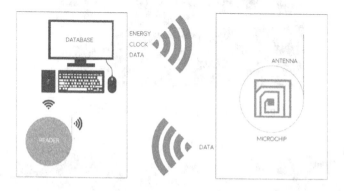

Fig. 3. The functioning of RFID technology.

They designed a desk for the person in charge of the instruments' count and a reader to be used just in case of loss items. Figures 4 and 5 below shows some sketches of the designed system.

Designing the smart desk, students took into account of the direct and indirect users' needs in the operating room. In fact, they choose a material that can be easily clean and sterilize, such as the Polyamide; the desk is white and the whole surface is polished. Moreover, it is suitable for a standing person because the work surface area is 91 cm high.

The reader must be used when a discrepancy in the count occurs and it is stored in a drawer at the back of the desk. It can be used with one hand. On the device top there is a button that must be clicked to turn it on. Once the system has been activated, the user has to scan the interested area, to detect the loss item.

The students also analyzed the visual and chromatic aspects of their project. In fact, they choose colors that are influenced by the context and by the healthcare: they choose a color range that is close to the "hospital green" (HEX # 2ab1bb). Moreover, the project logo is circular and divided into different parts, to recall their cyclical process. The project is named "No-Retech", is the meld of "No Retention" and "Technology".

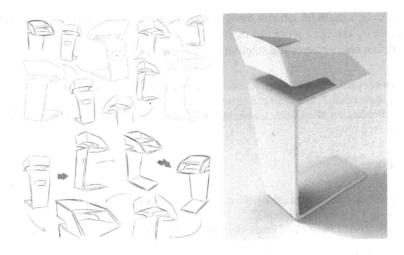

Fig. 4. The smart desk for the items' count

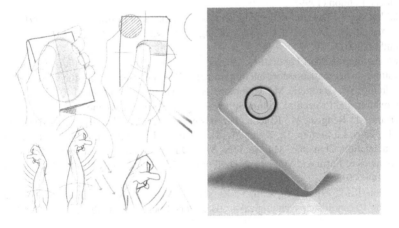

Fig. 5. The smart reader.

4   Conclusion

The described teaching and designing activities proves that a design approach is desirable in a field that involves sports' practice, wellbeing and healthcare. In such field, products are often complex and hard to use. Design research and its tools are useful to understand people and their needs in their everyday life context (such as workplace, home, gym and so on). Designers are able to understand the physical and psychological human needs, and to link them into positive experiences for their projects. A human centered design approach can be considered as suitable, in developing innovative products or systems.

Moreover, a multidisciplinary team represents an enrichment in the entire development process. The class proves its capability to research and examine in depth a topic and to define requirements and solution that take into account of the users' needs.

Acknowledgments. The Authors would like to thank all the students that took part to the "Disegno Industriale 2" Class, for their hard work. In particular, we would like to thank Eliana Martone, Daniela del Mar Gómez Guizo, Lorenzo Luchetti and Silvia Mascaretti, that allow us to present their projects.

References

1. International Council of Societies of Industrial Design, Definition of Industrial Design. http://www.icsid.org/about/definition/
2. Norman, D.A.: Living with Complexity. The MIT Press, Cambridge, Massachusetts, London (2010)
3. Green, W., Jordan, P.: Human Factors in Product Design. Taylor and Francis, London (1999)
4. Jordan, P.W.: Pleasure with Products: Human Factors for Body, Mind and Soul. Taylor & Francis, London (1999)
5. Maldonado, T.: Disegno industriale: un riesame. Feltrinelli Editore, Milano (1991)
6. Norman, D.A.: Design of Everyday Things. The MIT Press, Cambridge, Massachusetts, London (2002)
7. Engineering for Sport Laboratory – E4Sport Lab. http://www.polimi.it/it/ricerca-scientifica/strutture-di-ricerca/laboratori-interdipartimentali/e4sport-engineering-for-sport-laboratory/
8. Andreoni, G., Barbieri, M., Colombo, B.: Developing Biomedical Devices – Design, Innovation and Protection. Polimi Springer Briefs. Springer, Milano (2014)
9. Ferrara, M., Bengisu, M.: Kinetic materials experience. In: Chen, L.-L., T., Djajadiningrat, L.-L., Feijs, L., Steffen, D., Kyffin, S., Rampino, L., Rodriguez, E., Hu, J. (eds.) Aesthetics of interaction: Dynamic, Multisensory, Wise 9th International Conference on Design and Semantics of Form and Movement, DeSForM 2015, Milano, Italy, 13–17 October 2015, pp. 138–145 (2015)
10. Sheldon, K.M., Elliot, A.J., Kim, Y., Kasser, T.: What is satisfying about satisfying events? Testing 10 candidate psychological needs. J. Pers. Soc. Psychol. **80**, 325–339 (2001)

DIABESITY: A Study for mHealth Integrated Solutions

Italo Zoppis[1](✉), Giancarlo Mauri[1], Ferancesco Sicurello[1], Eugenio Santoro[2], Giada Pietrabissa[3,4], and Gianluca Castelnuovo[3,4]

[1] Department of Computer Science, University of "Milano-Bicocca", Milano, Italy
italo.zoppis@unimib.it
[2] Department of Epidemiology, IRCCS, Mario Negri, Milano, Italy
[3] Department of Psychology, Catholic University of Milan, Milano, Italy
[4] Psychology Research Laboratory, IRCCS Istituto Auxologico Italiano, Milano, Italy

Abstract. Obesity is now one of the most critical and demanding public health condition due to the correlation with many medical and psychological comorbidities, such as cardiovascular, orthopedic, pneumological, endocrinological, psychopathological complications, above all the type 2 diabetes. Obesity traditionally needs long and expensive treatments in a chronic care management approach. So clinical research has to develop, test and validate cheaper rehabilitation programs. For this reason, we developed the DIABESITY study, the design of a mHealth integrated platform to promote the empowerment of patients in self-monitoring and successfully managing their pathological conditions (focusing on obesity and type 2 diabetes) through the use of mobile devices. In this paper we report this study by discussing the following two important aspects of DIABESITY. (i) Dietary mHealth tools for home-patients; (ii) Measures to capture the psychological factors and processes which mediate change of behavior and affect initiation and maintenance phases.

Keywords: Type 2 diabetes · mHealth · Psychological questionnaires · Obesity

1 Introduction

Obesity and low level of physical activity are well known important public health problems that are typically correlated with many medical and psychological comorbidities, such as cardiovascular, orthopedic, pneumological, endocrinological, psychopathological complications, above all the type 2 diabetes. Obesity and its comorbidities traditionally need long treatments creating a very expensive chronic care management approach 1. Clinical research has to develop, evaluate and validate cheaper rehabilitation programs above all in out-patient settings. In order to manage these problems, we developed the DIABESITY project. DIABESITY is first of all an innovative approach in health care systems and behind this approach we planned a project with a clinical study that will test the technological platform developed in the project. Diabesity means a new approach,

© ICST Institute for Computer Sciences, Social Informatics and Telecommunications Engineering 2017
P. Perego et al. (Eds.): MobiHealth 2016, LNICST 192, pp. 195–199, 2017.
DOI: 10.1007/978-3-319-58877-3_26

a project but also a study and the platform we will develop in the study. In particular, in this paper, we will focus on how DIABESITY can help patients in maintaining lifestyle behavior changes, ensuring functional patient empowerment and engagement. With this aim, the following key-points will be discussed: (i) Dietary mHealth services for home-patients (Sect. 2.1) and (ii) Indexes to capture the psychological factors and processes which mediate change of behavior and affect initiation and maintenance phases (Sect. 2.2).

2 Functionality, Measures and Questionnaires

2.1 Functionality

The system is developed as integrable platform that should fit into existing diabetes health system functions and complement the health system goals of health service provision for overweight/obese people and patients with type 2 diabetes. Moreover DIABESITY follows current relevant standards, guidelines, and best practices[1]. Here we do not detail the technologies of DIABESITY, rather we discuss which functionality of DIABESITY can be applied in order for patients to maintain significant lifestyle behavior changes, improve health outcomes, and ensure functional empowerment and engagement. Specifically, we report in Table 1 the main functionality of the apps of this study.

2.2 Psychological and Behavioral Questionnaires

As suggested by Katan [9], cognition and feelings have a huge impact on behavior and may thus strength as well as disrupt adherence to treatment with clinical prescriptions. Psychological variables and processes influence every behavior change affecting the starting step and the following phases. DIABESITY program is designed to explore such factors in order to define which kind of patients could benefit from a mhealth based intervention. For this, we consider the indexes and questionnaires reported in Table 2. (taking into account that the psychological theory of change behind the DIABESITY approach is the *Transtheoretical Model of Change* [2–4,8,10]. This table is the same used in another previous project, TECNOB study, as reported in pages 5–6 of [1].

---

[1] In particular those concerning interoperability, minimum patient summary dataset to be shared across borders, standard on user safety (currently draft standard IEC 82304-1), app certification programs (e.g. NHS in the UK), apps as medical device (directive 93/42/EC under review) or in vitro diagnostic medical device (directive 98/79/EC under review) and compliance with personal data protection rules.

Table 1. Apps and functionality

App function	App contents	App specifications
Diet caloric restriction	Aiming to promote revolutionary principle approach of eating low calories density food, i.e. "eat more food while eating fewer calories and feeling the same degree of satiety" to maintain normal weight	(i) Consumer will get combinations of likely successful dietary treatments from a set of patients feature characteristics; (ii) Makes it easy to find a partner doctor in one of National's healthcare networks, and access to that doctor for advice; (iii) Book appointments at a Health Diabetes, Nutrition and Metabolic Diseases Center; (iv) Secure access to health data and logs via the app
Diet composition	Improvement in dietary patterns national diet (intervention pattern in fat, sugar intake and micronutrients intake)	(i) Tables and reports to suggest confidence to undergo specific dietary improvement; (ii) Makes it easy to find a partner dietician (a registered dietitian) in one of National's Health Diabetes Center; (iii) Dieticians can make personalized meal plan or can recommend standardized food portion size and can send images of the dietary patterns simply via the app; (iv) The app users will be able to create a personal patient record with standardized food portion size

Table 2. Scales and indexes (adapted from [1])

The self-report habit index (SRHI)	The SRHI is a measure of the development and strength of habits. It has a stem "[the behavior] is something that ..." followed by 12 items such as "I do without thinking"
Weight efficacy life style questionnaire (WELSQ)	The WELSQ is composed of 20 items that measure the confidence of the subjects about being able to successfully resist the desire to eat
Body uneasiness test (BUT)	The BUT is a self-report inventory that measures body uneasiness by a global severity index and five sub-scales: weight phobia, body image concerns, avoidance, compulsive self-monitoring, depersonalization
Binge eating scale (BES)	The BES is a short self-report questionnaire which measures severity of binge eating
Eating disorder inventory (EDI-2)	The EDI-2 is a widely used, standardized, self-report measure of psychological symptoms commonly associated with anorexia nervosa, bulimia nervosa and other eating disorders
Symptom check list (SCL-90)	The SCL-90 is a brief, multidimensional self-report inventory designed to screen for a broad range of psychological problems and psychopathological symptoms
Impact of weight on quality of life-lite (IWQOL-Lite)	IWQOL-lite is the short version of the original IWQOL and is composed by 31 items. The questionnaire is selfreport and consists of 5 scales assessing the impact of weight on QoL-related factors such as physical functioning, self-esteem, sexual life, public distress and work
The outcome questionnaire (OQ 45.2)	The OQ 45 items version is a measure of outcome and it is designed in order to collect repeated measures of patient progress during therapy and after its conclusion

3 Conclusions

The DIABESITY study integrates different solutions for the management and intervention of subjects with diabetes. This integration is designed to promote a stepped down intervention addressed to the behavior change [1]. As already indicated, ICT technologies may represent a functional integration to traditional treatments in order to reduce costs in chronic care management. Moreover ICT can enhance the adherence to prescribed treatments with the use of disappearing and real–time monitoring. In particular, social media [11] and specific analytical techniques [5–7], which share and integrate information, can improve the management of the pathologies e.g. by providing Internet-based spaces where patients can share experiences or by exploring the long-term intervention. Here, we focused on two main issues, which can support home-patients and capture the psychological factors affecting initiation and maintenance of the therapy.

The innovative features of the DIABESITY approach will be:

1. ORGANIZATIONAL INNOVATION: the out–patient step of the care will be provided in a new framework reducing hospital admissions and performing mobile and Internet based monitoring and treatment integrated protocols that will avoid high costs for the National Heath Services and waste of time for patients attending uselessly hospitals or clinics. This will also reduce the burden of disease of the patients, improving their quality of life.
2. TECHNOLOGICAL INNOVATION: the DIABESITY project will not produce new technological devices or biosensors, but it will use the gold–standard technology available on the market in a new user–friendly platform integrated in order to diagnose obesity and to assess severity or complications of it (above all type 2 diabetes).
3. CLINICAL INNOVATION: clinical units will manage obesity in a multidisciplinary approach, according to a chronic care management model, including biomedical, psychological, eating and physical activity data, improving the patients knowledge, empowerment, self–awareness and maximizing the rehabilitation impact.

References

1. Castelnuovo, G., Manzoni, G., Cuzziol, P., Cesa, G., Tuzzi, C., Villa, V., Liuzzi, A., Petroni, M., Molinari, E.: TECNOB: study design of a randomized controlled trial of a multidisciplinary telecare intervention for obese patients with type 2 diabetes. BMC Public Health **20**(1), 204 (2010)
2. Castelnuovo, G., Manzoni, G.M., Pietrabissa, G., Corti, S., Giusti, E.M., Molinari, E., Simpson, S.: Obesity and outpatient rehabilitation using mobile technologies: the potential mhealth approach. Front. Psychol. **5**, 559 (2014)
3. Castelnuovo, G., Pietrabissa, G., Manzoni, G.M., Corti, S., Ceccarini, M., Borrello, M., Giusti, E.M., Novelli, M., Cattivelli, R., Middleton, N.A., Simpson, S.G., Molinari, E.: Chronic care management of globesity: promoting healthier lifestyles in traditional and mHealth based settings. Front. Psychol. **6**, 1557 (2015)

4. Castelnuovo, G., Zoppis, I., Santoro, E., Ceccarini, M., Pietrabissa, G., Manzoni, G.M., Corti, S., Borrello, M., Giusti, E.M., Cattivelli, R., Melesi, A., Mauri, G., Molinari, E., Sicurello, F.: Managing chronic pathologies with a stepped mhealth-based approach in clinical psychology and medicine. Front. Psychol. **6**, 407 (2015)

5. Cava, C., Zoppis, I., Gariboldi, M., Castiglioni, I., Mauri, G., Antoniotti, M.: Copy–number alterations for tumor progression inference. In: Peek, N., Marín Morales, R., Peleg, M. (eds.) AIME 2013. LNCS, vol. 7885, pp. 104–109. Springer, Heidelberg (2013). doi:10.1007/978-3-642-38326-7_16

6. Cava, C., Zoppis, I., Gariboldi, M., Castiglioni, I., Mauri, G., Antoniotti, M.: Combined analysis of chromosomal instabilities and gene expression for colon cancer progression inference. J. Clin. Bioinform. **4**(1), 1 (2014)

7. Cava, C., Zoppis, I., Mauri, G., Ripamonti, M., Gallivanone, F., Salvatore, C., Gilardi, M.C., Castiglioni, I.: Combination of gene expression and genome copy number alteration has a prognostic value for breast cancer. In: 2013 35th Annual International Conference of the IEEE Engineering in Medicine and Biology Society (EMBC), pp. 608–611. IEEE (2013)

8. Ceccarini, M., Borrello, M., Pietrabissa, G., Manzoni, G.M., Castelnuovo, G.: Assessing motivation and readiness to change for weight management and control: an in-depth evaluation of three sets of instruments. Front. Psychol. **6**, 511 (2015)

9. Katan, M.B.: Weight-loss diets for the prevention and treatment of obesity. N. Engl. J. Med. **360**(9), 923–925 (2009)

10. Pietrabissa, G., Sorgente, A., Rossi, A., Simpson, S., Riva, G., Manzoni, G.M., Prochaska, J.O., Prochaska, J.M., Cattivelli, R., Castelnuovo, G.: Stages of change in obesity and weight management: factorial structure of the Italian version of the university of rhode island change assessment scale. Eat Weight Disord. (2016)

11. Santoro, E., Castelnuovo, G., Zoppis, I., Mauri, G., Sicurello, F.: Social media and mobile applications in chronic disease prevention and management. Front. Psychol. **6**, 567 (2015)

A Reference Framework of mHealth Patents
for Innovative Services

Massimo Barbieri[1] and Giuseppe Andreoni[2(✉)]

[1] Politecnico di Milano – Technology Transfer Office, P.zza L. Da Vinci 32, 20133 Milan, Italy
massimo.barbieri@polimi.it
[2] Dip. di Design, Politecnico di Milano, via G. Durando 38/A, 20158 Milan, Italy
giuseppe.andreoni@polimi.it

Abstract. mHealth is an emerging and rapidly developing field with huge exploitation expectancies both in improving life quality of patients and in market opportunities. Patents and innovations in mHealth represents a priority for companies to enter and exploit their know-how and market requests. This paper focuses on the analysis of the Intellectual Property Rights in the field of mHealth systems to draw a reference knowledge framework of the mHealth scenario. An up-to-date detailed categorization, the geographical distribution and the identification of top players in mHealth is presented.

Keywords: mHealth · IPR · Patent · Distribution · Companies · Exploitation

1 Introduction

In 2011 WHO stated that the use of mobile and wireless technologies to support the achievement of health objectives has the potential to transform the face of health service delivery across the globe. Mobile health (mHealth) covers "medical and public health practice supported by mobile devices, such as mobile phones, patient monitoring devices, personal digital assistants (PDAs), and other wireless devices [1]. Fourteen categories of mHealth services were identified by the WHO report: health call centres, emergency toll-free telephone services, managing emergencies and disasters, mobile telemedicine, appointment reminders, community mobilization and health promotion, treatment compliance, mobile patient records, information access, patient monitoring, health surveys and data collection, surveillance, health awareness raising, and decision support systems [1].

Also EU in its "Green Paper on mHealth" recognizes how mHealth is an emerging and rapidly developing field which has the potential to play a part in the transformation of healthcare and increase its quality and efficiency [2]. mHealth solutions cover various technological solutions, that among others measure vital signs such as heart rate, blood glucose level, blood pressure, body temperature and brain activities. Prominent examples of apps are communication, information and motivation tools, such as medication reminders or tools offering fitness and dietary recommendations. This means a huge market potential to be exploited through a widespread category of systems or devices

© ICST Institute for Computer Sciences, Social Informatics and Telecommunications Engineering 2017
P. Perego et al. (Eds.): MobiHealth 2016, LNICST 192, pp. 200–206, 2017.
DOI: 10.1007/978-3-319-58877-3_27

or software applications (or "apps"), that are considered to be a medical device according to the specific and corresponding regulation regulations [3, 4].

mHealth products are portable devices (such as smartphones or tablets), which use software applications (or "apps") for health monitoring purpose, prevention and detection of diseases and basic diagnosis [5]. mHealth apps are rapidly growing and evolving thanks to cloud computing and 4G technologies and are available in every area of healthcare such as physical activity, anti-obesity, diabetes and asthma self-management [6]. According to IMS Institute for healthcare informatics, more than 165,000 m-Health apps are available [7] and at the 2010 more than 200 million mHealth apps were downloaded [8].

New generation mobile/smartphones are equipped with embedded and advanced sensors such as accelerometers, gyroscopes, GPS, microphones (that can be used as stethoscopes to detect heart rate) and cameras. Techniques like ultrasound, fluorescence imaging and even a combination of imaging cytometry and fluorescent microscopy were developed using a smartphone. The computing capacity of smartphone/tablet PC is getting more and more high, as well as the quality of their components. Software platforms (iOS or Android or Windows), network protocol systems (3G, 4G, 5G), battery life of smartphones and graphical user interfaces (GUI) are the critical points to be faced and solved.

Innovation in the field of mHealth devices is rapidly growing and patents could be an indicator of these innovative activities. The purpose of this study is to evaluate the technology progress of mHealth devices and to analyze the patent data in more detailed way. For this reason this paper focuses on the analysis of the Intellectual Property Rights (IPR) in the field of mHealth systems to draw a reference knowledge framework of the mHealth scenario.

2 Materials and Methods

Patent searches can be carried out by means of keywords, classification symbols or a combination of both methods. Sometimes keyword searching is not effective because it's subjective and limited to the language used [9, 10]. These drawbacks can be overcome by using a classification tool. The patent classification systems are a language independent tools that help to retrieve patent information. The most worldwide used systems are IPC (*International Patent Classification*) and CPC (*Cooperative Patent Classification*). The IPC is used by more than 100 national and regional patent offices. It's a hierarchical classification system, revised annually, consisting of eight sections, which are divided into around 70,000 sub-divisions called classes, subclasses and groups. CPC is based on IPC and ECLA (the former European Classification). It's more frequently updated than IPC and has more detailed sub-divisions (around 200,000), useful for faster moving technology fields classification [11].

All patent searches were performed using Orbit database [12], which is a fee based patent database with a good data coverage.

3   Results

A search with the keywords ("mHealth" or "mobile health") in the "title/abstract/claims/ concepts/object of invention" search field showed 740 results. We performed a statistical analysis in order to retrieve the main IPC/CPC codes, as reported in Table 1. Patent applications relating medical information are generally classified in the generic subgroup G06F 19/00 of IPC.

Table 1.   Results of the quick search.

CPC codes	Definition	No. of inventions
G06F-019/3+	Medical informatics	107
A61B-005/00	Detecting, measuring or recording for diagnostic purposes	128
G06Q-050/22	Health care	98

A more precise and specific search was carried out using a quite complex query, which gave 6,550 results. The parameters of the query were: [(m_health OR (mobile 1w health) OR smartphone? OR (tablet 1w pc) OR PDA OR personal_digital_assistant OR phablet)/TI/AB/IW/CLMS/KEYW/OBJ AND (G06F-019/3+ OR G06Q-050/22 OR A61B-005+)/IPC/CPC]. The distribution of search results by publication years is shown in Fig. 1 below.

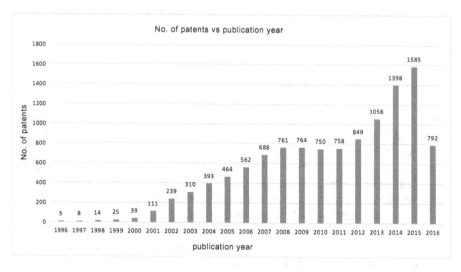

Fig. 1.   The evolution of patent number in the last 20 years by publication year.

Since patent applications are published 18 months after the filing date, it could be said that the number of patent applications grew rapidly from 2011, reaching its peak in

2013. The distribution of search results by Priority country reveals that most of inventions are generated in the United States of America (Fig. 2). The main patent applicants are reported in the Fig. 3 below.

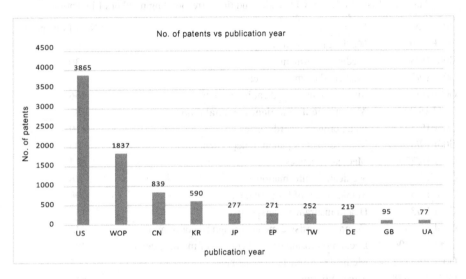

Fig. 2. The distribution of search results by priority country.

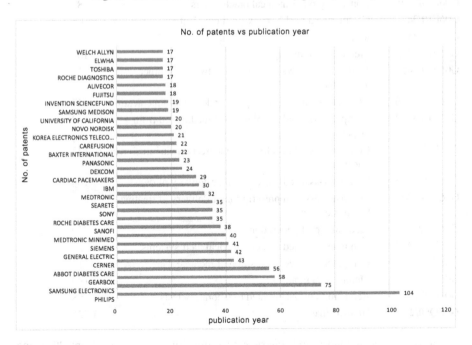

Fig. 3. List of top applicants.

A deeper analysis was performed on each relevant CPC code, using the same keywords (see Table 2, where in bold are evidenced the most populated fields).

Table 2. List of relevant CPC codes and the corresponding number of inventions.

CPC codes	Definition	No. of inventions
G06F-019/3+	Medical informatics	107
G06F19/30	Medical informatics	30
G06F19/32	Medical data management	10
G06F19/321	Management of medical image data	156
G06F19/322	**Management of patient personal data**	**583**
G06F19/323	on a portable record carrier	119
G06F19/324	Management of patient independent data	93
G06F19/325	Medical practices	73
G06F19/326	Medication information	76
G06F19/327	Management of hospital data	298
G06F19/328	Health insurance management	159
G06F19/34	Computer-assisted medical diagnosis or treatment	43
G06F19/3406	Local monitoring or local control of medical devices	482
G06F19/3412	Medical equipment management	93
G06F19/3418	**Telemedicine**	**819**
G06F19/3425	Consulting other medical practitioners	87
G06F19/3431	Calculating a health index for the patient	106
G06F19/3437	Medical simulation or modelling	90
G06F19/3443	Medical data mining	100
G06F19/345	Medical expert systems, neural networks or other automated diagnosis	312
G06F19/3456	Computer-assisted prescription or delivery of medication	347
G06F19/3462	Computer-assisted distribution of medication from dispensers	132
G06F19/3468	Computer-assisted delivery of medication via infusion or injection	147
G06F19/3475	Computer-assisted prescription or delivery of diets	168
G06F19/3481	Computer-assisted prescription or delivery of treatment by physical action	371
G06F19/3487	Medical report generation	229
G06F19/3493	Computer-assisted epidemiological alert systems	25
G06F19/36	Computer-assisted acquisition of medical data	19
G06F19/363	Manual data input	192
G06F19/366	Acquisition of data related to laboratory tests	58
G06Q50/22	**Health care**	**1,736**

Narrowing the second search query with a priority date starting from 2013 and G06F19/3+ sub-divisions, the search gave 926 results, and telemedicine and the management of patient personal data are the technical fields with more inventions.

4   Discussion

Data of publication year indicate the presence of different mHealth epochs: until 2001 there a few experiences and innovations probably due to the immaturity of technologies related to this field; with the diffusion of communication technologies, from 2002 to 2008 an increasing number of applications/inventions have been achieved. Another stability period started and lasted up to 2011, and since 2012 with the rapid introduction and global spreading of smartphone and related apps a new rapid development era is in progress.

About Top players data demonstrates that multinational biomedical companies cover the first position of ranking, but it is interesting to note the presence of big software developers and also one university.

Concerning the methodology, a big difference is noticeable in the results coming from other research engine or sources: using the search query "m-health or mobile health" Scopus provided 1.059 results, while Espacenet only 645 if analyzing the full text (57 if only in the title, or 106 including title and summary). This means that general data could be obtained by these sources, but the detail level provided by specific database is more relevant.

The technical fields in which innovation is more marked are: 1. Telemedicine; 2. Management of patient personal data (e.g. patient records); 3. Local monitoring of medical devices (e.g. graphical user interfaces); 4. Computer assisted prescriptions (e.g. prescription filling or compliance checking); 5. Medical expert systems (e.g. medical decision support systems).

5   Conclusion

This short IPR analysis demonstrated that mHealth is in the big expansion period. Technology is mature and related inventions start covering all the opportunities. A saturation and real discrimination of IPR is expected in the near future.

According to the responses to a European Commission public consultation, privacy and security, patient safety, a clear legal framework and better evidence on cost-effectiveness are all required to help mobile Health care ("mHealth") flourish in Europe [2].

References

1. World Health Organisation: mHealth – New horizons for health through mobile technologies, Global Observatory for eHealth series, vol. 3 (2011)
2. EU Commission: GREEN PAPER on mobile Health ("mHealth") (2014)
3. IEC 60601-1 Ed.3.1 (2013)
4. EU Commission, DG Health and Consumer: MEDICAL DEVICES: Guidance document - Classification of medical devices, Guidelines relating to the application of the Council Directive 93/42/EEC on Medical Devices, MEDDEV 2.4/1 Rev. 9 (2010)
5. Gagneja, A.P.S., Gagneja, K.K.: Mobile Health (mHealth) technologies. In: IEEE 17th International Conference on E_health Networking, Applications and Services (HealthCom), pp. 37–43 (2015)

6. Baig, M.M., GholamHosseini, H., Connolly, M.J.: Mobile healthcare applications: system design review, critical issues and challenges. Australas. Phys. Eng. Sci. Med. **38**, 23–38 (2015)
7. http://www.imshealth.com/en/about-us/news/ims-health-study:-patient-options-expand-as-mobile-healthcare-apps-address-wellness-and-chronic-disease-treatment-needs
8. Silva, B.M.C., Rodrigues, J.J.P.C., de la Torre Díez, I., López-Coronado, M., Saleem, K.: Mobile-health: a review of current state in 2015. J. Biomed. Inform. **56**, 265–272 (2015)
9. White, M.: Patent searching: back to the future – how to use patent classification search tools to create better searches. In: First Annual Conference of the Canadian Engineering Education Association, Kingston, Ontario (2010)
10. White, M.: Patent classification reform: implications for teaching, learning and using the patent literature. In: American Society for Engineering Education Annual Conference, San Antonio, Texas (2012)
11. List, J.: Editorial: on patent classification. World Pat. Inf. **41**, 1–3 (2015)
12. Questel Orbit Patent Search Database. http://www.orbit.com. Accessed 26 June 2016
13. Closa, D., Gardiner, A., Giemsa, F., Machek, J.: Patent Law for Computer Scientists. Springer, Heidelberg (2010). http://www.springer.com/us/book/9783642050770

Monitoring Patients in Ambulatory Palliative Care: A Design for an Observational Study

Vanessa C. Klaas[1(✉)], Alberto Calatroni[1], Michael Hardegger[1],
Matthias Guckenberger[2], Gudrun Theile[2], and Gerhard Tröster[1]

[1] ETH Zurich, Zurich, Switzerland
Vanessa.Klaas@ife.ee.ethz.ch
[2] University Hospital Zurich, Zurich, Switzerland
http://www.ife.ee.ethz.ch/people/vklaas

Abstract. We present the setup of an observational study that aims to examine the application of wearables in ambulatory palliative care to monitor the patients' health status – especially during the transition phase from hospital to home since this phase is critical and often patients are re-hospitalised. Following an user-centred design approach, we performed interviews with patients recruited at the Clinic of Radiation Oncology of the University Hospital Zurich, Switzerland. The patient group was perceived as very vulnerable and varied largely in physiological burden and mental aspects. Special needs concern primarily obtrusiveness of the system and sensitivity in the work with this vulnerable patient group.

Keywords: Palliative Care · User interviews · Remote monitoring systems · Real-world deployment · Wearable sensing

1 Introduction

Palliative care (PC) is a set of practices aiming at relieving patients with a life-threatening disease from physical symptoms (e.g., pain, fatigue, breathlessness, sleeplessness), and to support them in the perception of their psychosocial and spiritual needs [1].

Monitoring remotely PC patients would be beneficial in the transition phase from hospital to home, when the patients lose the continuous support of professional teams and have to adapt to changing conditions. A monitoring system would help physicians react in case of decline in patient conditions.

Since PC patients are a unique group combining physical and psychological weakness, existing monitoring systems for other patient groups may not be usable/accepted.

We present a patient-centric design of a new monitoring system tailored to PC patients, where the patients are fully involved in the design of the part of the system which affects them the most, i.e., the patient interface. The design process is carried out through guided interviews. The patient interface consists of

ⓒ ICST Institute for Computer Sciences, Social Informatics and Telecommunications Engineering 2017
P. Perego et al. (Eds.): MobiHealth 2016, LNICST 192, pp. 207–214, 2017.
DOI: 10.1007/978-3-319-58877-3_28

questionnaires and feedback mechanisms, while the monitoring system also logs various sensor data relevant for predicting changes in patient conditions. Sensor data are collected both through a smart-phone and an armband equipped with sensors. Since the system will be used in a future clinical trial, we involve patients for the system design with the same inclusion criteria as the future clinical trial, thereby maximising the representativeness of the outcome.

In this paper we present the patient-centric design procedure, the lessons learned and the final monitoring system, along with the protocol for the observational study which will be carried out.

2   Related Work

Mobile health, without the use of wearable sensors, has been explored in many diseases and patient groups, e.g., in cardiovascular diseases [2], mental disorders [3,4], stroke rehabilitation [5] and stressed persons [6]. The collection of patient subjective reported outcome using mobile health is already established in oncology and has been proven feasible in younger palliative care patients [7].

Monitoring systems including also wearable sensors have been developed for specific patient groups, e.g. patients who suffered from a heart failure [8], and to measure stress, activities or health status in less specific groups [9]. The application of monitoring systems has been proven beneficial for patients with schizophrenia [10] and heart failure [11], resulting in reduced hospitalisations and mortality.

For the specific case of PC patients, until now monitoring systems are limited to the digital collection of questionnaires or self reports through a smart-phone [12]. While the usability of smart-phone-based questionnaires was investigated [13], to our knowledge no study was conducted with a system including other wearable sensors, like an armband. Furthermore, it was not yet investigated which type of feedback (if any at all) would be desirable for PC patients.

We aim to fill this gap with an unobtrusive monitoring system designed specifically for and with the help of PC patients, using a patient-centric design approach. We advance the state of the art with an observational study to examine a real-world deployment of our system with this vulnerable patient group, which will lead to a future clinical study.

3   Procedure and System for the Observational Study

In this section we present the goals of the observational study with the resulting requirements for the monitoring system. Furthermore, we outline the procedure envisioned for the study.

Goals. The observational study aims to evaluate feasibility and acceptance of monitoring by means of wearable devices within the vulnerable palliative care patient group. The system should provide data whose analysis will allow to find correlations between subjective patient ratings concerning distress, quality of life and pain and objective measurements from the wearables in order to detect deterioration of symptoms.

Procedure. Similarly to related work [3,14], we choose a sample size of 30 participants. Patients will be recruited at the radio-oncology ward of the university hospital Zurich, Switzerland, under the condition that they are aged > 18 years, have an estimated life expectancy < 12 months (physician's estimation) and > 8 weeks, are able to de-ambulate and to perform all self-care. Patients may be unable to carry out any work activities for up to at least 50% of the time they are awake [15].

Study participants receive a smart-phone Samsung Galaxy S5 (if not already using an appropriate device) and a commercial armband, (i.e., non-obtrusive devices in contrast to e.g., chest belts or adhesive electrodes) to log their physical and social activity as well as vital parameters. For that purpose, the participants shall wear the devices with them all day long. They shall charge the smart-phone over night and the armband once a day. Once a day, the smart-phone will ask patients to rate their current level of distress according to the NCCN[1] distress thermometer ([16]) and their level of pain on visual scales from 0–10. Distress and pain mainly influence the quality of life of palliative patients and are also regularly assessed by physicians [17,18]. The design of the interface between the smart-phone app and the patient (patient interface) will be investigated thoroughly in Sect. 4, leading to a patient-centric design approach.

In case of consent, patients will receive the devices and will be introduced to them while still hospitalized. Three days after hospital discharge, a member of the scientific staff will visit patients at home to clarify questions of the patient and to ensure accurate data recording. We will call patients weekly for questionnaire-based interviews, e.g., EORTC QLQ-C30[2] and to verify device usage. Patients will be tracked over 12 weeks ending with a final interview about the device usage and their experiences.

System overview. Figure 1 sketches the technical system to be deployed in the study. The smart-phone provides sensor data (motion sensors) to monitor what patients are doing and how they are doing it as well as phone usage to monitor social activity. The armband, probably the Biovotion Everion, provides vital parameters, e.g., heart rate, stress from photoplethysmogram and galvanic skin response to monitor symptoms, e.g., pain, stress and anxiety.

4   Interviews with Palliative Patients and Resulting User Interface

Given the requirements outlined in Sect. 3, we now proceed with the patient-centric design of the patient interface and we define possible feedback channels.

---

[1] US National Comprehensive Cancer Network.

[2] EORTC: European Organization for Research and Treatment of Cancer, QLQ-C30: standardised questionnaire to measure quality of life of cancer patients.

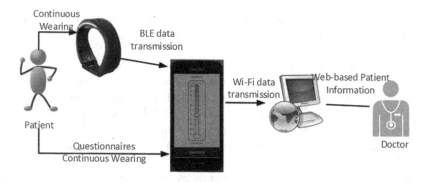

Fig. 1. System overview: body-worn, non-obtrusive sensors, regular encrypted data upload to a secured server, secured web interface for data analysis.

Since usability and convenience of the devices are crucial factors influencing the study, we involved potential users in our iterative system development. After receiving the ethical vote, we conducted qualitative interviews [19] in form of guided conversations. Furthermore, we showed patients different smart-phones of the Samsung Galaxy series and commercial armbands (Fitbit Charge HR and Angel Sensor, since Biovotion Everion was not available at that time) and let the patients choose between different design variants and control concepts. Finally, we asked them to use a prototype app on a Samsung Galaxy S5.

We present the observations in topical subsections together with our conclusions.

4.1 Characterization of Patients

We conducted interviews with 12 cancer patients between 49 and 80 years old (median: 63.5, standard deviation: 10.07). Table 1 shows descriptions of the patients. We encountered a broad spectrum of patients differing in many facets. Concerning the physiological aspects, the spectrum ranged from symptoms not observable by a non-expert to physiological burdens like tracheotomy. Concerning mental aspects, we encountered patients fully aware of their situations and patients blocking out that they are terminally ill. Also the mood of the patients varied strongly, from unhappy or depressed to happy and even euphoric.

4.2 Usability of the Smart-Phone App

- After a short introduction, all patients but one were able to use the smart-phone and to answer the questionnaire as shown in Fig. 2 autonomously – including patients who never used a smart-phone before (25% of the sample).
- Special needs came from co-morbidities or age (e.g., limited visual skills).
- Confirmatory gesture: All patients but one chose to have an extra confirmatory tap to save the questionnaire values. The confirmation dialogue was evaluated positively as providing reassurance and not as annoyance.

Table 1. List of interviewed patients; f=female, m=male

ID	Gender	Age	Interviewer's assessment
1	f	51	Autonomous and independent person; background in programming
2	f	71	Euphoric mood due to recovery from acute symptoms and aware about illness; technical background
3	f	80	Patient told off-topic stories, interview aborted after few questions about attitude toward smart-phones
4	m	68	Self-reported suffering from pain not noticeable during interview
5	m	72	Patient suffered from acute symptoms, interview aborted before talking about wristbands due to difficulties to speak
6	m	52	Very positive, optimistic despite progressive disease. Maybe blocking preoccupation with limited lifetime
7	m	50	Optimistic to recover; helpful despite critical towards research projects
8	m	68	Impressive entrepreneur with good profiling skills; handles his situation with humour in the outer world
9	m	63	Not that experienced with technology, but adventurous; hoping to have at least some years left despite divergent physician's guess
10	f	61	Values good quality and aesthetics – therefore critical; main symptoms: fatigue due to progressive disease, treatment and pain
11	m	49	Hopes for some years; very positive vibes despite of high symptom burden (weight loss of 25 kg, swollen belly, jaundice); interested to contribute to research
12	m	64	Fatigue due to disease and treatment

– Design: Patients of all ages preferred big numbers. The topic of smiley usage evoked emotional statements, e.g., *"I hate smileys."* (no. 8), *"I think smileys are sweet."* (no. 11). In our sample, all the patients who preferred smileys also preferred a colourful design of the distress thermometer and pain scale.

Conclusion: *Palliative care patients are willing and capable to use smartphones. Concerning the app design, we could not find any requirements constituted in the palliative situation. Based on the interviews, we finalized the design as illustrated in Fig. 2.*

4.3 Feedback Through the Smart-Phone App

– Eight out of 10 patients understood what is meant with feedback through the app.
– Three out of those 8 (no. 8, 11, 12) would be interested in feedback concerning their physical activity – but not more often than once a day. Those three patients already had experiences with fitness tracking apps.

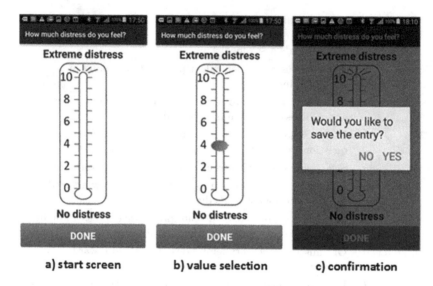

Fig. 2. Digital version of the NCCN distress thermometer: (a) graphical design is based on validated paper version of the NCCN Distress Thermometer [16], (b) value selection by tapping and sliding, (c) confirmation dialogue

- Depending on the patient, the feedback serves more for information and support and encouragement (no. 11, 12) or has an entertaining character (no. 8).

Conclusion: Most of the patients of our sample were not interested in direct feedback through the app – at least as long as it was not experienced before. However, feedback serves an informational, encouraging or entertaining purpose for some patients. Insensitive feedback could destabilize easily palliative patients since they carry already a high mental burden.

4.4   Motivation to Use a Monitoring System

- Nine out of 12 patients gave positive comments on the presented monitoring system, e.g., patient no. 2 said: *"I take the smart-phone always with me when I am leaving home. It gives me a more secure feeling, e.g., when driving alone. Such a system is useful, it makes me feel more safe."*
- Patients no. 7 and 10 were concerned about data security and privacy.
- Patients no. 10 and 12, suffering from fatigue (they are chronically exhausted) commented the task to take the phone with them the whole day long: *"I imagine it really cumbersome."*

Conclusion: In the sample, a positive attitude towards a monitoring system was dominant. Sceptical statements concerned mainly privacy issues. Comprehensibly, fatigue reduces the willingness to use the presented monitoring system. Important requirements towards the armband are easy to handle closing and charging mechanism and no user interaction in terms of buttons required.

4.5 Vulnerability and Sensitivity of Palliative Care Patients

– Not all patients are conscious about their health situation, e.g., patient no. 7 stated: *"I already survived cancer once and I am confident to recover again."* Thus, the monitoring system is not named as a system for palliative care, but as a system *for patients like you, when you leave hospital.*
– Interviewer and interviewees met for the first time. The exceptional situation of the patients and the chosen interview technique (guided conversation) yielded to a momentum in the relationship that required mindfulness and an open attitude and willingness to get involved in those relationships.
– Nevertheless, all patients with a severe cancer illness are in extreme and very demanding situations. Patient no. 10 stated: *"I would like to enjoy the time I have left and such stuff should not limit myself."*
– Some patients appreciated the opportunity to talk. When planning interviews with vulnerable user groups the aspect of "time to merely talk" should be taken into account (median of gross duration 62.5 min vs. 48 min net duration).

Conclusion: To equip palliative patients with tracking devices requires sensitivity. The goal of palliative care is to provide the best quality of life possible, not only with respect to medical, but also to psychosocial and spiritual needs. A monitoring system should not interfere with these profound human wants.

5 Conclusion and Outlook

In this work, we presented a monitoring system that was developed with early participation of vulnerable patients and that will be fully evaluated by means of an observational study. The interviews demonstrated the huge variety of the patient group. A first test with one patient delivered data and we were able to analyse the data manually. For trend detection, we need data of longer collection periods as will be provided by the main study. We will optimize the app with respect to battery consumption and memory needs by replacing the csv file based storage system through a binary file based system with buffered data queues reducing the file sizes and number of file accesses.

The next steps consist of patient recruitment and data collection. We will automate the data analysis using statistics and machine learning methods. Patients' experiences will be used to improve the monitoring system.

Based upon those results and the experiences gained through the observational study, we will develop a feedback strategy that respects the required sensitivity.

References

1. Stewart, B.W., Wild, C.P.: World Cancer Report 2014 (2014)
2. Urrea, B., Misra, S., Plante, T.B., et al.: Mobile health initiatives to improve outcomes in primary prevention of cardiovascular disease. Curr. Treat. Options Cardiovasc. Med. **17**(12), 1–12 (2015)

3. Grunerbl, A., Muaremi, A., Osmani, V., et al.: Smart-phone based recognition of states and state changes in bipolar disorder patients. IEEE J. Biomed. Health Inform. **19**(1), 140–148 (2014)
4. Saeb, S., Zhang, M., Karr, C.J., et al.: Mobile phone sensor correlates of depressive symptom severity in daily-life behavior: an exploratory study. J. Med. Internet Res. **17**(7), e175 (2015)
5. Seiter, J., Derungs, C., Schuster-Amft, C., et al.: Daily life activity routine discovery in hemiparetic rehabilitation patients using topic models. Methods Inf. Med. **54**, 248–255 (2015)
6. Muaremi, A., Arnrich, B., Tröster, G.: Towards measuring stress with smartphones and wearable devices during workday and sleep. Bionanoscience **3**(2), 172–183 (2013)
7. Lundström, S.: Is it reliable to use cellular phones for symptom assessment in palliative care? Report on a study in patients with advanced cancer. J. Palliat. Med. **12**(12), 1087 (2009)
8. Bhimaraj, A.: Remote monitoring of heart failure patients. Methodist Debakey Cardiovasc J. **9**(1), 26–31 (2013)
9. Incel, O.D., Kose, M., Ersoy, C.: A review and taxonomy of activity recognition on mobile phones. Bionanoscience **3**(2), 145–171 (2013)
10. Ben-Zeev, D., Wang, R., Abdullah, S., et al.: Mobile behavioral sensing for outpatients and inpatients with schizophrenia. Psychiatr. Serv. **67**(5), 558–561 (2016)
11. Abraham, W.T., Adamson, P.B., Bourge, R.C., et al.: Wireless pulmonary artery haemodynamic monitoring in chronic heart failure: a randomised controlled trial. Lancet **377**(9766), 658–666 (2011)
12. Allsop, M.J., Taylor, S., Mulvey, M.R., et al.: Information and communication technology for managing pain in palliative care: a review of the literature. BMJ Support. Palliat. Care **5**, 481–489 (2015)
13. Jaatun, E.A.A., Haugen, D.F., Dahl, Y., et al.: Designing a reliable pain drawing tool: avoiding interaction flaws by better tailoring to patients' impairments. Pers. Ubiquitous Comput. **19**(3–4), 635–648 (2015)
14. McCall, K., Keen, J., Farrer, K., et al.: Perceptions of the use of a remote monitoring system in patients receiving palliative care at home. Int. J. Palliat. Nurs. **14**(9), 426–431 (2008)
15. Oken, M.M., Creech, R.H., Tormey, D.C., et al.: Toxicity and response criteria of the Eastern Cooperative Oncology Group. Am. J. Clin. Oncol. **5**(6), 649–656 (1982)
16. Mehnert, A., Müller, D., Lehmann, C., et al.: The German version of the NCCN distress thermometer: validation of a screening instrument for assessment of psychosocial distress in cancer patients. Z. Psychiatr. Psychol. und Psychother. **54**(3), 213–223 (2006)
17. Peters, L., Sellick, K.: Quality of life of cancer patients receiving inpatient and home-based palliative care. J. Adv. Nurs. **53**(5), 524–533 (2006)
18. Cobb, M., Dowrick, C., Lloyd-Williams, M.: Understanding spirituality: a synoptic view. BMJ Support. Palliat. Care **2**(4), 339–343 (2012)
19. DiCicco-Bloom, B., Crabtree, B.F.: The qualitative research interview. Med. Educ. **40**(4), 314–321 (2006)

System for Fall Detection and Prediction

Fall Detection Using a Head-Worn Barometer

Guglielmo Cola[✉], Marco Avvenuti, Pierpaolo Piazza, and Alessio Vecchio

Dipartimento di Ingegneria dell'Informazione, University of Pisa,
Largo Lucio Lazzarino 1, 56122 Pisa, Italy
{guglielmo.cola,marco.avvenuti,alessio.vecchio}@iet.unipi.it

Abstract. Falls are a significant health and social problem for older adults and their relatives. In this paper we study the use of a barometer placed at the user's head (e.g., embedded in a pair of glasses) as a means to improve current wearable sensor-based fall detection methods. This approach proves useful to reliably detect falls even if the acceleration produced during the impact is relatively small. Prompt detection of a fall and/or an abnormal lying condition is key to minimize the negative effect on health.

Keywords: Accelerometer · Barometer · Fall detection · Head-worn device · Slow fall · Wearable sensor

1   Introduction and Related Work

A large fraction of older adults (about 30% at the age of 65+) are subject to a fall each year. Falls are one of the major causes of hospitalization and traumas at that age. Moreover, falls frequently represent the beginning of a sequence of physical and psychological problems for senior citizens. In fact, besides possible physical impairments, falls may bring reduced self-confidence and in some cases even depression [3]. The fear of falling again may also increase the chances of incurring in a more sedentary and less independent lifestyle. Notably, social and health problems caused by falls are going to increase because of our aging society.

Fall detection systems are aimed at automatically recognizing the occurrence of falls. Automatic detection is useful whenever the user who falls is subject to a loss of consciousness or a major trauma and he/she is thus unable to ask for help. In the context of fall detection, the term *long-lie* is typically used to refer to the condition of remaining on the floor for a prolonged time after a fall. It is also known that reducing the long-lie period has a positive impact on the outcomes of falls [12].

The majority of fall detection systems rely on wearable devices. In general, the worn device includes one or more sensors (usually accelerometers and gyroscopes) that can be used to recognize anomalous movements of the users [6,9,10]. In general, events characterized by values of acceleration above a given threshold are classified as falls. Some methods also include posture information to avoid raising false alarms [8].

© ICST Institute for Computer Sciences, Social Informatics and Telecommunications Engineering 2017
P. Perego et al. (Eds.): MobiHealth 2016, LNICST 192, pp. 217–224, 2017.
DOI: 10.1007/978-3-319-58877-3_29

More recently, a number of fall detection systems based on smartphones has been presented. Common smartphones include an accelerometer, a gyroscope, and a magnetic sensor to monitor the user's movements. In addition, smartphones are easily programmable and natively include a communication subsystem, which is mandatory for sending an alarm to the caregivers. The system presented in [1] extracts a set of features from acceleration-based information; then such features are provided as input to a classification module able to recognize not only falls, but also other activities of daily living (ADLs) such as walking, sitting, and lying.

Fall detection methods based on acceleration suffer from the problem of being unable to recognize "slow falls", which occur when the subject uses the hands to soften the impact or in case of a non-instantaneous loss of consciousness. In fact, such falls may be characterized by acceleration values that are generally smaller than the threshold used to discriminate falls from ADLs (note that the threshold cannot be lowered, to avoid an unbearable number of false alarms during normal activities).

In fall detection methods based on a wearable device, the latter is generally placed at the user's waist. The rationale for this choice is twofold: a waist-mounted device is in proximity of the center of mass of the user; waist is less subject to spurious movements with respect to other parts of the body (e.g., arms). Nevertheless, we believe that studying the use of head-worn devices deserves more attention with respect to existing literature. Practically, the hardware needed for detecting falls could be embedded in headwear, glasses, or an ear-worn device[1]. This would free the user from wearing an additional device in case he/she is already using one of these accessories.

The work presented in this paper contributes to existing literature as follows: (i) for the first time the use of a head-worn barometer is proposed and studied in the context of fall detection, as a means to improve detection accuracy even in the case of slow falls; (ii) changes in pressure detected by the barometer are used not only for detecting falls, but also other simple postures (standing and sitting); this is achieved combining the output of the barometer with acceleration information.

2   Method

The main idea behind the proposed method is to combine accelerometric and barometric information to improve the reliability of a fall detection system, even when the fall produces relatively small accelerations (*slow fall* hereafter). In particular, the barometer is used to measure the pressure variation associated to a particular user's movement, the latter being detected with the accelerometer. The pressure variation is caused by the vertical displacement experienced by the sensor, for example when the user sits or falls down. Such pressure variation can be used to discriminate whether the movement led to a safe postural change

---

[1] For example, an ear-worn device embedding an accelerometer has been used for detecting anomalies in gait [4].

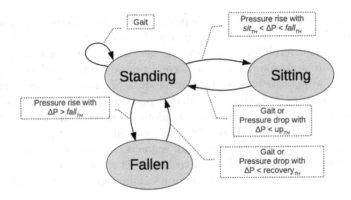

Fig. 1. State diagram representation of the proposed method.

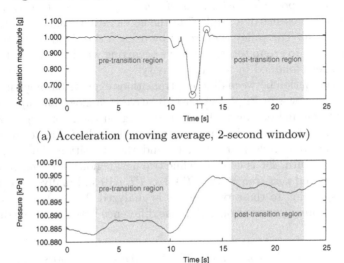

(a) Acceleration (moving average, 2-second window)

(b) Barometric pressure (moving average, 2-second window)

Fig. 2. Slow fall example, finding pre and post-transition regions. (Color figure online)

(such as sitting down on a chair), or to a potentially dangerous situation like being lying on the floor. The proposed technique assumes that the barometer has been placed near to the user's head. As previously mentioned, this position can be conveniently used if the sensor is embedded in headwear, glasses, or a hearing aid device. An additional motivation is represented by the fact that the user's head experiences the highest vertical displacement (and thus the highest pressure variation) during a fall.

The way we aim to combine acceleration and barometric pressure is described in Fig. 1, using a finite state machine (FSM) representation. Each state in the FSM represents a particular *posture*. For the sake of simplicity, in this study we considered only three possible postures: *standing*, *sitting*, and *fallen*.

Fallen actually means that the user is lying on the floor, whatever the acceleration that produced the transition to such posture. In the typical context of fall detection (an older adult living alone), the fact that the user's head is close to ground level can be reasonably used as a condition to trigger an alarm, especially if such condition persists for a significant amount of time (e.g., one minute).

When the system is started, the current posture is unknown and fall detection is based on accelerometric analysis alone. However, the FSM enters the *standing* state as soon as a short interval of walking activity (gait) is detected (e.g., six consecutive steps). To detect gait segments, the acceleration-based technique described in [8] was used. Such technique is sufficiently *lightweight* to be implemented and executed in real time on a miniaturized device with limited resources [7].

After the standing posture has been detected, the system starts to monitor acceleration for a possible *posture transition*. A possible posture transition is triggered by the presence of a "valley" in the acceleration magnitude (Euclidean norm) signal [1,5]. The valley is detected by using a threshold ($valley_{TH}$), with an additional test to group together valleys occurring within a short interval and to discard valleys followed by walking activity.

The discrimination between different transitions exploits barometric analysis. An example is shown in Fig. 2, which is relative to a slow fall happened from standing position and ending with the user lying on the floor. Figure 2a shows the acceleration signal, which is used to detect the valley. The local minimum and maximum (red circles) are used to find the transition time TT (dotted vertical line). In turn, TT is used to define two new regions: *pre-transition* $[TT - 10\ s, TT - 3\ s]$ and *post-transition* $[TT + 3\ s, TT + 10\ s]$. Finally, the barometric signal corresponding to these two regions is analyzed (Fig. 2b). More precisely, it is found the pressure variation ΔP as the difference between the median value in each region:

$$\Delta P = median(\text{post-transition}) - median(\text{pre-transition}).$$

A positive ΔP like in Fig. 2b, clearly indicates that the user's head has moved towards the ground. Conversely, when pressure drops the user is moving the head upward, for example because of standing up from sitting position.

Posture transitions are recognized by comparing ΔP against a set of thresholds. When the user is standing, a positive ΔP leads to the *sitting* state if the pressure variation is within sit_{TH} and $fall_{TH}$. Instead, the FSM moves to the *fallen* state state if ΔP is higher than $fall_{TH}$. The rationale is that the pressure variation is higher when the user falls to the ground, with respect to sitting on a chair. Pressure variation is also exploited to promptly detect recovery from fall, by comparing a negative ΔP (*pressure drop*) against a negative threshold ($\Delta P < recovery_{TH}$). Recovery is also detected if the user walks.

Besides activity recognition purposes, the recognition of the *sitting* state represents a useful information even for fall detection. In particular, while sitting down the user is closer to the ground with respect to the standing posture, and the system may produce false negatives (i.e., falls that are not detected) if a

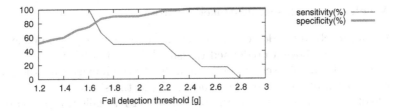

Fig. 3. Sensitivity and specificity when varying the acceleration threshold.

pressure variation above $fall_{TH}$ is required to detect a fall from a chair. As a solution, the system may temporarily disable the use of barometric pressure for fall detection while the user is sitting. Transition from sitting to *standing* is recognized either by pressure analysis ($\Delta P < up_{TH}$) or by detecting gait.

3   Experimental Setting

We used a Shimmer 3 device, equipped with a TI MSP430 MCU, an ST Micro LSM303DLHC accelerometer, and a Bosch BMP180 pressure sensor [11]. The accelerometer was set to operate within ± 8 g range. The barometer was operated in ultra-high resolution mode (0.03 hPa RMS noise). Acceleration and pressure were sampled with ~ 50 Hz frequency and stored on the persistent storage of the device. To reduce noise, both acceleration and pressure were low-pass filtered using a moving average with a 2-second window. The Shimmer 3 was attached on a pair of common glasses, in proximity of the user's temple.

Six volunteers agreed to participate to a supervised experiment. The experiment consisted in a predefined sequence of transitions between the postures to be recognized by the proposed method. More precisely, each volunteer performed the following actions: (a) walk for about 30 s; (b) sit down on a chair; (c) stand up; (d) short walk; (e) sit down on a different chair; (f) stand up; (g) walk for about 20 s; (h) lie down on the floor (slow fall); (i) stand up. Volunteers remained in each posture (standing, sitting, fallen) for at least 10 s. Experiments were recorded with a video camera in order to facilitate manual labeling of posture transitions.

4   Results and Discussion

In this section the performance achieved by the proposed method is presented and discussed. The evaluation starts by describing the results achieved by a system based on a simple accelerometric threshold, in order to highlight the contribution introduced by the combined use of acceleration and barometric pressure.

4.1   Acceleration Threshold-Based System

A typical approach to fall detection consists in searching for peaks in the acceleration magnitude above a predefined threshold. Indeed, a fall produces one or more sharp peaks in the acceleration signal, due to the impact with the ground of different parts of the body. The choice of the threshold is determined by the trade-off between *sensitivity* (the proportion of real falls that are correctly detected) and *specificity* (the proportion of normal activities that are correctly ignored by the fall detection system). If the threshold is too high, there is a risk of missing real falls (low sensitivity). On the other hand, if the threshold is too low, the system is likely to produce frequent false alarms throughout the day (low specificity) [2]. Threshold values used in the literature ranged from 2 to 3 g.

In our experiment, for each volunteer, there is one *positive* (a slow fall from standing position), and some normal activities that can lead to false positives (walking, standing, sitting). Each of these activities can be considered as a *negative* instance, which can be used to find the specificity (proportion of negatives that are correctly ignored). In total there are 11 negative instances per user (6 walking intervals, 2 sitting transitions, 3 standing transitions). We applied different threshold values to verify the performance in terms of sensitivity and specificity. The average result is shown in Fig. 3. It is clearly visible that the detection of slow falls by means of a simple accelerometric threshold would lead to an unbearable number of false alarms during normal activities. For example, the highest threshold that would allow the detection of all the falls is 1.6 g – such threshold leads to a specificity as low as 75%, meaning that about 3 false alarms per user were produced during our experiment.

4.2   Proposed Method Results and Future Work

The first step of the proposed method consists in finding possible *transitions*, which are identified by the presence of a valley in the acceleration magnitude. We verified that all the effective transitions were detected by the system. In addition to real transitions, the system occasionally detected valleys produced during walking activity. However, such transitions were filtered out by means of walking detection (a possible transition is discarded if it occurs during walking activity).

After a transition is found, the system finds the ΔP value in order to determine the transition type. Table 1 shows per-user and average results in terms of the ΔP measured during a specific posture transition. More specifically, for each user it is shown his/her height, and the average ΔP measured while sitting down, standing up (from sitting), falling down, and standing up after a fall. The measured ΔP is not always consistent with the effective vertical displacement (e.g., for user 6 there is a significant difference, in terms of absolute ΔP, between sitting down and standing up from a chair). However, for the purpose of this study, the most important result is that for all the users there is a measurable difference between sitting and falling, in terms of ΔP. In the worst case (user 5),

Table 1. ΔP [Pa] measured for each posture transition – per-user and average results.

User ID	height [m]	stand → sit [Pa]	sit → stand [Pa]	stand → fall [Pa]	fall → stand [Pa]
1	1.63	3.1	−5.8	14.3	−16.3
2	1.75	3.4	−3.8	15.5	−12.1
3	1.90	6.7	−5.1	18.6	−18.4
4	1.73	3.5	−4.2	12.1	−15.9
5	1.90	9.0	−8.6	15.9	−16.0
6	1.75	3.9	−6.7	17.1	−18.9
Average	1.78	4.9	−5.7	15.6	−16.3

the "gap" between falling and sitting was 6.9 Pa (ΔP=15.9 Pa after falling, and ΔP=9.0 Pa after sitting).

The thresholds required to discriminate different transitions were set using a leave-one-user-out cross-validation strategy and taking into account users' height. The cross-validation procedure consists in leaving one user out for validation, while other users' results are used to find the thresholds. In particular, we used the average pressure variation per meter of height displacement to estimate all of the other thresholds. For example, the threshold used to detect a fall ($fall_{TH}$) was set – with a conservative approach – to 70% of the expected pressure variation. The result of cross-validation was that all the transitions (posture changes) were recognized correctly. Therefore, the system was able to detect the slow falls without producing false alarms (100% sensitivity and specificity). This promising result confirms that barometric information can successfully enhance an acceleration-based fall detection system, enabling the detection of slow falls while keeping a low false positive rate.

Future work will address some scenarios that have not been considered in this preliminary study. For example, it will be evaluated whether the same approach could be used to reliably distinguish lying on a bed from lying/falling on the floor. Another interesting scenario is the possible presence of stairs. Walking down a flight of stairs produces a pressure rise that may lead to a false alarm when the user stops walking. However, acceleration and pressure information could be used to detect walking on stairs and temporarily disable the use of pressure for fall detection purposes. The use of pressure is then re-enabled as soon as the user walks on level ground. In future research, we will also investigate if pressure variation thresholds can be tuned automatically to the user, by using a semi-supervised training phase based on just normal activities. Different thresholding methods will be considered, including the use of estimated vertical displacement derived from pressure variation. Finally, it will be evaluated the use of a barometer embedded in a wrist-worn device.

5   Conclusions

A barometer, embedded in headwear, glasses, or an ear-worn device, can be successfully used to detect posture transitions and improve the reliability of a

fall detection system. Whenever a possible transition is detected by acceleration analysis, the event can be safely classified as a non-fall in case the pressure variation observed by the barometer is not compatible with a fall. The
barometer could be particularly helpful in recognizing slow falls, which are frequently undetected in acceleration-based methods. Future work will concern a
long-term experimentation with a larger number of subjects and in uncontrolled
environment.

Acknowledgements. This research was supported by the PRA 2016 project "Analysis of sensory data: from traditional sensors to social sensors", funded by the University
of Pisa.

References

1. Abbate, S., Avvenuti, M., Bonatesta, F., Cola, G., Corsini, P., Vecchio, A.: A
   smartphone-based fall detection system. Pervasive Mob. Comput. **8**(6), 883–899
   (2012)
2. Abbate, S., Avvenuti, M., Cola, G., Corsini, P., Light, J.V., Vecchio, A.: Recognition of false alarms in fall detection systems. In: Proceedings of the IEEE Consumer
   Communications and Networking Conference (Workshops), Las Vegas, NV, USA,
   pp. 538–543, January 2011
3. World Health Organization. WHO Global Report on Falls Prevention in Older
   Age. World Health Organization (2007)
4. Atallah, L., Aziz, O., Lo, B., Yang, G.Z.: Detecting walking gait impairment with
   an ear-worn sensor. In: Proceedings of the Sixth International Workshop on Wearable and Implantable Body Sensor Networks, pp. 175–180, June 2009
5. Bieber, G., Koldrack, P., Sablowski, C., Peter, C., Urban, B.: Mobile physical activity recognition of stand-up and sit-down transitions for user behavior analysis. In:
   Proceedings of the 3rd International Conference on Pervasive Technologies Related
   to Assistive Environments. ACM (2010)
6. Bourke, A., O'Brien, J., Lyons, G.: Evaluation of a threshold-based tri-axial
   accelerometer fall detection algorithm. Gait Posture **26**(2), 194–199 (2007)
7. Cola, G., Avvenuti, M., Vecchio, A., Yang, G.Z., Lo, B.: An on-node processing
   approach for anomaly detection in gait. IEEE Sens. J. **15**(11), 6640–6649 (2015)
8. Cola, G., Vecchio, A., Avvenuti, M.: Improving the performance of fall detection
   systems through walk recognition. J. Ambient Intell. Humanized Comput. **5**(6),
   843–855 (2014)
9. Kangas, M., Konttila, A., Lindgren, P., Winblad, I., Jms, T.: Comparison of low-
   complexity fall detection algorithms for body attached accelerometers. Gait Posture **28**(2), 285–291 (2008)
10. Li, Q., Stankovic, J.A., Hanson, M.A., Barth, A.T., Lach, J., Zhou, G.: Accurate,
    fast fall detection using gyroscopes and accelerometer-derived posture information.
    In: Proceedings of the International Workshop on Wearable and Implantable Body
    Sensor Networks, pp. 138–143, June 2009
11. Shimmer (2016). http://www.shimmersensing.com
12. Tinetti, M., Liu, W., Claus, E.: Predictors and prognosis of inability to get up after
    falls among elderly persons. JAMA **269**(1), 65–70 (1993)

Investigation of Sensor Placement for Accurate Fall Detection

Periklis Ntanasis[1(✉)], Evangelia Pippa[1], Ahmet Turan Özdemir[2], Billur Barshan[3], and Vasileios Megalooikonomou[1]

[1] Department of Computer Engineering and Informatics, University of Patras, Rion, Patras, Greece
{ntanasis,pippa,vasilis}@ceid.upatras.gr
[2] Department of Electrical and Electronics Engineering, Erciyes University, Melikgazi, 38039 Kayseri, Turkey
aturan@erciyes.edu.tr
[3] Department of Electrical and Electronics Engineering, Bilkent University, Bilkent, 06800 Ankara, Turkey
billur@ee.bilkent.edu.tr

Abstract. Fall detection is typically based on temporal and spectral analysis of multi-dimensional signals acquired from wearable sensors such as tri-axial accelerometers and gyroscopes which are attached at several parts of the human body. Our aim is to investigate the location where such wearable sensors should be placed in order to optimize the discrimination of falls from other Activities of Daily Living (ADLs). To this end, we perform feature extraction and classification based on data acquired from a single sensor unit placed on a specific body part each time. The investigated sensor locations include the head, chest, waist, wrist, thigh and ankle. Evaluation of several classification algorithms reveals the waist and the thigh as the optimal locations.

Keywords: Fall detection · Fall classification · Wearable sensors · Sensor placement · Machine learning · Classification · Accelerometers · Gyroscopes

1 Introduction

Falls are a common cause of injury among elderly people. According to the World Health Organization, 28–35% of people aged 65 and over fall at least once a year with serious consequences such as heavy injuries and even death. Additionally, the moments after a fall are very critical. Many people experience what is called the "long lie," a long period of immobility after a fall that can have serious complications in a person's health. Unless precautions are taken, the number of injuries and the costs associated with fall-related trauma will double in the near future [1]. Fall detection is therefore considered an extremely important aspect of healthcare.

The most challenging aspect of fall detection is the distinction between falls and Activities of Daily Living (ADLs) such as sitting, standing and walking since falls typically occur while performing daily activities. In particular, ADLs with high acceleration

© ICST Institute for Computer Sciences, Social Informatics and Telecommunications Engineering 2017
P. Perego et al. (Eds.): MobiHealth 2016, LNICST 192, pp. 225–232, 2017.
DOI: 10.1007/978-3-319-58877-3_30

are often confused with falls. Misinterpreting a fall as an ADL can have serious effects on the subject's health [2]. Therefore, a fall detection system should be able to accurately and immediately distinguish falls from ADLs when they occur. This requires falls to be automatically detected in real time. Another challenge is to make the system as simple as possible, with low false-alarm rates. Subjects using the system should feel comfortable and their quality of everyday life should not be affected. Accurate, reliable and real time fall detection systems are therefore essential.

Significant research has been conducted in this field and various fall detection systems have been proposed in the recent years. Noury et al. [3] and Yu et al. [4] have investigated the principles of fall detection and reviewed early works on the subject. Fall detection approaches can be divided into two main categories: vision-based and wearable device (motion sensor)-based systems.

Several context aware systems that use devices such as cameras or infrared sensors to detect falls within an environment have been developed. Rougier et al. [5] used human shape deformation to track the person's silhouette in recordings taken from four cameras. Falls and ADLs were classified with 98% accuracy. In [6], a human 3D bounding box was created and the Kinect infrared sensor was used to accurately detect falls without any prior knowledge of the environment. Olivieri et al. [7] used motion templates taken from a camera to recognize certain ADLs and detect falls, achieving 99% recognition rate. However, these approaches have certain limitations; the system can only monitor activities within the environment and thus, outdoor activities are excluded, restricting the mobility of the user. Also, other people moving within the same environment might also confuse the system and trigger false alarms in some cases.

The use of wearable motion sensors has been preferred by many researchers. With the advances in micro electro-mechanical systems (MEMS) technology, sensors such as accelerometers, gyroscopes and magnetometers have been integrated within small motion sensor units. The units that contain the above sensors can be used to collect movement data and detect falls. They are compact, light, inexpensive and have low power consumption. They can be placed in the subject's pockets or be easily attached at different body parts without making the subject uncomfortable; thus, they make the analysis of outdoor activities possible. Different body parts have been proposed for the sensor placement that improve the accuracy with minimum intrusion to the subject's everyday life. Yang and Hsu [8] have examined the fundamentals of such sensors as well as the optimal position on the human body for sensor placement.

In fall detection studies, typically simple thresholding is used. A fall is detected when the acceleration suddenly increases due to the change in orientation from upright to lying position [9]. In [10], the results of certain threshold-based methods that consider fall impact, velocity and posture have been assessed and tested on elderly subjects, achieving 94.6% sensitivity. Thresholding methods sometimes tend to miss "soft falls," meaning falls that might not exceed the threshold. Also, certain ADLs with high acceleration may exceed the threshold and be misclassified as falls.

The main classification problem is to distinguish falls from ADLs. Machine learning techniques have been used to achieve more reliable results. Every recorded movement in the fall and activity database [11] has its own pattern. By extracting features from the raw data, these patterns can be classified by different classification methods. Before raw data are given to different classifiers, they must be pre-processed using a windowing technique. Such a technique divides the sensor signal into smaller time segments (i.e., windows) and a classification algorithm is applied separately to each window, producing a classification result. After pre-processing, features from the time or spatial domain are extracted to feed trained classifiers such as artificial neural (ANN) or Bayesian networks (BN), support vector machines (SVMs), decision trees, k-nearest neighbors (k-NN), etc. Kerdegari et al. [12] used statistical features such as maximum, minimum, mean, range, variance and standard deviation extracted from a waist-worn tri-axial accelerometer to investigate the performance of various classifiers on fall detection. The multilayer perceptron yielded the best sensitivity (90.15%). Özdemir and Barshan [11] added auto-correlation coefficients and discrete Fourier transform (DFT) coefficients extracted from data acquired by sensors placed at different body parts. Six classifiers (k-NN, SVM, ANN, least-squares method, Bayesian decision making, dynamic time warping) were used to assign a fall or ADL class label to the feature vectors concatenated from all sensors. All methods achieved higher than 97.47% and 93.44% sensitivity and specificity, respectively. Yuwono et al. [13] obtained data from a single waist-worn tri-axial accelerometer and extracted features using the Particle Swarm Optimization (PSO) clustering method. Then, they proceeded to classify the data, achieving above 98.6% sensitivity in detecting falls.

Earlier studies report conflicting results on the best location to carry a single fall detection device on the human body. Some studies report that the waist is the best place since it is close to the body's center of gravity [10, 14], while some claim that the chest or the head is better [9, 15–17]. Several studies consistently agree that the arms and the legs are not suitable parts of the body to carry a fall detection device since they are usually associated with higher accelerations [16, 18]. Resolving this issue through experiments that follow standardized procedures will be a valuable contribution. Özdemir and Barshan [11] acquired data from sensors placed on six body parts including the head, chest, waist, wrist, thigh and ankle. In order to proceed with classification, the features extracted from each location are concatenated to a single feature vector leading to a high-dimensional feature space. However, fall detection often needs to be performed in real time which requires lighter processing that can be achieved either through dimensionality reduction or selection of a single sensor unit located at the optimal position.

In this work, we attempt to determine the optimal location for the sensor placement on the human body. To achieve this, we evaluate the activity and fall dataset acquired by Özdemir and Barshan [11] with respect to several classification algorithms using only the data acquired from a single sensor location each time. The classification performance in terms of accuracy is used as the criterion to reveal the optimal sensor location. Since data from a single sensor unit are used, there is no need for dimensionality reduction, making the proposed methodology computationally efficient and thus, more capable of real-time fall detection.

The rest of the paper is organized as follows. In Sect. 2, we provide details on the dataset and the classification methodology. In Sect. 3, we present and discuss the achieved results. Finally, Sect. 4 concludes this work.

2   Materials and Methods

2.1   Dataset

With Erciyes University Ethics Committee approval, seven males (24 $\pm$ 3 years old, 67.5 $\pm$ 13.5 kg, 172 $\pm$ 12 cm) and seven females (21.5 $\pm$ 2.5 years old, 58.5 $\pm$ 11.5 kg, 169.5 $\pm$ 12.5 cm) healthy volunteers participated in the study with informed written consent. We tightly fitted six wireless sensor units with special strap sets to the subjects' heads, chests, waists, right wrists, right thighs, and right ankles. Each unit comprises three tri-axial devices (accelerometer, gyroscope, and magnetometer/compass) with respective ranges of $\pm$120 m/s^2, $\pm$1200°/s, and $\pm$1.5 Gs, and an atmospheric pressure meter with 300–1100 hPa operating range, which we did not use. We recorded raw motion data along three perpendicular axes (x, y, z) from each unit with a sampling frequency of 25 Hz [11]. A set of trials consists of 20 fall actions (front-lying, front-protection-lying, front-knees, front-knees-lying, front-right, front-left, front-quick-recovery, front-slow-recovery, back-sitting, back-lying, back-right, back-left, right-sideway, right-recovery, left-sideway, left-recovery, syncope, syncope-wall, podium, rolling-out-bed) and 16 ADLs (lying-bed, rising-bed, sit-bed, sit-chair, sit-sofa, sit-air, walking-forward, jogging, walking-backward, bending, bending-pick-up, stumble, limp, squatting-down, trip-over, coughing-sneezing). We adopted these from [19] and each lasted about 15 s on the average. The 14 volunteers repeated each test for five times. Thus, we acquired a considerably diverse dataset comprising 1400 falls (20 tasks × 14 volunteers × 5 trials) and 1120 ADLs (16 tasks × 14 volunteers × 5 trials), resulting in 2520 trials. Many of the non-fall actions included in the dataset are high-impact events that may be easily confused with falls.

2.2   Feature Extraction

Before we train the classifiers, we need to identify and isolate the actual experimental events since raw data acquired from the sensors include several time points that correspond to immobility before and after the detected fall event. In order to identify the fall event, we detect the peak of the total acceleration vector. Total acceleration is defined as:

$$A_T = \sqrt{A_x^2 + A_y^2 + A_z^2} \tag{1}$$

where A_x, A_y and A_z are the accelerations along the x, y and z axis, respectively.

In contrast to [11] which considers the waist accelerometer as reference, we measure the total acceleration on each sensor unit separately. For each sensor type on the same unit, we keep two seconds of the sequence before and after the peak acceleration, that is, 50 values before and after the peak given the sampling frequency of 25 Hz. Therefore, for each test, we obtain six arrays of size 9 × 101, one for each of the six sensor units.

We parameterize each one of the nine measured events using the features proposed in [11]: minimum, maximum and mean values, skewness, kurtosis, the first 11 values of the autocorrelation sequence and the first five frequencies with maximum magnitude of the DFT along with the five corresponding amplitudes, resulting in a feature vector of dimensionality 234 (26 features for each one of the nine measured signals) for each test.

2.3 Classification

We evaluate the ability of the above features to discriminate between falls and ADLs using several classification algorithms implemented by the WEKA machine learning toolkit [20] including J48 decision tree, k-nearest neighbors algorithm with value of k = 7 (IBk) [21], Random Forest (RF) [22, 23], Random Committee (RC) and SVM [24] with RBF Kernel (SMO). The classifiers in our study are selected in an attempt to evaluate representative algorithms for each one of the main categories of machine learning classifiers including decision trees (J48), support vector machines (SMO), ensemble classifiers (RF, RC) but also simple methods such as k-NN (IBk).

3   Results

We evaluated binary classification performance using accuracy, sensitivity and specificity. Evaluation was performed in a 10-fold cross validation setting.

Table 1 shows the achieved results in terms of accuracy, sensitivity and specificity for each sensor location for the J48, IBk, RC, RF and SMO algorithms, respectively. The position resulting in the best accuracy is highlighted in boldface fonts in the table. Figure 1 shows a comparative diagram across different body locations for each classifiers.

We achieve the overall highest accuracy (99.48%) for the thigh sensor location using the SMO classifier. For this case, the obtained sensitivity, that is, the fraction of actual falls which are correctly identified as such is 99.21% and the specificity, that is, the proportion of ADLs that were correctly classified as such is 99.82%. It seems that thigh-attached sensors can significantly reflect gait-related features during the performance of falls and ADLs, making their discrimination more accurate. The waist sensor location follows by achieving the highest accuracy values for the RF (99.28%), RC (98.89%) and k-NN, IBk (98.61%) classifiers. These results agree with our intuition for the superiority of the waist location based on the fact that it is near the body's center of gravity. Finally, for the J48 classifier, the most accurate sensor location is the thigh, reaching 98.24% accuracy.

To summarize, the waist and thigh sensors achieve the highest accuracies for all classifiers, followed by the chest and ankle sensors. The wrist sensor is the one with the lowest accuracy for all classifiers, followed by the head. It is noteworthy, however, that all sensors achieve accuracies higher than 90% and there are cases where the differences among the sensors are not significant, especially when comparing the most accurate sensor locations such as the thigh and the waist.

Table 1. Evaluation of the classifiers considered in this study

Classifier	Sensors	Accuracy (%)	Sensitivity (%)	Specificity (%)
(a) J48	Head	96.48	91.06	95.76
	Chest	97.53	97.70	97.31
	Waist	97.96	97.99	97.94
	Wrist	93.71	94.78	92.37
	Thigh	**98.24**	98.71	97.67
	Ankle	97.45	97.49	97.40
(b) IBk	Head	93.70	92.84	94.77
	Chest	97.45	97.28	97.67
	Waist	**98.61**	98.85	98.30
	Wrist	89.74	84.13	96.77
	Thigh	96.42	94.20	99.19
	Ankle	95.58	93.34	98.39
(c) RC	Head	97.17	98.57	95.41
	Chest	98.61	99.07	98.03
	Waist	**98.89**	99.28	98.39
	Wrist	94.63	96.35	92.47
	Thigh	98.77	99.00	98.48
	Ankle	98.77	98.85	98.66
(d) RF	Head	96.77	99.36	93.51
	Chest	98.61	99.28	97.76
	Waist	**99.28**	99.64	98.84
	Wrist	95.62	98.28	92.29
	Thigh	99.20	99.43	98.93
	Ankle	98.77	99.07	98.39
(e) SMO	Head	97.29	97.92	96.49
	Chest	98.89	99.28	98.39
	Waist	99.36	99.50	99.19
	Wrist	96.78	97.71	95.61
	Thigh	**99.48**	99.21	99.82
	Ankle	98.57	98.85	98.21

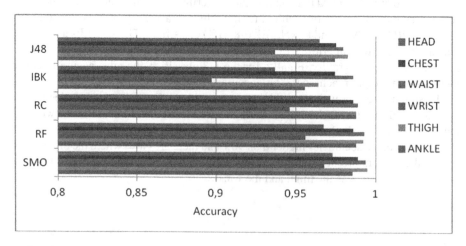

Fig. 1. Bar graph showing the accuracy of the classifiers considered for each sensor unit.

4   Conclusion

In this paper, we investigated optimal sensor placement location for accurate fall detection based on feature extraction and classification. Evaluation of several classifiers reveals the superiority of thigh and waist locations. However, the differences on sensitivity and accuracy among the different sensor locations are relatively low and sometimes negligible, especially for the best performing waist and thigh sensors. Finally, since our method proposes the utilization of a single sensor unit, it keeps the feature vector dimensionality rather low, providing the means for real-time fall detection, even when using mobile devices with limited computational capabilities. In future work, a cross analysis can be conducted using actigraphy, to monitor daily activities and to detect and classify falls.

Acknowledgements. This work was supported by the FrailSafe project funded from the European Union's Horizon 2020 research and innovation programme under grant agreement No. 690140. The paper reflects only the view of the authors and the Commission is not responsible for any use that may be made of the information it contains.

References

1. World Health Organization: Global report on falls prevention in older age. http://www.who.int/ageing/publications/Falls_prevention7March.pdf
2. Gurley, R.J., Lum, N., Sande, M., Lo, B., Katz, M.H.: Persons found in their homes helpless or dead. N. Engl. J. Med. **334**, 1710–1716 (1996)
3. Noury, N., Fleury, A., Rumeau, P., Bourke, A.K., Laighin, G.O., Rialle, V., Lundy, J.E.: Fall detection—principles and methods. In: Proceedings of the 29th Annual International Conference of the IEEE Engineering in Medicine and Biology, Lyon, France, pp. 1663–1666 (2007)
4. Yu, X.: Approaches and principles of fall detection for elderly and patient. In: 10th International Conference on e-health Networking, Applications and Services, HealthCom, Singapore, pp. 42–47 (2008)
5. Rougier, C., Meunier, J., St-Arnaud, A., Rousseau, J.: Robust video surveillance for fall detection based on human shape deformation. IEEE Trans. Circuits Syst. Video Technol. **21**, 611–622 (2011)
6. Mastorakis, G., Makris, D.: Fall detection system using Kinect's infrared sensor. J. Real-Time Image Proc. **9**, 635–646 (2012)
7. Olivieri, D.N., Conde, I.G., Sobrino, X.A.V.: Eigenspace-based fall detection and activity recognition from motion templates and machine learning. Expert Syst. Appl. **39**, 5935–5945 (2012)
8. Yang, C., Hsu, Y.: A review of accelerometry-based wearable motion detectors for physical activity monitoring. Sensors **10**, 7772–7788 (2010)
9. Bourke, A.K., O'Brien, J.V., Lyons, G.M.: Evaluation of a threshold-based tri-axial accelerometer fall detection algorithm. Gait Posture **26**, 194–199 (2007)

10. Bourke, A.K., van de Ven, P., Gamble, M., O'Connor, R., Murphy, K., Bogan, E., McQuade, E., Finucane, P., Laighin, G., Nelson, J.: Assessment of waist-worn tri-axial accelerometer based fall-detection algorithms using continuous unsupervised activities. In: Annual International Conference of the IEEE Engineering in Medicine and Biology, Buenos Aires, Argentina, pp. 2782–2785 (2010)
11. Özdemir, A.T., Barshan, B.: Detecting falls with wearable sensors using machine learning techniques. Sensors **14**, 10691–10708 (2014)
12. Kerdegari, H., Samsudin, K., Ramli, A.R., Mokaram, S.: Evaluation of fall detection classification approaches. In: 4th International Conference on Intelligent and Advanced Systems (ICIAS), Kuala Lumpur, Malaysia, pp. 131–136 (2012)
13. Yuwono, M., Moulton, B.D., Su, S.W., Celler, B.G., Nguyen, H.T.: Unsupervised machine-learning method for improving the performance of ambulatory fall detection systems. Biomed. Eng. Online **11**, 1–11 (2012)
14. Özdemir, A.T.: An analysis on sensor locations of the human body for wearable fall detection devices: principles and practice. Sensors **16**, 1161 (2016)
15. Kangas, M., Konttila, A., Lindgren, P., Winblad, I., Jamsa, T.: Comparison of low-complexity fall detection algorithms for body attached accelerometers. Gait Posture **28**, 285–291 (2008)
16. Kangas M., Konttila A., Winblad I., Jamsa T.: Determination of simple thresholds for accelerometry-based parameters for fall detection. In: 29th Annual International Conference of the IEEE Engineering in Medicine and Biology Society, Lyon, France, pp. 1367–1370 (2007)
17. Bourke, A.K., Lyons, G.M.: A threshold-based fall-detection algorithm using a bi-axial gyroscope sensor. Med. Eng. Phys. **30**, 84–90 (2008)
18. Bianchi, F., Redmond, S.J., Narayanan, M.R., Cerutti, S., Lovell, N.H.: Barometric pressure and triaxial accelerometry-based falls event detection. IEEE Trans. Neural Syst. Rehabil. Eng. **18**, 619–627 (2010)
19. Abbate, S., Avvenuti, M., Corsini, P., Vecchio, A., Light, J.: Monitoring of human movements for fall detection and activities recognition in elderly care using wireless sensor network: a survey. In: Merret, G.V., Tan, Y.K. (eds.) Wireless Sensor Networks: Application-Centric Design, pp. 147–166. InTech, Rijeka (2010). Chapter 9
20. Hall, M., Frank, E., Holmes, G., Pfahringer, B., Reutemann, P., Witten, I.H.: The WEKA data mining software: An update. SIGKDD Explor. Newsl. **11**, 10–18 (2009)
21. Aha, D.W., Kibbler, D., Albert, M.K.: Instance-based learning algorithms. Mach. Learn. **6**, 37–66 (1991)
22. Liaw, A., Wiener, M.: Classification and regression by randomForest. R news **2**, 18–22 (2002)
23. Breiman, L.: Random forests. Mach. Learn. **45**, 5–32 (2001)
24. Keerthi, S.S., Shevade, S.K., Bhattacharyya, C., Murthy, K.R.K.: Improvements to Platt's SMO algorithm for SVM classifier design. Neural Comput. **13**, 637–649 (2001)

Fall Detection with Orientation Calibration Using a Single Motion Sensor

Shuo Yu[✉] and Hsinchun Chen

Department of Management Information Systems, University of Arizona, Tucson, AZ, USA
shuoyu@email.arizona.edu, hchen@eller.arizona.edu

Abstract. Falls are a major threat for senior citizens living independently. Sensor technologies and fall detection algorithms have emerged as a reliable, low-cost solution for this issue. We proposed a sensor orientation calibration algorithm to better address the uncertainty issue faced by fall detection algorithms in real world applications. We conducted controlled experiments of simulated fall events and non-fall activities on student subjects. We evaluated our proposed algorithm using sequence matching based machine learning approaches on five different body positions. The algorithm achieved an F-measure of 90 to 95% in detecting falls. Sensors worn as necklace pendants or in chest pockets performed best.

Keywords: Fall detection · Sensor orientation calibration · Machine learning

1 Introduction

People are enjoying longer lives due to advances in medicine and technology. Senior citizens are facing challenges to their independent living, e.g., chronic health conditions that compromise their ability to maintain their independence. Among those conditions, falls have been a major cause of fatal injury and create a serious obstruction to independent living. According to a report from the World Health Organization [1], approximately 28 to 35% of people aged 65 and over fall each year, and this proportion increases to 32 to 42% for those over 70 years of age. Falls threaten senior citizens' autonomous living both physically and psychologically. On one hand, in addition to the direct injuries from the fall, many who fall are unable to get up again without assistance, which can lead to hypothermia, dehydration, bronchopneumonia and pressure sores, which increases the severity of consequences [2]. On the other hand, senior citizens with a history of falling live in fear of future falls, which has been shown to be associated with negative consequences such as avoiding or reducing physical activity, falling, depression, decreased social contact, and lower quality of life [3].

The consequences of falling can be severe. Nevertheless, obtaining quick assistance after a fall reduces the risk of hospitalization by 26% and the risk of death by 80% [4]. For senior citizens living alone, automatic fall detection systems with motion sensors are necessary for requesting prompt care after falls. Those mini-sized sensors are placed on the body and track the activities performed by the sensor wearer. When the sensor

© ICST Institute for Computer Sciences, Social Informatics and Telecommunications Engineering 2017
P. Perego et al. (Eds.): MobiHealth 2016, LNICST 192, pp. 233–240, 2017.
DOI: 10.1007/978-3-319-58877-3_31

detects a fall, caregivers will be dispatched accordingly, even if the wearer becomes unconscious after the fall.

The effectiveness of an automatic fall detection system depends in large part on the fall detection algorithms as well as sensor positions. In this paper, we propose an approach using a single accelerometer for detecting falls in home settings to deal with the sensor orientation issue, which has been little addressed by former fall detection researchers.

This paper is organized as follows. The next section reviews the literature in acceleration signal processing. Section 3 presents our research design for applying sensor orientation calibration. Section 4 provides evaluations and discussions of experiment results. The final section concludes the study and suggests future directions.

2   Literature Review and Research Gaps

The data collected by the wearable motion sensors, or accelerometers, are acceleration signals. Therefore, we reviewed past studies related to acceleration signal processing, specifically, sensor orientation calibration and fall detection.

2.1   Sensor Orientation Calibration

Three-axial accelerometers are typically used for tracking the motion of the human body. The acceleration signals are described by tuples of three orthogonal acceleration components (x, y, z) in the sensor reference system. However, the sensor reference system is not always well-aligned with the body reference system denoted by the vertical (VT), medio-lateral (ML) and antero-posterior (AP) directions. This inconsistency provides much complexity in data processing, in that two series of signals may not be directly comparable without prior knowledge of sensor orientation, common in real world scenarios. Kale et al. [5] concluded that the classification algorithm can only achieve an accuracy of less than 50% if the sensor is misoriented for more than 15° on any axis.

According to Henpraserttae et al. [6], we can calibrate the signals to a unified reference system before feature extraction to solve this issue. A transformation matrix is applied on the raw acceleration signals for calibration. This approach can provide acceptable consistency across the signal sequences without losing direction information. We further investigated studies in sensor orientation calibration.

Mizell [7] proposed an approach to calibrate the acceleration signals implicitly, without extra device support or human effort. Since the accelerometer is constantly measuring the gravity, it acts as a clue for the direction of VT axis in the body reference system. By taking the average of acceleration signals over a reasonable time period, the approach produces a good estimate of the gravity (i.e., the VT axis) in the sensor reference system, and then the vertical components can be isolated. Yang [8] estimated the horizontal components of the acceleration signals after removing the vertical components from the raw signals. They utilized the magnitude of horizontal components to avoid identifying AP and ML axes. Henpraserttae et al. [6] further estimated the AP axis from the horizontal components by performing eigen-decomposition on the covariance matrix, assuming that most of the activities were done along a certain direction (e.g., the AP axis). Morales et al. [9] directly applied principal component analysis (PCA) on the acceleration signals without estimating the gravity. Features were extracted from the PCA-transformed signals for classification algorithms. Those studies mainly focused on activity recognition. Although none of them were conducted in the context of fall detection, they provide a solid foundation of techniques for addressing the sensor orientation issue.

2.2 Fall Detection

A fall is an event which results in a person inadvertently coming to rest on the ground or floor or other lower level [10]. The goal of fall detection algorithms is to distinguish fall events from non-fall activities with high precision and recall rates, since false alarms can be noisy, and failing to capture a fall event will be very costly and potentially dangerous. Compared to regular activities of daily living, fall events contain multiple special characteristics. Three phases occur sequentially during a fall event, which are collapse, impact, and inactivity. In the collapse phase, the faller accelerates towards the floor. Various rule-based thresholds were proposed to identify the three phases, including impact detection, vertical velocity detection, and posture monitoring [11, 12], among which impact detection is the most prevalent approach. When the faller approaches the floor, a very large magnitude of acceleration would be recorded by the accelerometer, which can be used as an identifier for a fall. Subjects were asked to wear the sensors on the upper body in fixed initial sensor orientations, and performed simulated fall events and non-fall daily activities. Past studies reported 85 to 100% of fall detection accuracies based on simulated falls. However, Bagalà et al. [13] applied several rule-based algorithms on a real world dataset with real falls, reporting that the detection accuracies were considerably lower (57 to 83%), and the number of false alarms generated by the algorithms during one-day monitoring of three representative fallers ranged from 3 to 85. Rule-based methods also suffer from the ad hoc nature of setting the thresholds, in that researchers set the thresholds to best fit their own datasets, with a concern of generalizability.

Machine learning approaches are also applied for fall detection. They can be further categorized as feature based and sequence matching based algorithms. Özdemir and Barshan [14] investigated fall detection with wearable sensors using various machine feature based learning techniques. Sequence matching based methods do not extract features from signal sequences. Instead, sequence matching directly compares the similarity between two signal sequences using certain metrics. Two popular metrics include Euclidean distance [15], and dynamic time warping [16]. A k-Nearest Neighbor (k-NN) classifier is applied on the distance metrics, with k typically set to 1. Unfortunately, most of the machine learning approaches did not discuss the sensor orientation issue explicitly, assuming the sensor orientation is given and fixed. It remains to be studied how the sensor orientation calibration would affect the accuracies of fall detection.

2.3 Research Gaps

As is discussed above, most prior studies on machine learning based activity recognition and fall detection assumed that the sensor orientations were given and fixed across different acceleration signal sequences. However, this assumption can hardly be held in real world applications. Each time the sensor is unequipped and re-equipped, a new arbitrary orientation will be set for the sensor, which cannot be predicted. Furthermore, failing to align the sensor orientation will lead to a decrease in activity recognition and fall detection accuracies. The sensor orientation issue needs to be addressed properly. Hence, we propose the following research question:

- Can sensor orientation calibration techniques be leveraged to improve the precision, recall rates for sensor-based fall detection?

3   Research Design

3.1 Data Collection

Five student subjects (aged 23 to 29) participated in our controlled experiments. We used MetaWear C sensors, measuring between ±4G at a sampling frequency of 12.5 Hz. The goal for this relatively low sampling rate is to save the battery power as much as possible without losing necessary information for classification. Although we aim to detect falls using a single motion sensor, we attached five sensors simultaneously on subjects' bodies to investigate the influence of different positions. The five positions we attached sensors to were neck, waist keychain, left chest pocket, right pants pocket, and right shoe. The necklace sensor was set in the pendant. The keychain sensor was clipped on the belt on the waist. The right shoe sensor was clipped on the shoe. Note that none of the sensors were attached firmly to subjects' body. Pocket sensors may be rolling, and keychain sensors may be dangling throughout the experiment. The initial sensor orientations were arbitrarily chosen by the subjects without our control. This setting is very unique compared to prior studies where the sensor orientations were pre-set and fixed by researchers, as we would like to mimic the real usage scenarios as much as possible.

Four simulated fall events were performed by each subject. The subject intentionally falls onto a large mattress from a static upright posture in four directions (once for each), namely, forward, backward, left laterally, and right laterally. Eight non-fall activities of daily living were performed, including quiet sitting, quiet standing, 10-meter walk, timed up and go, 5-time sit-to-stand, sit-stand-walk mixture, collapsing onto a chair (sit down on a soft armchair with a certain acceleration), and collapsing onto a mattress (sit down and then lie down on a mattress with a certain acceleration). The last two events were introduced because they tend to be misclassified by traditional threshold-based impact detection algorithms. Overall, 20 fall samples and 40 non-fall samples were collected for each sensor. The samples are transmitted to a desktop computer via Bluetooth Low Energy (BLE) for further processing.

3.2 Signal Preprocessing

Each signal sample, S, is an $n \times 3$ matrix, consisting of n acceleration vectors. Since we focus on fall detection, we extracted the acceleration signals around a potential shock or impact [14]. The potential shock is identified by the maximum magnitude of acceleration.

After the potential shock is identified, 2-second intervals both before it and after it (included) are extracted, generating 4-second time windows with signal samples of 50 data points (12.5×4). This 4-second time window is considered to be sufficient to cover the entire fall procedure, including the collapse, impact and inactivity phases, and also simplifies the comparison across signal samples.

3.3 Sensor Orientation Calibration

To completely transform the sensor reference system (x, y, z) to the human reference system (VT, AP, ML), we need to express two orthogonal axes in the sensor reference system. The third axis can be delivered by a cross product of the two known axes. Taking the average of acceleration signals over a reasonable time period (e.g., t_0 to t_1) can produce a good estimate of the gravity, and thus the VT axis, a_V [7, 8]. The amplitude of vertical component, v, in the acceleration vector, a, is extracted by:

$$v = |a| cos\theta = a \frac{a_V^T}{|a_V|}$$

Note that v can be negative. The horizontal acceleration component, c, is orthogonal to the direction of vertical component, which is given by:

$$c = a - v \frac{a_V}{|a_V|}$$

Now, if it is known that most of the activity is in a particular direction, e.g., AP direction in walking scenarios, the AP axis, a_P, may also be estimated by proper operations on c. However, in our case that deals with static activities, the estimation of a_P may be less meaningful. Instead, Yang [8] suggested to extract the features from the magnitude of the horizontal component, $|c|$. By this approach, the acceleration vectors are expressed in a combination of vertical amplitude and horizontal magnitude. Each calibrated signal sample, S', is then expressed in a 50×2 matrix.

3.4 Fall Classification

We implemented sequence matching based machine learning approaches on our sensor orientation calibration algorithm (CAL). Euclidean distance (EUC) and dynamic time warping (DTW) were chosen to be used as distance metrics. Given two time series, $X = (x_1, x_2, \ldots, x_n), Y = (y_1, y_2, \ldots, y_n)$,

$$\text{EUC}(X, Y) = \sum_{i=1}^{n} ||x_i - y_i||$$

Dynamic time warping is a method that calculates an optimal match between two given sequences (e.g., time series) with certain restrictions. The sequences are "warped" non-linearly in the time dimension to determine a measure of their similarity independent of certain non-linear variations in the time dimension. Further discussion can be found in [16].

A k-NN classifier was applied on the distances. k was set to 1 as in prior studies [15, 16]. The leave-one-out cross-validation method was applied to avoid over-fitting. We compared our approach with two benchmarks, which are raw tri-axial acceleration signals (RAW), S_1, and acceleration magnitude (MAG), S_2. Both benchmarks have been widely used by prior fall detection and activity recognition studies. All 5 sensor positions were evaluated separately.

4   Evaluation and Discussion

Figure 1 plots the precision, recall and F-measure for the sequence matching based algorithms. In terms of precision, all three algorithms performed reasonably well. The MAG benchmark outperformed the others by achieving 100% precision for all sensor positions. However, MAG performed relatively poorly in the recall rates. All three tests with recall rates greater than or equal to 85% were achieved by CAL. Similarly, all three tests with F-measures greater than or equal to 90% were achieved by CAL. Although MAG seems to reduce the false alarm rate, the poor recall rates led to the more severe consequence of fall events not being recognized properly. CAL with EUC metric at the position of chest pocket achieved an F-measure of 95%, outperforming all the other experiments conducted in this study.

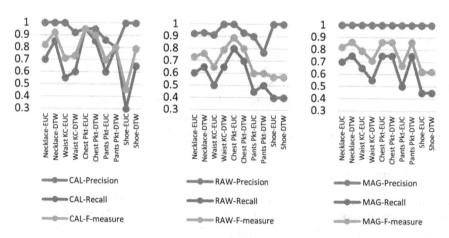

Fig. 1. Precision and recall and F-measure for sequence matching based algorithms

The sensor positions on the human body seem to influence the precision and recall rates of fall detection for sequence matching based algorithms. Consistent with the literature, the sensors set on the upper body (necklace and chest pocket) achieved relatively satisfactory results. Although the waist is typically regarded as a legitimate position to place the sensor, one potential issue for waist keychain sensors is that the dangling sensors may produce more random and complex patterns across experiment trials, increasing the difficulty of sequence matching. Pants pocket sensors and shoe sensors may encounter the issue that they are set on the lateral side of body and/or are too far away from the center of mass, which cannot properly reflect the body movement.

5   Conclusion

In this study, we proposed an orientation calibration algorithm to improve the precision and recall rates for fall detection. This algorithm aims to eliminate the influence of arbitrary sensor orientation issue in real world scenarios, improving the effectiveness and robustness of fall detection. F-measures of 90 to 95% have been achieved for sensors positioned in necklace pendants and chest pockets using a sequence matching based machine learning approach, which seems promising for real life applications.

We need to address several related directions in future works. First, we need to study feature based machine learning approaches to assess the proposed sensor orientation calibration algorithm more extensively. Feature based approaches may be able to provide high level abstraction from acceleration signals, and may perform differently from sequence matching approaches. Second, we may consider combining multiple approaches in practice. For instance, we can construct a classifier that first filters out stationary activities, and then applies a trained classifier to detect falls. This approach may consume fewer computational resources for large-scale applications.

One limitation to this study is that the data samples were collected from young healthy student subjects in a small sample size, as experiments of simulated falls by senior citizens may be improper and dangerous. Although conventional in literature, this setting may not necessarily reflect senior citizens' activities. Data samples from senior citizens in real life scenarios need to be investigated in the future to identify any potential discrepancies.

Acknowledgement. This study was supported by USA NSF SES-1314631, DUE-1303362, and STTR-1622788. Also, the authors thank Cathy Larson for the proofreading and suggestions.

References

1. World Health Organization: Ageing and Life Course Unit, "WHO Global Report on Falls Prevention in Older Age", World Health Organization (2008)
2. Tinetti, M.: Predictors and prognosis of inability to get up after falls among elderly persons. JAMA **269**(1), 65 (1993)

3. Scheffer, A., Schuurmans, M., van Dijk, N., van der Hooft, T., de Rooij, S.: Fear of falling: measurement strategy, prevalence, risk factors and consequences among older persons. Age Ageing 37(1), 19–24 (2007)
4. Stevens, J.: Falls among older adults—risk factors and prevention strategies. J. Saf. Res. 36(4), 409–411 (2005)
5. Kale, N., Lee, J., Lotfian, R., Jafari, R.: Impact of sensor misplacement on dynamic time warping based human activity recognition using wearable computers. In: Proceedings of the Conference on Wireless Health. ACM (2012)
6. Henprasertttae, A., Thiemjarus, S., Marukatat, S.: Accurate activity recognition using a mobile phone regardless of device orientation and location. In: 2011 International Conference on Body Sensor Networks (2011)
7. Mizell, D.: Using gravity to estimate accelerometer orientation. In: Proceedings of the 7th IEEE International Symposium on Wearable Computers, ISWC 2003. IEEE Computer Society (2003)
8. Yang, J.: Toward physical activity diary. In: Proceedings of the 1st International Workshop on Interactive Multimedia for Consumer Electronics - IMCE 2009 (2009)
9. Morales, J., Akopian, D., Agaian, S.: Human activity recognition by smartphones regardless of device orientation. In: Mobile Devices and Multimedia: Enabling Technologies, Algorithms, and Applications 2014 (2014)
10. "WHO|Falls", Who.int. http://www.who.int/violence_injury_prevention/other_injury/falls/en/. Accessed 11 May 2016
11. Bourke, A., O'Brien, J., Lyons, G.: Evaluation of a threshold-based tri-axial accelerometer fall detection algorithm. Gait Posture 26(2), 194–199 (2007)
12. Lee, J., Robinovitch, S., Park, E.: Inertial sensing-based pre-impact detection of falls involving near-fall scenarios. IEEE Trans. Neural Syst. Rehabil. Eng. 23(2), 258–266 (2015)
13. Bagalà, F., Becker, C., Cappello, A., Chiari, L., Aminian, K., Hausdorff, J., Zijlstra, W., Klenk, J.: Evaluation of accelerometer-based fall detection algorithms on real-world falls. PLoS ONE 7(5), e37062 (2012)
14. Özdemir, A., Barshan, B.: Detecting falls with wearable sensors using machine learning techniques. Sensors 14(6), 10691–10708 (2014)
15. Lan, M., Nahapetian, A., Vahdatpour, A., Au, L., Kaiser, W., Sarrafzadeh, M.: SmartFall: an automatic fall detection system based on subsequence matching for the smartcane. In: Proceedings of the 4th International ICST Conference on Body Area Networks (2009)
16. Paiyarom, S., Tangamchit, P., Keinprasit, R., Kayasith, P.: Fall detection and activity monitoring system using dynamic time warping for elderly and disabled people. In: Proceedings of the 3rd International Convention on Rehabilitation Engineering & Assistive Technology - ICREATE 2009 (2009)

A Neural Network Model
Based on Co-occurrence Matrix
for Fall Prediction

Masoud Hemmatpour$^{(\boxtimes)}$, Renato Ferrero, Bartolomeo Montrucchio,
and Maurizio Rebaudengo

Politecnico di Torino, Torino, Italy
{masoud.hemmatpour,renato.ferrero,
bartolomeo.montrucchio,maurizio.rebaudengo}@polito.it

Abstract. Fall avoidance systems reduce injuries due to unintentional falls, but most of them are fall detections that activate an alarm after the fall occurrence. Since predicting a fall is the most promising approach to avoid a fall injury, this study proposes a method based on new features and multilayer perception that outperforms state-of-the-art approaches. Since accelerometer and gyroscope embedded in a smartphone are recognized to be precise enough to be used in fall avoidance systems, they have been exploited in an experimental analysis in order to compare the proposal with state-of-the-art approaches. The results have shown that the proposed approach improves the accuracy from 83% to 90%.

1 Introduction

Falls are one of the causes of hospitalization that mostly increases health service costs [1]. In particular, since the risk of falling increases progressively with age, the United Nations advises improving health care for elderly people and creating a supportive environment for them. Fall detection systems have been massively studied [2–5], but they only notify user's acquaintance after a fall occurrence. As such, they do not avoid the fall, whereas this is the goal of Fall Prediction Systems (FPSs). FPSs usually follow a common procedure: first, they collect data from sensors, then, the collected data are analyzed to extract an appropriate feature set. Afterwards, a classification algorithm is applied on the feature set. In this study, new features with combination of a multilayer perceptron neural network are proposed and they are compared with different state-of-the-art approaches.

Most of FPSs analyze user's posture or gait variables. Kinematic-based solutions usually exploit sensors to investigate the characteristics of the movement, in particular accelerometer (for measuring acceleration, i.e., the rate of change of the velocity of an object) and gyroscope (it measures angular rate around one or more axes of the space). Real-time kinematic-based FPSs avoid a fall by alerting the user [6–8] or by using an external aid such as a walker or robot [9,10]. This study investigates kinematic-based FPSs, considering in particular data acquired with gyroscope and accelerometer sensors.

© ICST Institute for Computer Sciences, Social Informatics and Telecommunications Engineering 2017
P. Perego et al. (Eds.): MobiHealth 2016, LNICST 192, pp. 241–248, 2017.
DOI: 10.1007/978-3-319-58877-3_32

After obtaining signals from accelerometer and gyroscope, appropriate features should be extracted. Since data collected from sensors contain undesired information, filtering techniques eliminate some frequencies from the original signal to attenuate the background noise and to remove the undesired frequencies. After filtering the collected data, appropriate features should be selected. Afterwards, classification algorithm applied on the feature set to recognize the abnormal walking.

The remainder of the paper is organized as follows. The main features selected in the literature are reviewed in Sect. 2. The set of proposed features is described in Sect. 3. Experimental setup, and the results are presented in Sect. 4. Finally, some conclusions are written in Sect. 5.

2   Related Work

The measurements performed for recognizing a fall usually regard the *acceleration* and *tilt* change. The main features extrapolated from these measurements are reviewed in the following.

Acceleration. While a fall occurs, the acceleration of the body movement changes, so this parameter is investigated in FPSs to determine an abnormal walking [11–13]. Features frequently extrapolated from the acceleration are described in the following. In the presented formulas, $A(t)$ indicates the acceleration and $A_x(t)$, $A_y(t)$, $A_z(t)$ refer to the components of the acceleration in the 3 axes. Furthermore, A_{xi}, A_{yi} and A_{zi} are the discrete i-th acceleration samples in the 3 axes.

- Signal Magnitude Area (SMA)
   SMA can be used to classify the activities of the user [11]. It is computed as:

$$SMA = \frac{1}{T} \left(\int_0^T |A_x(t)| dt + \int_0^T |A_y(t)| dt + \int_0^T |A_z(t)| dt \right) \quad (1)$$

   where T is the monitored interval.
- Signal Magnitude Vector (SMV)
   SMV is adopted to calculate the resultant of the signal:

$$SMV = \frac{1}{n} \Sigma_{i=1}^n \sqrt{A_{xi}^2 + A_{yi}^2 + A_{zi}^2} \quad (2)$$

   SMV specifies the degree of the movement intensity and it can be a metric in FPSs [6,7,11,13].
- Derivative ($A'(t)$)
   The derivative ($A'(t)$) of the acceleration indicates the vibration of the movement and it is evaluated in FPSs [11].

- Hjorth parameters
  Hjorth parameters are statistical measures of the signal in time domain [14]. They use the variance of the signal $var(A(t))$ in their computation: $Hjorth\ activity = var(A(t))$, which indicates the signal power. $Hjorth\ mobility = \sqrt{\frac{var(A'(t))}{var(A(t))}}$, it is an indicator of the smoothness of the signal curve. $Hjorth\ complexity = \frac{mobility(A'(t))}{mobility(A(t))}$, it effectively measures the irregularities in the frequency domain. The Hjorth parameters are utilized to analyze accelerometer and gyroscope signals in FPSs [7].
- Peak and peak-to-peak
  Peak and peak-to-peak are simple and useful measurements of data changing over time. The peak is the maximum value of the signal over the period of time, and the peak-to-peak is the difference between the minimum and the maximum value of the signal over the period of time. The acceleration amplitude and derivative of peak-to-peak are two features used to predict a fall [15].
- Energy
  The energy of the acceleration signal specifies the amount of activity in the vertical and horizontal directions. It can determine the strength of the contact with the floor, so it can be used to recognize abnormal walking pattern such as stumbling [6,8]. The energy of the signal can be computed as follows:

$$E_x = \int_{-\infty}^{\infty} |A(t)|^2 dt, \tag{3}$$

Tilt. When a user significantly tilts in a direction, he assumes an abnormal posture and this can lead to a fall. So, the user tilt can be a factor to assess the risk of a fall. User tilt can be estimated with the combination of gyroscope and accelerometer by means of a tilt vector [6–8]. The average of N instances of the acceleration data vectors is computed as follows:

$$\vec{B}(t) = \frac{1}{N} \Sigma_{t=1}^{N} \vec{A}_0(t) \tag{4}$$

The tilt angles are found as:

$$\theta_1 = \arctan\left(\frac{B_y}{B_z}\right), \theta_2 = \arctan\left(\frac{B_x}{B_y \sin(\theta_1) + B_z \cos(\theta_1)}\right) \tag{5}$$

The tilt acceleration is computed as follows:

$$\vec{A}_1(t) = \begin{bmatrix} \cos(\theta_2)\sin(\theta_1)\sin(\theta_2) & -\cos(\theta_1)\sin(\theta_2) \\ 0 & \cos(\theta_1) & -\sin(\theta_1) \\ \sin(\theta_2)\sin(\theta_1)\cos(\theta_2) & \cos(\theta_1)\cos(\theta_2) \end{bmatrix} \times \vec{A}_0(t) \tag{6}$$

The tilt gyroscope $\vec{G}_1(t)$ is computed similarly to $\vec{A}_1(t)$. Subsequently, the gravity vector is removed from the accelerometer data:

$$\vec{A}_2(t) = \left[\vec{A}_1x(t), \vec{A}_1y(t), \vec{A}_1z(t) - \frac{1}{N}\Sigma_{t=1}^{N}\vec{A}_1z(t)\right] \tag{7}$$

Finally, a general tilt vector is created by computing the magnitude of the horizontal acceleration and combining it with the measurement of the gyroscope.

$$\overrightarrow{A_h}(t) = \sqrt{A_{2x}(t)^2 + A_{2y}(t)^2}, \ \overrightarrow{G_t}(t) = \sqrt{G_{1p}(t)^2 + G_{1r}(t)^2} \tag{8}$$

Energy and Hjorth parameters of the tilt vector are used as feature of the tilt to recognize the abnormal walking [6–8].

3   Proposed Features

In this section, six gait features are proposed. A group of five features are obtained from co-occurrence matrix and another feature is obtained from relative frequencies of different samples.

Co-occurrence Matrix Features. A co-occurrence matrix shows the scattering of similar adjacent values at a given offset. Normally, it is applied to images [16], but in this study it is used to analyze the acceleration and gyroscope values. In order to create the co-occurrence matrix of the data: first, the acceleration and gyroscope data are stored in a matrix. Each column of the matrix presents a sample in a specific time. Then, each couple of consecutive cells is analyzed to find the number of similar pattern in the whole matrix. Afterwards, the number of similar pattern is presented in the co-occurrence matrix with the index of cell contents. Let p_{ij} be the $(i, j)th$ element of the co-occurrence matrix divided by the sum of all the elements of the co-occurrence matrix. The following features are computed:

1. Contrast
   It is the measure of the intensity between a value and its neighbor cells over the entire obtained matrix:

   $$Contrast = \sum_{i=1}^{K}\sum_{j=1}^{K}(i-j)^2 p_{ij} \tag{9}$$

2. Homogeneity
   It measures the spatial closeness of the distribution of the elements to the diagonal in co-occurrence matrix:

   $$Homogeneity = \sum_{i=1}^{K}\sum_{j=1}^{K}\frac{p_{ij}}{1+|i-j|} \tag{10}$$

3. Correlation
   It shows how a value is correlated to its neighbor over the entire matrix:

   $$Homogeneity = \sum_{i=1}^{K}\sum_{j=1}^{K}\frac{(i-m_r)(j-m_c)p_{ij}}{\sigma_r \ \sigma_c}\sigma_r \neq 0; \sigma_c \neq 0 \tag{11}$$

where m_r, m_c, σ_r and σ_s are computed as follows:

$$m_r = \sum_{i=1}^{K}\sum_{j=1}^{K} ip_{ij}, \quad m_c = \sum_{j=1}^{K}\sum_{i=1}^{K} jp_{ij} \tag{12}$$

$$\sigma_r = \sum_{i=1}^{K}\sum_{j=1}^{K}(i - m_r)^2 p_{ij}, \quad \sigma_c = \sum_{j=1}^{K}\sum_{i=1}^{K}(i - m_c)^2 p_{ij} \tag{13}$$

4. Uniformity

It specifies the uniformity of elements in the co-occurrence matrix:

$$Uniformity = \sum_{i=1}^{K}\sum_{j=1}^{K} p_{ij}^2 \tag{14}$$

5. Maximum probability

It measures the highest value of the co-occurrence matrix. Simply, it can be computed by $\max(p_{ij})$.

Standard Deviation of Relative Frequency. Relative frequency presents the distribution of the data. In order to compute the relative frequency, firstly, range of values are ordered in different intervals from minimum to maximum. Then, a histogram based on the repetition of the values is computed. Finally, relative frequency is computed by histogram divided by range of values. After computing the relative frequency, the standard deviation of the relative frequency distribution can be computed as a feature to classify the normal and abnormal walking.

4   Experimental Setup and Results

In this study, an experiment was performed with 22 users walking 10 s through two paths. The first path was along a flat area, while obstacles were put along the second path. Users couldn't look at obstacles and this can be a good simulation of abnormal walking [11].

In this section, firstly, proposed features of real-time data are analyzed on normal and abnormal walking then, different state-of-the-art approaches are implemented and evaluated. Analyzing the average values of features obtained from the co-occurrence matrix in normal and abnormal walking cases shows that *Homogenity*, *Uniformity* and *Correlation* of the normal walking are higher than the ones of the abnormal walking. On the contrary, the *Contrast* of the abnormal walking is higher than normal walking. Also, on average *Maximum* in normal walking is higher than in abnormal walking. Moreover, Fig. 1 shows the regression of the standard deviation of the relative frequencies. Since the standard deviation of abnormal walking is higher than normal walking in most of the cases, standard deviation of relative frequency can be a good classifier

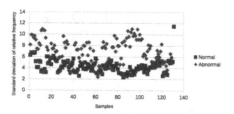

Fig. 1. Standard deviation of relative frequency.

for the normal and abnormal walking. In the following, combination of the co-occurrence matrix features and standard deviation of the relative frequency are used to classify the abnormal and normal walking. Two state-of-the-art methods are selected for a comparison. The first method [6] analyzes the tilt, and it is a basic algorithm exploited in future studies [7,8]. The second method [11] uses different acceleration features such as SMA, SMV, acceleration derivatives, peak-to-peak acceleration amplitude, and peak-to-peak acceleration derivative. The main classification methods of the abnormal and normal walking pattern are decision tree (DT) and support vector machine (SVM), and multilayer percepteron (MLP). For both algorithms different classifiers are evaluated and the best results are presented.

In this study, MLP with one hidden layer is used. Each neural node uses the following computation function:

$$CF = \phi(\sum_{i=1}^{n}(w_i x_i + b)), \tag{15}$$

where ϕ is the sigmoid activation function $\frac{1}{(1+e^{-x})}$, activation function helps to specify the output of node, w_i is the weight of each link, x_i is the input to the node, and b is the bias. Bias is a link with input one to the node.

Table 1. Results of different approaches.

Measures	Tilt	Acceleration	Proposed method
	DT	DT	MLP
Accuracy	83.88	81.42	90.82
Error rate	16.11	18.57	9.17
Sensitivity	0.88	0.78	0.87
Generality	0.21	0.15	0.06
Precision	0.81	0.83	0.93
Recall	0.88	0.78	0.87
F-measure	0.84	0.82	0.90
ROC area	0.86	0.82	0.96

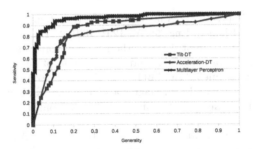

Fig. 2. ROC curves of different approaches.

The accuracy of the six proposed features with one layer MLP reaches 90.82%, which outperforms the other two state-of-the-art methods. Table 1 shows the result of different approaches.

The ROC curve is a graphical plot that illustrates the performance of a classifier [17]. The generality and sensitivity are plotted on x and y axes of the ROC plot, respectively. The best classifier is located at the top left corner of the ROC graph, which represents 100% sensitivity and 100% specificity.

The ROC curves allow to accurately compare the methods. As it can be seen in Fig. 2, the ROC curve of the proposed method outperforms the other two methods, because the area under the ROC curve of the proposed method is higher. Moreover, it increases the accuracy up to 7%.

5   Conclusion

This paper analyzed various fall factors and described corresponding features. New gait features based on acceleration data are proposed: five statistical features of the co-occurrence matrix and the standard deviation of relative frequency. Furthermore, state-of-the-art fall prediction algorithms have been experimentally evaluated. Based on the presented results, the proposed features in combination with a neural network present the best performance among the other fall prediction algorithms.

Acknowledgement. This work was partially supported by the grant "Bando Smart Cities and Communities", OPLON Project (OPportunities for active and healthy LONgevity) funded by the Italian Ministry for University.

References

1. Alexander, B.H., Rivara, F.P., Wolf, M.E.: The cost and frequency of hospitalization for fall-related injuries in older adults. Am. J. Public Health **82**(7), 1020–1023 (1992)
2. Shen, V.R.L., Lai, H.-Y., Lai, A.-F.: The implementation of a smartphone-based fall detection system using a high-level fuzzy Petri net. Appl. Soft Comput. **26**, 390–400 (2015)

3. Li, Y., Ho, K.C., Popescu, M.: A microphone array system for automatic fall detection. IEEE Trans. Biomed. Eng. **59**(5), 1291–1301 (2012)
4. Zigel, Y., Litvak, D., Gannot, I.: A method for automatic fall detection of elderly people using floor vibrations and sound-proof of concept on human mimicking doll falls. IEEE Trans. Biomed. Eng. **56**(12), 2858–2867 (2009)
5. Bian, Z.-P., Hou, J., Chau, L.-P., Magnenat-Thalmann, N.: Fall detection based on body part tracking using a depth camera. IEEE J. Biomed. Health Inform. **19**(2), 430–439 (2015)
6. Majumder, A.J.A., Rahman, F., Zerin, I., Ebel Jr., W., Ahamed, S.I.: iPrevention: towards a novel real-time smartphone-based fall prevention system. In: 28th Proceedings of the ACM Symposium on Applied Computing, pp. 513–518. ACM (2013)
7. Majumder, A.J.A., Zerin, I., Uddin, M., Ahamed, S.I., Smith, R.O.: Smartprediction: a real-time smartphone-based fall risk prediction and prevention system. In: Proceedings of the Research in Adaptive and Convergent Systems, pp. 434–439. ACM (2013)
8. Majumder, A.J.A., Zerin, I., Ahamed, S.I., Smith, R.O.: A multi-sensor approach for fall risk prediction and prevention in elderly. ACM SIGApp Appl. Comput. Rev. **14**(1), 41–52 (2014)
9. Hirata, Y., Muraki, A., Kosuge, K.: Motion control of intelligent passive-type walker for fall-prevention function based on estimation of user state. In: Proceedings IEEE International Conference on Robotics and Automation (ICRA) (2006)
10. Di, P., Huang, J., Sekiyama, K., Fukuda, T.: A novel fall prevention scheme for intelligent cane robot by using a motor driven universal joint. In: International Symposium on Micro-NanoMechatronics and Human Science (MHS), pp. 391–396. IEEE (2011)
11. Weiss, A., Shimkin, I., Giladi, N., Hausdorff, J.M.: Automated detection of near falls: algorithm development and preliminary results. BMC Res. Notes **3**(1), 1–8 (2010)
12. Horta, E.T., Lopes, I.C., Rodrigues, J.J.P.C., Misra, S.: Real time falls prevention and detection with biofeedback monitoring solution for mobile environments. In: 15th International Conference on e-Health Networking, Applications & Services (Healthcom), pp. 594–600. IEEE (2013)
13. Tong, L., Song, Q., Ge, Y., Liu, M.: HMM-based human fall detection and prediction method using tri-axial accelerometer. IEEE Sens. J. **3**(5), 1849–1856 (2013)
14. Hjorth, B.: Eeg analysis based on time domain properties. Electroencephalogr. Clin. Neurophysiol. **29**(3), 306–310 (1970)
15. Guimarães, V., Teixeira, P.M., Monteiro, M.P., Elias, D.: Phone based fall risk prediction. In: Nikita, K.S., Lin, J.C., Fotiadis, D.I., Arredondo Waldmeyer, M.-T. (eds.) MobiHealth 2011. LNICSSITE, vol. 83, pp. 135–142. Springer, Heidelberg (2012). doi:10.1007/978-3-642-29734-2_19
16. Gonzalez, R.C., Woods, R.E.: Digital image processing. Nueva Jersey (2008)
17. Fawcett, T.: An introduction to ROC analysis. Pattern Recogn. Lett. **27**(8), 861–874 (2006)

Machine Learning in mHealth Applications

Using Smartwatch Sensors to Support the Acquisition of Sleep Quality Data for Supervised Machine Learning

Cinzia Bernardeschi, Mario G.C.A. Cimino, Andrea Domenici[✉], and Gigliola Vaglini

Department of Information Engineering, University of Pisa, 56122 Pisa, Italy
{c.bernardeschi,m.cimino,a.domenici,g.vaglini}@ing.unipi.it

Abstract. It is a common practice in supervised learning techniques to use human judgment to label training data. For this process, data reliability is fundamental. Research on sleep quality found that human sleep stage misperception may occur. In this paper we propose that human judgment be supported by software-driven evaluation based on physiological parameters, selecting as training data only data sets for which human judgment and software evaluation are aligned. A prototype system to provide a broad-spectrum perception of sleep quality data comparable with human judgment is presented. The system requires users to wear a smartwatch recording heartbeat rate and wrist acceleration. It estimates an overall percentage of the sleep stages, to achieve an effective approximation of conventional sleep measures, and to provide a three-class sleep quality evaluation. The training data are composed of the heartbeat rate, the wrist acceleration and the three-class sleep quality. As a proof of concept, we experimented the approach on three subjects, each one over 20 nights.

Keywords: Sleep monitoring · Smartwatch · Sleep quality estimation

1 Introduction

Supervised learning is a promising approach to a wide range of problems related to monitoring health conditions and diagnosing pathologies [1]. This work is part of a research effort aimed at designing a supervised learning architecture to detect sleep behavior shift. Behavior shift is a pattern used in broad-spectrum assessment of initial signs of disease or deviations in performance [2,3]. The availability of labeled training data is fundamental for supervised learning [4]. In the case of sleep behavior, the training data are sets of sensor data, each labeled with the related sleep quality. The objective of this study is to propose a support to the collection of per-night sleep quality data. In the literature it is well known that, besides the sleep state, other events and cognitive experiences may influence the judgment, resulting in a cognitive bias [5]. The aim of this study is to support human judgment by collecting additional data during the

© ICST Institute for Computer Sciences, Social Informatics and Telecommunications Engineering 2017
P. Perego et al. (Eds.): MobiHealth 2016, LNICST 192, pp. 251–259, 2017.
DOI: 10.1007/978-3-319-58877-3_33

monitored nights, via a familiar device, and to extract three-class sleep quality evaluations to be compared to those reported by the subject.

Polisomnography is a standard approach to sleep monitoring. It involves recording multiple physiologic variables at specialized centers, scored by human examiners on the basis of standardized criteria. It can be used for a few nights, which are insufficient for sleep habits. It is intrusive, which may disturb sleep. Consequently, it is not accurate for sleep behavior [6]. The diagnosis may vary depending on the examiner with a 20% variance [7]. Another approach is *actigraphy*, which is based on a watch-like device equipped with motion accelerometer, to monitor motion-related sleep disorders. Normal subjects show more than 90% correlation between actigraphy and polisomnography [6].

In the literature, there is a growing interest in the possibility of gathering sleep data from wearable devices. Recently developed smartwatches have been used for monitoring sleep patterns variation, because they can also feature sensors such as heartbeat rate monitor, wrist acceleration recorder, pedometer, magnetometer, barometer, ambient thermometer, oxymeter, skin conductance and temperature sensors, and GPS locator [8]. More specifically, heart rate and body movement are known to vary greatly during sleep and have a close relationship with sleep stages. Indeed, the autonomic nervous system significantly affects heart rate, and body movement is linked to sleep level [6]. It is known that wrist watch-shaped devices monitoring motion and pulse can measure sleep quality with sufficient accuracy. For example in [7] the authors evaluate a good correlation between sleep stages estimated using a wrist device and using polysomnography, by observing 45 subjects.

In this paper, smartwatches are used to gather data on individuals' physiological parameters. The main contribution of this preliminary work is a method and a software prototype to derive an identification of sleep stages as *wake*, *rapid eye movement* (REM), and *non rapid eye movement* (NREM), which are used to rate subject's sleep quality into three classes: *Normal*, *mediocre* and *scarce*. This way, human judgment can be supported by software-driven evaluation in order to identify the final training data set used for supervised learning.

This method is implemented by a *sleep stage estimator* (SSE), a Matlab application that analyzes smartwatch recordings of *heartbeat rate* (HBR) and *acceleration* of the subject's wrist. As a first step, the algorithm produces a simplified hypnogram from such recordings.

The SSE design is based on basic notions about sleep stages. During wake, body movement, as recorded by electromyography, is frequent, voluntary, and continuous. During REM sleep, movement is nearly absent, as it is potentially directed by dream activity but inhibited. During NREM sleep, movement occurs in episodic and involuntary posture shifts [9]. The use of heartbeat, recorded by electrocardiography, is a recurrent subject in the sleep staging literature. Heart rate variability (HRV) is significantly higher in REM sleep than in NREM sleep [10]. HRV has been also used to understand autonomic changes during different sleep stages in [11]. Moreover, a decision support system for sleep classification based on HRV has been presented in [12]. The process of falling asleep presents fluctuation in vigilance. Autonomic function changes during the wake-to-sleep transition, as reflected by the instantaneous HRV, are studied in [13]. Sleep staging is also performed in [14] on the basis of two channels of EEG.

The majority of the studies in the literature use clinical monitoring equipment and a very constrained experimental setting. In contrast, the present proposal has been conceived for a non-intrusive monitoring method, based on a general-purpose wearable device and minimally affecting the subject's everyday life. Clearly, the proposed sleep stage estimation provided by a smartwatch can deliver a broad-spectrum score of sleep quality, and not a precise evaluation of medical symptoms.

The paper is organized as follows: Sect. 2 covers materials and methods, Sect. 3 describes synthetically the SSE prototype design, Sect. 4 illustrates the sleep quality model, and discusses how the approach supports the selection of a training set. Section 5 draws conclusions and future work.

2   Materials and Methods

Figure 1 represents the overall method, from left to right. During physiological sleep, both subject perception and device sensing-logging contribute to the data acquisition.

On the side of the subject's judgment, sleep/wake perception is a process of discrimination that involves cognitive interpretation of physiological and psychological data [5]. According to this assumption, unreliable perception may occur when heterogeneous, incomplete, dynamic, uncertain aspects of experience are taken into consideration. The major events are manually annotated, either at the moment or later. In the next morning, an overall judgment of the night's sleep quality is given, scored as *normal, mediocre* and *scarce*.

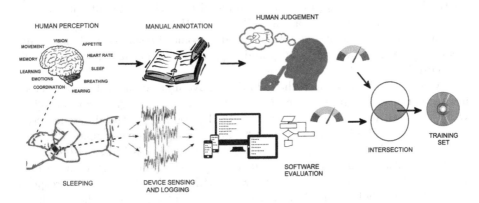

Fig. 1. Representation of the overall method.

On the side of computerized evaluation, the smartwatch senses physiological data with a heartrate monitor and an accelerometer that measures the acceleration in ms^{-2}. The smartwatch used to collect data was an LG Watch Urbane (LG-W150). The heart rate monitor uses an optical sensor to detect peaks in blood flow and computes the heart rate over an interval of time established by the constructor. The computed heart rate value is updated every tenth of a second, and the resulting time series is sampled by the SSE at one-second intervals. The acceleration data are sampled at 10 Hz. The SSE produces as an output: standard deviation of the acceleration magnitude (σ_a), variance of the heartbeat rate (σ^2_{hbr}), and approximate sleep staging. Also the respective plots are produced. Subsequently, a sleep quality evaluation is carried out, to produce a score with the above mentioned categories. The result can be sent to a mobile application and to a desktop application via Bluetooth and USB, respectively.

Finally, the resulting scores are compared: any night log whose computed score matches the perceived sleep quality becomes an entry of the final training set. Discordant scores are not considered for the training set. The method has been applied to three subjects of different age for 20 nights.

3   A Sleep Stage Estimator

This section illustrates the criteria adopted by the SSE to estimate sleep stages. In essence, the subject is considered: (i) in WAKE stage, when motion level is high; (ii) in a REM stage, when motion level is low and pulse level and variability are both high; (iii) otherwise it is considered in a NREM stage.

Starting from the three above criteria, the automatic evaluation of sleep stages is made according the following rules. First, the standard deviation of the acceleration magnitude (σ_a) is computed over a three-second sliding window. The variance is used in order to reduce the influence of the constant component due to gravity and of accelerometer noise. The mean values ($\bar{\sigma}_a$) of σ_a and HBR ($\bar{h}$) are computed over the complete series. Then, average m_{hbr} and variance σ^2_{hbr} for HBR and average m_{asd} for σ_a are computed for each five-minute interval.

Each interval is marked as a wake, REM, or NREM period, by comparing the computed values of mean and variance against some thresholds: m^{th}_{hbr} for HBR mean, v^{th}_{hbr} for HBR variance, m^u_{asd} and m^l_{asd} for the upper and lower limits of standard deviation of the acceleration.

The criterion for staging is the following: a five-minute interval is considered a wake period if the difference δ_{asd} between m_{asd} and $\bar{\sigma}_a$ is greater than m^u_{asd}. Otherwise, the interval is considered a REM period if (i) the difference δ_{hbr} between m_{hbr} and $\bar{h}$ is greater than m^{th}_{hbr}, and (ii) σ^2_{hbr} is greater than v^{th}_{hbr}, and (iii) δ_{asd} is smaller than m^l_{asd}. Otherwise, the interval is marked as NREM.

The resulting marks are then recorded and plotted as a hypnogram, assigning the numerical values of 3, 2, and 1 to wake, REM, and NREM periods, respectively. The threshold values have been chosen so as to maximize the matching between the stages identified by a human observer applying the three above criteria, and those generated by the SSE.

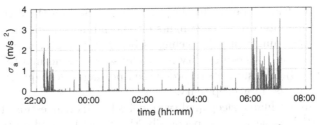

(a) Standard deviation of acceleration magnitude.

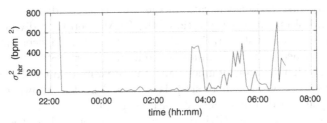

(b) Variance of heart beat rate.

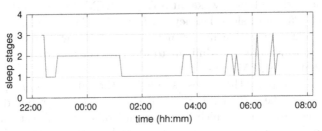

(c) Hypnogram (3: wake, 2: REM, 1: NREM).

Fig. 2. Recording of a sample night (Sept 4, 2015).

Figure 2 shows the plots of the standard deviation of the acceleration magnitude, the HBR variance, and the estimated hypnogram of a sample night of a subject, respectively. After a short NREM sleep, the hypnogram shows a two-hour REM stage, followed by fairly long periods of NREM sleep separated by REM stages.

4   Sleep Quality Evaluation

The data used in the experiment were collected from three subjects of different age: a healthy man aged 22 (subject A), a man aged 72 (subject B), affected by minor age-related ailments, and a woman aged 88 (subject C), affected by arterial hypertension.

Human judgment on per-night sleep quality is based on three cognitive criteria: (i) the time interval between lights off and falling asleep; (ii) the number of nocturnal awakenings; (iii) the feeling of being rested after sleep. An overall judgment of the night's sleep quality is usually scored as normal (N), mediocre (M) and scarce (S). The subjects recorded their per-night sleep quality, according to the above criteria, in a sleep diary.

The software-evaluated sleep quality model is based on an estimation of wake, REM, and NREM stages. More specifically, the model is based on the following criteria: (i) sleep latency, defined as the time interval between lights off and the fall asleep; (ii) wake ratio is the ratio of the wake time divided by total time in bed; (iii) REM sleep ratio is the ratio of the REM sleep time divided by total time in bed; (iv) NREM sleep ratio is the ratio of the NREM sleep time divided by total time in bed. All these values are computed by the SSE.

We remark that human judgment and the software-evaluated sleep quality model share two criteria, namely sleep latency and nocturnal awakenings. But they also depend on two independent features, namely feeling rested after sleep and the ratio of REM and NREM stages, respectively. Thus, they are both incomplete when taken separately.

Table 1 shows the values of wake ratio W (%), REM sleep ratio R (%), NREM sleep ratio NR (%), and sleep latency SL (min) for the three subjects and for each night N. We remark that no distinction is made between wake and shallow NREM phases, which are very difficult to identify. For this reason, the value of W includes shallow NREM phases.

The table also reports the scores assigned by the subject (*diary quality*, DQ) and computed by the software (*computed quality*, CQ). Computed scores are evaluated using thresholds, which may vary for different subjects as shown in Table 2, where W_{min}^{th} and W_{max}^{th} are the lower and upper thresholds for the wake time ratio and R^{th} and SL^{th} are for the REM sleep time ratio and sleep latency. Note that R is not considered for the elderly subjects, since it decreases with age and in practice disappears. The calculation of CQ is made according tho the following rules. Classes are ordered for decreasing quality, i.e., N, M, S.

1. CQ is initially set to the best quality, i.e., N.
2. for each W, SL, R:
   - If $W > W_{max}^{th}$, CQ is set to the next lower class.
   - If $W < W_{min}^{th}$, CQ is set to the next higher class.
   - If $SL > SL^{th}$, CQ is set to the next lower class.
   - If $R < R^{th}$, CQ is set to the next lower class.

The values causing CQ to move to the next lower and higher class are highlighted with minus and plus signs, respectively, in Table 1.

As a result, by comparing the values of DQ and CQ, we note that: (i) Subject A has 4 discordant cases on 20, i.e., nights 4, 13, 15, and 17); (ii) Subject B has 5 discordant cases on 20, i.e., nights 1, 4, 5, 14, and 16; (iii) Subject C has 12 cases of discordance on 20.

Table 1. Summary data.

N	Subject A						Subject B						Subject C					
	W	R	NR	SL	DQ	CQ	W	R	NR	SL	DQ	CQ	W	R	NR	SL	DQ	CQ
1	−51	41	59	25	M	M	+24	0	100	5	M	N	+50	75	25	10	M	N
2	+27	−5	95	10	N	N	+34	0	100	10	N	N	70	30	70	60	N	N
3	39	24	76	15	N	N	−49	11	89	10	M	M	+58	89	11	15	M	N
4	+19	17	83	5	M	N	40	5	95	10	M	N	+59	29	71	10	M	N
5	+28	18	82	5	N	N	−57	3	97	25	N	M	+38	9	91	15	N	N
6	40	39	61	5	N	N	37	14	86	10	N	N	+53	84	16	10	S	N
7	+32	−9	91	5	N	N	39	2	98	20	N	N	+52	96	4	5	M	N
8	+25	32	68	10	N	N	35	2	98	5	N	N	61	7	93	10	M	N
9	38	19	81	5	N	N	−45	15	85	10	M	M	−85	13	87	35	M	M
10	+30	−0	100	15	N	N	−61	0	100	25	M	M	−76	50	50	10	S	M
11	35	11	89	5	N	N	33	31	69	10	N	N	63	23	77	5	N	N
12	+14	65	35	5	N	N	−61	0	100	20	M	M	+37	76	24	−75	M	M
13	−47	−0	100	5	N	S	−72	5	95	15	M	M	+54	100	0	15	N	N
14	+21	18	82	5	N	N	−54	0	10	30	N	M	68	16	84	15	N	N
15	+28	−0	100	15	M	N	−68	4	96	15	M	M	+19	33	67	10	M	N
16	35	20	80	5	N	N	−56	3	97	10	N	M	−80	41	59	25	N	M
17	42	−0	100	10	N	M	31	0	100	20	N	N	+46	54	46	40	M	N
18	+28	−0	100	15	N	N	42	0	100	5	N	N	+45	35	65	15	M	N
19	+19	−8	92	10	N	N	−60	0	100	10	M	M	70	33	67	10	M	N
20	+31	31	69	10	N	N	41	13	88	10	N	N	+57	5	95	10	N	N

Table 2. Thresholds for CQ quality assessment.

Subject	W_{min}^{th}	W_{max}^{th}	R^{th}	SL^{th}
A	35	45	10	30
B	35	45	−	30
C	60	70	−	60

A closer look at the discordant cases of Subject C can be usefully made, to obtain a better insight of sleep quality. The diary score is always lower than the software-computed one, and it can be ascribed to a potential cognitive bias.

5 Conclusions

Generating a reliable set of training data for sleep quality evaluation is a challenging problem, mainly due to misperceptions by a subject's judgment. In this paper we propose a novel approach to identify a reliable sleep quality data set for supervised machine learning by comparing sleep quality estimates derived from computation on physiological parameters and from human judgment. The approach is based on a software sleep stage estimator which exploits a subject's physiological parameters provided by commercially available smartwatches. Training data can be selected considering the subset of data for which the human judgment and the computed estimation concur. The experimental study on three subjects shows the viability of the approach. As a future work, the system will be cross-validated on a higher number of subjects. Further, information provided by the pedometer can be exploited to improve the software-driven evaluation.

Acknowledgements. This work was partially supported by the PRA 2016 project "Analysis of Sensory Data: from Traditional Sensors to Social Sensors" funded by the University of Pisa. The authors thank Giovanni Pollina, Silvio Bacci and Silvia Volpe for their work on the subject during their thesis.

References

1. Redmond, S.J., Lee, Q.Y., Xie, Y., Lovell, N.H.: Applications of supervised learning to biological signals: ECG signal quality and systemic vascular resistance. In: 2012 Annual International Conference of the IEEE Engineering in Medicine and Biology Society, pp. 57–60, August 2012
2. Aztiria, A., Farhadi, G., Aghajan, H.: User behavior shift detection in ambient assisted living environments. JMIR Mhealth Uhealth **1**(1), e6 (2013)
3. Barsocchi, P., Cimino, M.G.C.A., Ferro, E., Lazzeri, A., Palumbo, F., Vaglini, G.: Monitoring elderly behavior via indoor position-based stigmergy. Pervasive Mob. Comput. **23**, 26–42 (2015)
4. Cimino, M.G.C.A., Lazzeri, A., Vaglini, G.: Improving the analysis of context-aware information via marker-based stigmergy and differential evolution. In: Rutkowski, L., Korytkowski, M., Scherer, R., Tadeusiewicz, R., Zadeh, L.A., Zurada, J.M. (eds.) ICAISC 2015. LNCS, vol. 9120, pp. 341–352. Springer, Cham (2015). doi:10.1007/978-3-319-19369-4_31
5. Weigand, D., Michael, L., Schulz, H.: When sleep is perceived as wakefulness: an experimental study on state perception during physiological sleep. J. Sleep Res. **16**(4), 346–353 (2007)
6. Nam, Y., Kim, Y., Lee, J.: Sleep monitoring based on a tri-axial accelerometer and a pressure sensor. Sensors **16**(5), 750 (2016)
7. Suzuki, T., Ouchi, K., Kameyama, K.-I., Takahashi, M.: Development of a sleep monitoring system with wearable vital sensor for home use. In: BIODEVICES 2009 International Conference on Biomedical Electronics and Devices, pp. 326–331 (2009)
8. Guiry, J.J., van de Ven, P., Nelson, J.: Multi-sensor fusion for enhanced contextual awareness of everyday activities with ubiquitous devices. Sensors **14**(3), 5687–5701 (2014)
9. Hobson, J.A.: Sleep and dreaming. J. Neurosci. **10**(2), 371–382 (1990)
10. Versace, F., Mozzato, M., De Min, G., Tona, C.C., Stegagno, L.: Heart rate variability during sleep as a function of sleep cycle. Biol Psychol. **63**(2), 149–162 (2003)
11. Stein, P.K., Yachuan, P.: Heart rate variability, sleep and sleep disorders. Sleep Med. Rev. **16**(1), 47–66 (2012)
12. Mendez, M.O., Matteucci, M., Castronovo, V., Ferini-Strambi, L., Cerutti, S., Bianchi, A.M.: Sleep staging from heart rate variability: time-varying spectral features and hidden markov models. Int. J. Biomed. Eng. Technol. **3**(3/4), 246–263 (2010)

13. Shinar, Z., Akselrod, S., Daga, Y., Baharav, A.: Autonomic changes during wake-sleep transition: a heart rate variability based approach. Auton. Neurosci. **130**(12), 17–27 (2006)

14. Imtiaz, S.A., Rodriguez-Villegas, E.: Automatic sleep staging using state machine-controlled decision trees. In: Proceedings of the IEEE Engineering in Medicine and Biology Society, pp. 378–381. IEEE (2015)

Multilayer Radial Basis Function Kernel Machine

Mashail Alsalamah[✉] and Saad Amin

Faculty of Engineering and Computing, Coventry University, Priory Street,
Coventry CV1 5FB, UK
alsalam2@coventry.ac.uk

Abstract. Radial Basis Function (RBF) Kernel Machines have become commonly used in Machine Learning tasks, but they contain certain flaws (e.g., some suffer from fast growth in the number of learning parameters while predicting data with large number of variations). Besides, Kernel Machines with single hidden layers lack mechanisms for feature selection in multidimensional data space, and machine learning tasks become intractable. This paper investigates "deep learning" architecture composed of multilayered adaptive non-linear components – Multilayer RBF Kernel Machine – to address RBF limitations. Three different approaches of features selection and dimensionality reduction to train RBF based on Multilayer Kernel Learning are explored, and comparisons made between them in terms of accuracy, performance and computational complexity. Results show that the multilayered system produces better results than single-layer architecture. In particular, developing decision support system in term of data mining.

Keywords: Machine learning · Classification · Unsupervised regression · Supervised regression · Principal component analysis

1 Introduction

In the recent decades, a number of techniques for different machine learning tasks, including classification, regression, function approximation clustering and feature transformation were developed with help of the class of non-linear functions – radial basis functions (rbf) [1, 2]. One of the interesting ideas is radial basis functions networks and their generalization kernel networks. In this work, special emphasis is given to the application of these networks to the problem of data classification.

Radial basis functions are a special kind of function which has a characteristic feature to monotonically decrease or increase with increase of the distance from the central point. The center, the distance scale and particular shape could vary for different models [1]. The most commonly used example is the Gaussian function:

$$f(x) = e^{-\frac{(x - c)^2}{r^2}}$$

and multi-quadratic function

© ICST Institute for Computer Sciences, Social Informatics and Telecommunications Engineering 2017
P. Perego et al. (Eds.): MobiHealth 2016, LNICST 192, pp. 260–268, 2017.
DOI: 10.1007/978-3-319-58877-3_34

$$f(x) = \frac{\sqrt{r^{2+(x-c)^2}}}{r}$$

while, of course, a lot of variations possible. Another way to think about rbf networks is as kernel machines with specific type of kernel. Kernel machines are special machine learning methods which allow the use of regular machine learning techniques developed to learn linear functions in the problems with non-linear dependencies. This goal is achieved via transformation (mapping) of input feature space into the Hilbert space. The first kernel machines were a natural extension of the Support Vector Machine proposed by Vapnik for classification of the linearly separable data points. The goal of the algorithm was to find the hyperplane which will divide two datasets and will have maximum distance (margin) between itself and closest points from two classes. This hyperplane can be presented as the linear combination of the training samples lying on that margin (support vectors):

$$H(x) = \sum_i (\alpha_i y_i \langle x_i, x \rangle) + \alpha_0.$$

The algorithm finds the optimal values for the parameters α. The extension for the non-linear separable case exploits so called feature mapping function g with the hyperplane of the form:

$$H(x) = \sum_i (\alpha_i y_i \langle g(x_i), g(x) \rangle) + \alpha_0.$$

The function

$$K(x_i, x)$$

which satisfy the conditions of the Mercer's theorem can be presented in the form

$$K(x_i, x) = \langle g(x_i), g(x) \rangle$$

in the Hilbert space is called kernel. If the kernel function is selected appropriately the data points can become separable in the new feature space can become separable. This method is usually referred to in the literature as the "kernel trick". In this case the method for linear SVM training could be applied. The Gaussian radial basis function is one of this kernels, so the support vector learning could be applied as learning method for radial basis function network with support vectors being the centers of radial basis functions [7, 8].

The term of "deep" learning was coined in the contrast to the "shallow" learning algorithms which have fixed usually single layer architecture. The "deep" learning architectures are compositions of many layers of adaptive non-linear components [27].

Several attempts to combine the deep-learning approach with kernel based method were made in the past. For instance, method proposed in [29, 34] mimics the behavior of the multilayer neural network via single layer kernel network with specifically generated kernel functions (arc-cosine kernels). Arc-cosine kernels are produced with recursive substitutions of the output of the kernel function. This action is equivalent to the non-linear transformation of the feature maps. In [35] the notion of the hierarchical feature invariance is proposed.

This paper provides three different approaches of features selection and dimensionality reduction to train RBF kernel based on the idea of MLK, and makes a comparison between them in terms of accuracy, the effect of changing the number of layers on the performance and computational complexity.

2   Deep RBF Kernel Machine

2.1   Multilayer RBF machine based on Kernel PCA

Below is a summary on how we implemented the Multilayer RBF machine based on Kernel PCA and shown in Fig. 2.

1. Let N be the number of layers we would like to use.
2. Prune the features by ranking method removing redundant features.
3. Select appropriate kernels and kernel parameters (cross-validation or otherwise) – not described in the Cho's work.
4. Apply kernel PCA algorithm and make the result be next layer set of features.
5. Determine number of features to extract (not described how), prune the redundant features from the resulting set – optional step.
6. If number of iterations exceeds N go to step 6, otherwise go to step 2.
7. Feed the feature representations to the classifier to make final decision.

2.2   Multilayer RBF machine based on supervised kernel regression

Below is a summary on how we implemented the Multilayer RBF machine based on supervised kernel regression and shown in Fig. 2.

1. Let N be the number of layers we would like to use.
2. Select appropriate kernels and kernel parameters (cross-validation or otherwise) – not described in the work.
3. Apply supervised regression to extract next feature value and corresponding eigen value.
4. If eigen value is greater than selected threshold go to step 3 otherwise use all the extracted features as input to the next layer.
5. If number of iterations exceeds N go to step 6, otherwise go to step 2.
6. Feed the feature representations to the classifier to make the final decision.

2.3 Multilayer RBF machine based on unsupervised kernel regression

Below is a summary of how we implement the Multilayer RBF machine based on unsupervised kernel regression and shown in Fig. 2.

1. Let N be the number of layers we would like to use.
2. Apply unsupervised regression to extract latent variables which better represent the input parameters. (Kernel parameters selection and dimensionality selection is embedded in this step) based on the ideas described in the Memisevic work: http://www.iro.umontreal.ca/~memisevr/pubs/ukr.pdf
   - Learning of optimal latent space representation with input data.
   - Learning of transformation from observable to latent space.
   - Selection of the kernel parameters and optimal dimensionality of the latent space.
3. Use extracted latent variables as input to the next step.
4. If number of iterations exceeds N go to step 6, otherwise go to step 2.
5. Feed the feature representations to the classifier to make the final decision (Fig. 1).

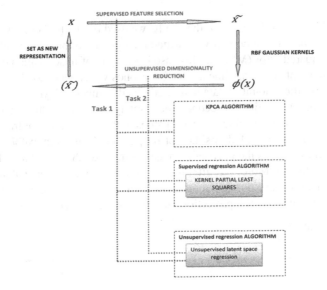

Fig. 1. Multilayer kernels machine (MKMs) for the three different transformation

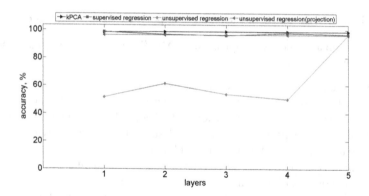

Fig. 2. Accuracy % with different methods

3   Results

In order to achieve the robustness of the results we used the 10-fold cross validation.

Accuracy is the ratio of correctly classified data points to the total number of data points. Mean squared error (MSE) in this case is the ratio of misclassified data to total number of data point. Training time is time in seconds which were solely used to train the model on specific amount of data with predefined number of layers.

Prediction time is the time in seconds spent solely on the prediction step with pre-trained model containing specific number of steps with fixed amount of training data.

The dataset is the MNIST digits dataset (http://yann.lecun.com/exdb/mnist/). The data there are presented as the grayscale images of the size 28 × 28 pixels. The values can vary from 0 to 255. Moreover, after trained and evaluated the three algorithms the unsupervised method gave not that good accuracy and in order to improve it the Unsupervised latent regression with projection method is suggested (Figs. 3 and 4).

(1)   Dataset result.

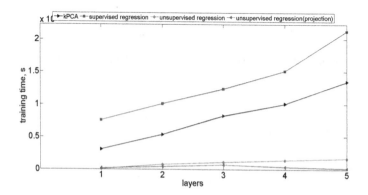

Fig. 3. Training time with different methods

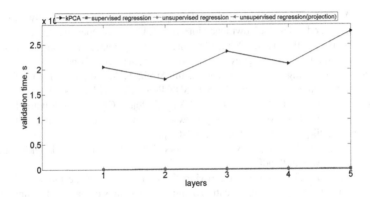

Fig. 4. Validation time with different methods

4 Discussion

The most stable results were shown by the supervised regression method for both balanced and unbalanced datasets. This is the only algorithm which shows continuous improvement in sensitivity and specificity with the increasing number of layers. Other algorithms show the tendency to stabilize results very quickly. That means that in practice it makes sense to test these algorithms only on small number of layers to understand whether they are sufficient for the current dataset or not. The worst time results were shown for the kPCA algorithms for both validation and training phases. It is caused by the large number of features selected at the projection step which are then transferred to the feature selection algorithm and knn-classifier. The time parameters can be improved by the limit on the number of features selected after projection. However, that might affect the accuracy in some cases.

5 Conclusion

In conclusion, the multilayered systems generally show relatively better results with large and highly varied data, as compared with "shallow learning" algorithms with usually single layer architecture. Moreover, amongst the multilayer algorithms, it show the ability of pattern and relationship discovery within large data sets. It holds promise in many area of the data application to quality assurance as found its way into data mining application and decision support system.

References

1. Orr, M.J.L.: Introduction to radial basis function network (1996). http://www.cc.gatech.edu/~isbell/tutorials/rbf-intro.pdf
2. Orr, M.J.L.: Recent advances in radial basis function networks (1999). http://www.anc.ed.ac.uk/rbf/papers/recad.ps

3. Kubat, M.: Decision trees can initialize radial basis function networks. http://citeseerx.ist.psu.edu/viewdoc/download?doi=10.1.1.43.6674&rep=rep1&type=pdf

4. Schwenker, F., Kestler, H.A., Palm, G.: Three learning phases for radial-basis-function networks (2001). http://sci2s.ugr.es/keel/pdf/specific/articulo/skg01.pdf

5. Kohonen, T.: Learning vector quantization. In: Arbib, M.A. (ed.) The Handbook of Brain Theory and Neural Networks, pp. 537–540. MIT Press, Cambridge (1995)

6. Schwenker F., Kestler H.A., Palm, G.: 3-D Visual Object Classification with Hierarchical Radial Basis Function Networks. http://www.uni-ulm.de/fileadmin/website_uni_ulm/iui/Ulmer_Informatik_Berichte/2001/UIB_2001-02.pdf

7. Cortes, C., Vapnik, V.: Support-vector networks (1995). http://image.diku.dk/imagecanon/material/cortes_vapnik95.pdf

8. Wettschereck, D., Dietterich, D.: Improving the performance of the radial basis function networks by learning center locations. http://papers.nips.cc/paper/544-improving-the-performance-of-radial-basis-function-networks-by-learning-center-locations.pdf

9. Chen, S., Grant, P.M., Cowan, C.F.N.: Orthogonal least-squares algorithm for training multi-output radial basis function networks (1992). https://cours.etsmtl.ca/sys828/REFS/B3/Chen_IEEE1992.pdf

10. Gomm, B.J., Yu, D.L.: Selecting radial basis function network centers with recursive orthogonal least-squares training (2000). http://ieeexplore.ieee.org/xpl/login.jsp?tp=&arnumber=839002

11. De Castro, L.N., Von Zuben, F.J.: An immunological approach to initialize centers of radial basis function neural networks (2001). http://www.dca.fee.unicamp.br/~vonzuben/research/lnunes_dout/artigos/cbrn01.pdf

12. Yousef, R., el Hindi, K.: Training radial basis function networks using reduced sets as center points. http://citeseerx.ist.psu.edu/viewdoc/download?doi=10.1.1.131.4275&rep=rep1&type=pdf

13. Vachkov, G., Stoyanov, V., Christova, N.: Growing RBF network models for solving nonlinear approximation and classification problems (2015). http://www.scs-europe.net/dlib/2015/ecms2015acceptedpapers/0481-is_ECMS2015_0053.pdf

14. Billing, A.S., Zheng, G.L.: Radial basis function network configuration using genetic algorithms. http://www.sciencedirect.com/science/article/pii/089360809500029Y

15. Fasshauer, G.E., Zhang, J.G.: On choosing "optimal" shape parameters for RBF approximation. http://www.math.iit.edu/~fass/Dolomites.pdf

16. Hoffmann, G.A.: Adaptive transfer functions in radial basis function (RBF) networks. In: Bubak, M., Albada, G.D., Sloot, Peter M.A., Dongarra, J. (eds.) ICCS 2004. LNCS, vol. 3037, pp. 682–686. Springer, Heidelberg (2004). doi:10.1007/978-3-540-24687-9_102. http://www.citemaster.net/get/a719201c-fb59-11e3-8a7f-00163e009cc7/hoffmann04adaptive.pdf

17. Duch, W., Jankowski, N.: Transfer functions: hidden probabilities for better neural networks. https://www.elen.ucl.ac.be/Proceedings/esann/esannpdf/es2001-400.pdf

18. Dorffner, G.: A unified framework for MLPs and RBFNs: introducing conic section functions networks. http://citeseerx.ist.psu.edu/viewdoc/download?doi=10.1.1.49.7264&rep=rep1&type=pdf

19. Mongillo, M.: Choosing basis functions and shape parameters for radial basis function methods. https://www.siam.org/students/siuro/vol4/S01084.pdf

20. Webb, R.A., Shennon, S.: Shape-adaptive radial basis functions. http://ieeexplore.ieee.org/xpl/login.jsp?tp=&arnumber=728359

21. Bengio, Y., Courville, A., Vincent, P.: Representation learning: a review and new perspectives. http://www.cl.uni-heidelberg.de/courses/ws14/deepl/BengioETAL12.pdf

22. Wang, X.: The application of deep kernel machines to various types of data. https://uwaterloo.ca/computational-mathematics/sites/ca.computational-mathematics/files/uploads/files/shirly_project.pdf

23. Bengio, Y., LeCun, Y.: Scaling learning algorithms towards AI. http://cseweb.ucsd.edu/~gary/cs200/s12/bengio-lecun-07.pdf

24. Bengio, Y.: Learning deep architecture for AI. http://www.iro.umontreal.ca/~bengioy/papers/ftml_book.pdf

25. Cho, Y.: Kernel methods for deep learning. http://citeseerx.ist.psu.edu/viewdoc/download?doi=10.1.1.387.4491&rep=rep1&type=pdf

26. LeCun, Y., Bengio, Y.: Convolutional networks for images, speech and time-series. http://yann.lecun.com/exdb/publis/pdf/lecun-bengio-95a.pdf

27. Vincent, P., Larochelle, H., Lajoie, I., Bengio, Y., Manzagol, P.A.: Stacked denoising auto-encoders: learning useful representations in a deep network using local denoising criteria. http://www.jmlr.org/papers/volume11/vincent10a/vincent10a.pdf

28. Hinton, G.E., Osindero, S., Teh, Y.-W.: A fast learning algorithm for deep-belief nets. https://www.cs.toronto.edu/~hinton/nipstutorial/nipstut3.pdf

29. Cho, Y., Saul, K.: Large margin classification in infinite neural networks. http://cseweb.ucsd.edu/~yoc002/paper/neco_arccos.pdf

30. Bouvrie, J., Rosasco, L., Poggio, T.: On invariance in hierarchical models. http://papers.nips.cc/paper/3732-on-invariance-in-hierarchical-models.pdf

31. Bo, L., Ren, X., Fox, D.: Kernel descriptors for visual recognition. http://www.cs.washington.edu/robotics/postscripts/kdes-nips-10.pdf

32. Bo, L., Lai, K., Ren, X., Fox, D.: Object recognition with hierarchical kernel descriptors. http://www.cs.washington.edu/robotics/postscripts/hkdes-cvpr-11.pdf

33. Mairal, J., Koniusz, P., Harchaoui, Z., Schmid, C.: Convolutional kernel networks. http://arxiv.org/pdf/1406.3332v2.pdf

34. Zhuang, J., Tsang, I.W., Hoi, S.C.H.: Two-layer multiple kernel learning. http://jmlr.csail.mit.edu/proceedings/papers/v15/zhuang11a/zhuang11a.pdf, http://www.di.ens.fr/~fbach/skm_icml.pdf

35. Huang, P.-S., Avron, H., Sainath, T.N., Sindhvani, V., Ramabhadran, B.: Kernel methods match deep neural networks on TIMIT. http://www.ifp.illinois.edu/~huang146/papers/Kernel_DNN_ICASSP2014.pdf

36. Jose, C., Goyal, P., Aggrwal, P., Varma, M.: Local deep kernel learning for efficient non-linear SVM prediction. http://research.microsoft.com/en-us/um/people/manik/pubs%5Cjose13.pdf

37. Yger, F., Berar, M., Gasso, G., Rakotomamonjy, A.: A supervised strategy for deep kernel machine. https://www.elen.ucl.ac.be/Proceedings/esann/esannpdf/es2011-21.pdf

38. Schölkopf, B., Smola, A., Müller, K.-R.: Kernel principal component analysis. In: Gerstner, W., Germond, A., Hasler, M., Nicoud, J.-D. (eds.) ICANN 1997. LNCS, vol. 1327, pp. 583–588. Springer, Heidelberg (1997). doi:10.1007/BFb0020217. http://www.ics.uci.edu/~welling/classnotes/papers_class/Kernel-PCA.pdf

39. Ng, A.Y., Jordan, M.I., Weiss, Y.: On spectral clustering analysis and an algorithm. http://ai.stanford.edu/~ang/papers/nips01-spectral.pdf

40. Welling, M.: Kernel canonical correlation analysis. http://www.ics.uci.edu/~welling/classnotes/papers_class/kCCA.pdf

41. Wiering, M.A., Schutten, M., Millea, A., Meijster, A., Schomaker, L.R.B.: Deep support vector machines for regression problems. http://www.ai.rug.nl/~mwiering/GROUP/ARTICLES/DSVM_extended_abstract.pdf

42. Takeda, H., Farsiu, S., Milanfar, P.: Kernel regression for image processing and reconstruction. http://people.duke.edu/~sf59/KernelRegression_Final.pdf

43. Unsupervised kernel regression for non-linear dimensionality reduction. http://www.iro.umontreal.ca/~memisevr/pubs/ukr.pdf

44. Memisevic, R.: Unsupervised kernel dimension reduction. http://www.cs.berkeley.edu/~jordan/papers/wang-sha-jordan-nips11.pdf

45. http://deeplearning.net/datasets/

46. https://archive.ics.uci.edu/ml/datasets.html,   https://physionet.org/physiobank/database/#multi

Improving the Probability of Clinical Diagnosis of Coronary-Artery Disease Using Extended Kalman Filters with Radial Basis Function Network

Mashail Alsalamah$^{(\boxtimes)}$ and Saad Amin

Faculty of Engineering and Computing, Coventry University,
Priory Street, Coventry CV1 5FB, UK
alsalam2@coventry.ac.uk

Abstract. Kalman filters have been popular in applications to predict time-series data analysis and prediction. This paper uses a form of Extended Kalman Filter to predict the occurrence of CAD (Coronary Artery Disease) using patients data based on different relevant parameters. The work takes a novel approach by using different neural networks training algorithms Quasi-Newton and SCG with combination of activation functions to predict the existence/non-existence of CAD in a patient based on patient's data set. The prediction probability of this combination is resulted in accuracy of about 92% or above, using cross validation and thresholding to remove the limitation of time-series prediction introduced because of the Extended Kalman filter behavior.

Keywords: Coronary artery disease · Extended kalman filter · Radial basis function · Quasi-Newton and Scaled Conjugate Gradient

1 Introduction

Medical diagnosis is a vast subject and there have been several ways and methodologies, which are pure medical and depend upon the physicians. However, with advancement in computing technologies and artificial intelligence lot have been done to diagnose complex diseases using available data and patient information and symptoms. CAD is one such disease, which is a complex condition of artery blockage with high mortality figures [1] and it is not straight forward for ordinary staff to detect this disease.

A host of factors are used in the diagnosis of CAD, and these include patient's blood pressure, cholesterol, sugar levels, high BMI (overweight/obese), physical inactivity, unhealthy eating, and smoking [2]. Other factors such as age, gender, and family history of heart disease are also likely risk factors for CAD (British Heart Foundation, 2015; National Heart, Lung and Blood Institute, 2015) [3].

This research explores the application of a data fusion algorithm (Kalman filtering) in diagnosing CAD, as well as in the prediction of the need to conduct a Coronary Artery Bypass Graft (CABG) in patients identified as having CAD.

© ICST Institute for Computer Sciences, Social Informatics and Telecommunications Engineering 2017
P. Perego et al. (Eds.): MobiHealth 2016, LNICST 192, pp. 269–277, 2017.
DOI: 10.1007/978-3-319-58877-3_35

Kalman filters (KF) [4] are generally used for applications such as navigation, as their ability to accurately predict next points based on the history of tracking and travel; the success of these algorithms lie in the fact that the model considers measurement noise between present and future points. The novel application of data fusion algorithm in this research precisely entails the derivation of Kalman filter equations that facilitate the recursive calculation of two terms/factors of interest stated earlier (i.e., CAD status and CABG requirement). This process uses a combination of knowledge/observations/measurements from patients, predictions from systems models and inherent noise in the observations/measurements.

The rest of the paper is divided into four sections; Sect. 2 covers the literature review to describe the work done in detection of CAD and use of Kalman Filtering in disease diagnosis; Sect. 3 will discuss the methodology and principles of this novel approach of the Extended Kalman filtering and radial basis functions. Section 4 will enlighten with the procedure of the testing and verification of the patient data set. Section 5 will present the results and analysis of the test runs and the combinations of different training and activation algorithms. Finally Sect. 6 summarizes the work and gives pointers towards the future work.

2 Literature Review

Nonetheless, over the years, Automatic Computer-Assisted Detection processes have been used in the diagnosis of CADs. With linear and logistic regression model frequently used [6–10]. Other commonly used predictive models are the Linear Discriminant Analysis, K-nearest Neighbor Classifier, Artificial Neural Network and Support Vector Machine [11–13]. These models have to some extent been shown to be of some predictive value. For example, [16] showed that the prediction accuracy of training and test sets of Linear Discriminant Analysis could be as high as 90.6% and 72.7% respectively, while [11] showed that Artificial Neural Networks could produce accuracy in test set that is as high as 81.2%. In spite these reasonable results; there are apparent limitations in most of these learning algorithms. The Linear Regression and the Linear Discriminant Analysis are both linear techniques and cannot be extended to consider non-linear modalities (variables) which are inevitable in the proper diagnosis of CAD. As a way of circumventing this issue, research in this field has also considered the use of more complex models such as the combination of Support Vector Machine with a Radial Basis Function (RBF) Kernel, Support Vector Machine optimized by particle swarm optimization or other forms of integration of two individual approaches to generate a non-linear technique [14–16]. The result of this is an improvement in the prediction accuracy of training and test sets (for example, as high as 96.9% [11]).

These facts show that there are obviously more room for improvements. One important way of going about this process of improvement, which is yet to be well exploited, is by enhancing the quality of the data sets used in the prediction. This could be done by developing novel means that reduce noise and inconsistency in data. Measures of capability or predictability of algorithms such as validation error are affected by the variations in data (e.g., high level of missing data, which is inherent in the sets of data often used in CAD diagnosis/prediction as these data sets come from multiple sources – oral interviews, doctors' examinations and technical measurements with different instruments). A potential candidate for improving data quality is the Matrix Completion, which is a process that entails the addition of entries to a matrix which contains some unknown/missing values. Research has shown that how the Matrix Completion could greatly help enhance the accuracy of prediction [17, 18].

Furthermore, another step in the advancement of this realm of research could also be in the potentially novel adoption and application of hybrid Extended Kalman Filter (EKF) in the prediction/diagnosis of CAD. The Kalman Filter (KF) is a well-established estimation theory that has been in existence since the 1960 s. Though the initially designed filter provides recursive solution through a linear optimal filtering for estimating desired parameters, the extended version of the filter (i.e., Extended Kalman Filter – EKF) has the capability to handle non-linear systems/conditions [19].This learning algorithm has been used in diverse research realms and has shown excellent results in terms of prediction accuracy [21, 22]). Nonetheless, the EKF's alluring capabilities are yet to be explored in the area of Coronary Artery Disease prediction. This is most likely due to the lack of awareness about its existence, as majority of researchers in this realm of research and beyond are more familiar with the KF which can only provide a recursive solution through a linear means.

3 Methodology

The suitability of the RBF (Radial Basis Function) Neural network models for classification problems such as detection of diseases, in our case occurrence of CAD. There has been several steps involved in the determination of this classification problem, in this section a brief on the methodology steps is provided (Fig. 1).

A. Data set Classification

The study is based on Saudi Arabia population, in King Abdullah Medical City (KAMC). The obtained data set needs to be classified and pre-processed before been applied to the RBF network. The purpose of this work is to find a relationship between existence/non-existence of CAD based on the variables; namely, demographic variables like age, gender, occupation, physical variables like height, weight, smoking habit, medical history among others. There were 59 independent variables in the data. The frequency distribution of each of them were studied to ensure further modifications, if any, to fit in the model and to eliminate data entry errors. Mismatched entries were found and were considered as "no information" and tagged as 0 in required cases. The details of the analysis and classification of data based on their statistics is author's work in [19].

B. Matrix Completion

Matrix completion has been used as secondary techniques to condition the patient data. Due to several recording, interview and manual entry deficiencies the patient data has some anomalies, in certain cases missing of several or one of the major contributing fields. One of the possible solution so that the erroneous or missing data does not disturb the estimation process a simpler way is to discard the patients information,

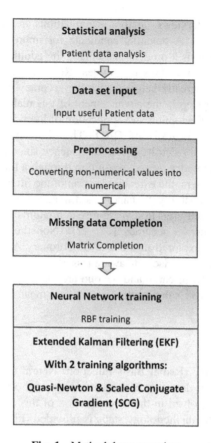

Fig. 1. Methodology overview

however due to scarcity of the patient information from the source (check acknowledgement section), there was a requirement not to discard any such data. Therefore Matrix completion techniques were used to improve the prediction efficiency. Although this has not provided a high percentage of accuracy, though helped to use patient information with less number of missing fields and higher confidence in the MC results have been included in the study. Exact Matrix Completion via Convex Optimization is used in this work to improve the data quality and availability.

C. Kalman Matrix

The Kalman Filter gain is a time-varying gain matrix. It is given by the algorithm presented below. In the expressions below the following matrices are used and shown in Fig. 2.

- Auto-covariance matrix (for lag zero) of the estimation error of the corrected estimate:
- Auto-covariance matrix (for lag zero) of the estimation error of the predicted estimate:

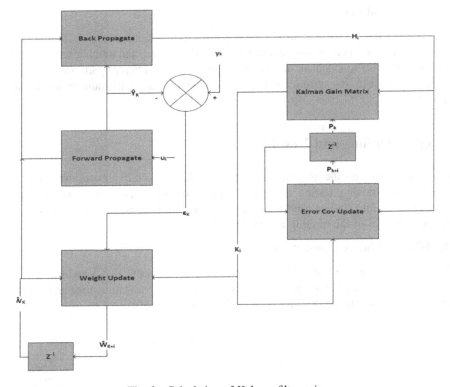

Fig. 2. Calculation of Kalman filter gain

- The transition matrix A of a linearized model of the original nonlinear model calculated with the most recent state estimate, which is assumed to be the corrected estimate xc(k):
- Given the continuous-time nonlinear process model. Linearize it at the operating point to obtain
- Then calculate A = A discrete as the discretized version of A continuous. Forward method of discretization in manual calculations can be used; however in this case Matlab is used to discretize this function.

4   Procedure

The main theme of this classification solution is to optimize the network and then validate the results. This is mainly divided into three steps i.e. train test and validate.

If enough data is available then we can divide the data for training and testing based on the inputs and the outputs. This way several models trained on the training set will be available to be applied on the test set. The best result on the test set based on these several trained models is then considered as the optimal simulation.

D. Cross Validation

The discussed above can introduce a bias towards a particular data set. Therefore, in this case the data set can be portioned and swapped as testing and training sets to negate this bias and also to calculate an average based on these different partitions.

The data set in this system has been divided to three sections training, testing and validation.

5   Observations and Results

The experiment uses the hospital data set and makes three different combinations, by swapping the training, testing and validation sets. In this experiment the two different training algorithms will be used with the different combinations of the data sets to see the performance of the training algorithms

E. Without Matrix Completion

The results of the four different combinations are given in the Fig. 3 and the Table 1 shows the details, including training errors, testing errors, validation error and the best iteration in each training algorithm for each of the three sets.

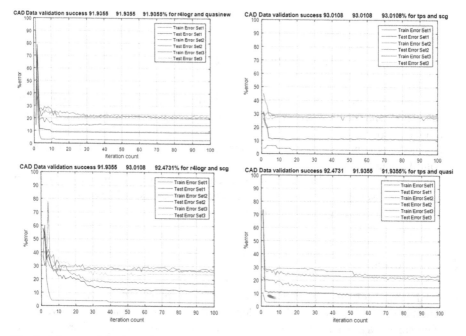

Fig. 3. Three combinations of data sets and 4 different training and activation functions without matrix completion

Table 1. Summary of the best result obtained from the observations shown for Fig. 1

Combinations of training algorithms & activation functions		Best results of Data sets														
		Set No 1					Set No 2					Set No 3				
Training Algo	Act Fcn	Train Error %	Test Error %	Valid Error %	Accuracy %	Best Iter	Train Error %	Test Error %	Valid Error %	Accrcy %	Best Iter	Train Error %	Test Error %	Valid Error %	Accuracy %	Best iter
Quasi New	R4R	21.33	3.00	8.06	91.9%	4	14.67	21	8.06	91.9%	15	9.00	21.00	8.06	91.9%	13
Quasi New	Tps	26.33	3.00	7.53	92.47%	3	15.00	23.00	8.06	91.9%	22	9.00	23.00	8.06	91.9%	90
SCG	R4R	27.33	3.00	6.99	93.01%	30	27.33	3.00	8.06	91.4%	39	12.00	26.00	7.53	92.47%	58
SCG	Tps	27.67	3.00	6.99	93.01%	17	19.00	26.00	6.99	93.01%	3	11.67	28.00	6.99	93.01%	5

*Training Algo: Training Algorithm
*Act Fcn: Activation Function
*Valid Error: Validation error
*Best iter: Best Iteration

F. With Matrix Completion

The results of the four different combinations are given in the Fig. 4 and the Table 2 shows the details, including training errors, testing errors, validation error and the best iteration in each training algorithm for each of the three sets after Matrix completion.

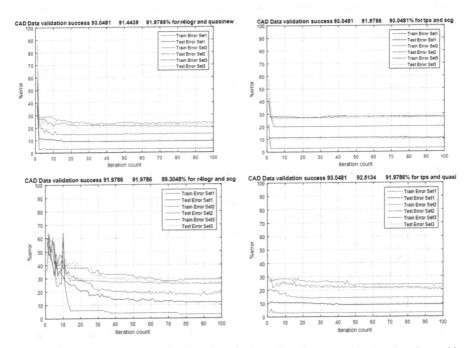

Fig. 4. Three combinations of data sets and 4 different training and activation functions with matrix completion

Table 2. Summary of the Best result obtained from the observations shown for Fig. 2

Combinations of training algorithms & activation functions		Best results of Data sets															
		Set No 1					Set No 2					Set No 3					
Training Algo	Act Fcn	Train Error %	Test Error %	Valid Error%	Accuracy %	Iter no	Train Error %	Test Error %	Valid Error%	Accuracy %	Iter no	Train Error %	Test Error %	Valid Error %	Accuracy %	Best iter
Quasi New	R4R	28.33	3.00	6.95	93.0%	2	20.00	21.00	8.56	91.4%	3	9.00	23.00	8.02	91.9%	29
Quasi New	Tps	28.67	3.00	10.70	93.0%	1	14.67	22.00	7.49	92.5%	21	9.00	23.00	8.02	91.9%	49
SCG	R4R	26.00	3.00	8.02	91.9%	76	11.33	27.00	8.02	91.9%	81	12.33	28.00	10.70	89.3%	66
SCG	Tps	27.67	3.00	6.95	93.0%	2	23.67	25.00	8.02	91.9%	3	11.33	27.00	6.95	93.0%	3

*Training Algo: Training Algorithm
*Act Fcn: Activation Function
*Valid Error: Validation error
*Best iter: Best Iteration

6 Conclusion

This work deals with the prediction of Coronary artery disease by applying the patient information as a set of data feed to the RBF neural network. The training of these neural networks is based on the prediction strength of Extended Kalman filters and combination of training algorithms. The work still need to be investigated and that suggests that it's possible that ensemble of the classifiers trained on different part of the dataset might have a greater performance.

Acknowledgment. We are very thankful to King Abdullah Medical City in Saudi Arabia for providing the patient data to be used in this study.

References

1. WHO: WHO World Health Organization, January 2015. http://www.who.int/mediacentre/factsheets/fs317/en/. Accessed 6 Mar 2016
2. NIH: What is Coronary Heart Disease, National Institute of Health, 3 October 2015. http://www.nhlbi.nih.gov/health/health-topics/topics/cad. Accessed 6 Mar 2016
3. British Heart Foundation: Risk factors (2015). https://www.bhf.org.uk/heart-health/risk-factors. Accessed 6 Mar 2016
4. Wan, E.A., Van Der Merwe, R.: The unscented Kalman filter for nonlinear estimation. In: The IEEE Conference on Adaptive Systems for Signal Processing, Communications, and Control Symposium 2000, AS-SPCC (2000)
5. Julier, S.J., Uhlmann, J.K.: New extension of the Kalman filter to nonlinear systems. In: AeroSense 1997 International Society for Optics and Photonics (1997)
6. Genders, T.S.S., Steyerberg, E.W., Hunink, M.G.M., Nieman, K.: Prediction model to estimate presence of coronary artery disease: Retrospective pooled analysis of existing cohorts. Br. Med. J. **344**, 1–13 (2012)
7. Yamada, H., Do, D., Morise, A., Atwood, J.E., Froeliche, V.: Review of studies using multivariable analysis of clinical and exercise test data to predict angiographic coronary artery disease. Prog. Cardiovasc. Dis. **39**, 457–481 (1997)

8. Pryor, D.B., Harrell, F.E., Lee, K.L., Califf, R.M., Rosati, R.A.: Estimating the likelihood of significant coronary artery disease. Am. J. Med. **75**, 771–780 (1983)
9. Diamond, G.A., Forrester, J.S.: Analysis of probability as an aid in the clinical diagnosis of coronary artery disease. N. Engl. J. Med. **300**, 1350–1358 (1979)
10. Kalman, R.: A new approach to linear filtering and prediction problems. J. Basic Eng. **83**, 35–45 (1960). Transaction of the ASME
11. Heydari, S.T., Ayatollahi, S.M.T., Zare, N.: Comparison of artificial neural networks with logistic regression for detection of obesity. J. Med. Syst. **36**(4), 2449–2454 (2012)
12. Hongzong, S., Tao, W., Xiaojun, Y., Huanxiang, L., Zhide, H., Mancang, L., BoTao, F.: Support vector machines classification for discriminating coronary heart disease patients from non-coronary heart disease. West Indian Med. J. **56**(5), 451–457 (2007)
13. Hedeshi, N.G., Abadeh, M.S.: Coronary artery disease detection using a fuzzy-boosting PSO approach. Comput. Intell. Neurosci 6 (2014)
14. Karabulut, E.M., İbrikçi, T.: Effective diagnosis of coronary artery disease using the rotation forest ensemble method. J. Med. Syst. **36**, 3011–3018 (2012)
15. Oh, S.: Matrix Completion: Fundamental Limits and Efficient Algorithms. Stanford University, California (2010)
16. Wu, T.T., Lange, K.: Matrix completion discriminant analysis. Comput. Stat. Data Anal. **92**, 115–125 (2015)
17. Arif, M., Malagore, I.A., Afsar, F.A.: Detection and localization of myocardial infarction using K-nearest neighbor classifier. J. Med. Syst. **36**, 279–289 (2010)
18. Comak, E.: A biomedical decision support system using LS-SVM classifier with an efficient and new parameter regularization procedure for diagnosis of heart valve diseases. J. Med. Syst. **36**, 549–556 (2010)
19. Salamah, M.: The Statistic analysis Study of Coronary-Artery Disease Data Based on King Abdullah Medical City in Saudi Arabia (KAMC-CAD). Coventry (2016)
20. Haykin, S.: Kalman Filtering and Neural Networks. Wiley, New York (2001)
21. Sepasi, S., Ghorbani, R., Liaw, B.Y.: Improved extended kalman filter for state of charge estimation of battery pack. J. Power Sources **255**, 368–376 (2014)
22. Sun, X., Jin, L., Xiong, M.: Extended Kalman filter for estimation of parameters in nonlinear state-space models of biochemical networks. PLoS ONE **3**(11), 1–13 (2008)

A Hypothetical Reasoning System for Mobile Health and Wellness Applications

Aniello Minutolo[✉], Massimo Esposito, and Giuseppe De Pietro

Institute for High Performance Computing and Networking, ICAR-CNR,
Via P. Castellino, 111, 80131 Naples, Italy
{aniello.minutolo,massimo.esposito,
giuseppe.depietro}@icar.cnr.it

Abstract. In the last years, rule-based systems have been used in mobile health and wellness applications for embedding and reasoning over domain-specific knowledge and suggesting actions to perform. However, often, no sufficient information is available to infer definite indications about the action to perform and one or more hypothesis should be formulated and evaluated with respect to their possible impacts. In order to face this issue, this paper proposes a mobile hypothetical reasoning system able to evaluate set of hypotheses, infer their outcomes and support the user in choosing the best one. In particular, it offers facilities to: (i) build specific scenarios starting from different initial hypothesis formulated by the user; (ii) optimize them by eliminating common domain-specific elements and avoiding their processing more than once; (iii) efficiently evaluate a set of logic rules over the optimized scenarios directly on the mobile devices and infer the logical consequences by providing timely responses and limiting the consumption of their resources. A case study has been arranged in order to evaluate the system's effectiveness within a mobile application for managing personal diets according to daily caloric needs.

Keywords: Hypothetical reasoning · Rule-based systems · Mobile health and wellness applications

1 Introduction

In the last years, the growing availability of mobile phones and wearable devices has enabled the development of new mobile health and wellness applications able to continuously support individuals anywhere and anytime. These applications are often designed on the top of rule-based systems, since these latter enable the reproduction of explicit deductive reasoning mechanisms on the basis of the explicit formalization of logic production rules built on the top of domain-specific knowledge.

A production rule is usually made of a conjunction of condition elements to satisfy, in its left-hand side (LHS), and a set of action elements in its right-hand side (RHS), respectively. A rule-based system checks whether LHSs hold against a knowledge base including a representation of domain-specific elements, named facts, and, in case the LHS of a rule is satisfied, the corresponding RHS of the rule is inferred. Thanks to these

© ICST Institute for Computer Sciences, Social Informatics and Telecommunications Engineering 2017
P. Perego et al. (Eds.): MobiHealth 2016, LNICST 192, pp. 278–286, 2017.
DOI: 10.1007/978-3-319-58877-3_36

capabilities of embedding and reasoning over domain-specific knowledge, rule-based systems have been profitably used in mobile health and wellness applications to suggest actions to perform with the aim of enhancing quality of care, improving adherence to therapies and supporting wellness and healthy lifestyles.

However, often, missing knowledge can arise and rule-based systems embedded in mobile applications are not able to suggest a specific indication to follow or action to perform. Indeed, no sufficient domain-specific elements are available to prove truth or falsity of the condition elements of their rules and, thus, to infer definite suggestions. In such cases, the user is directly asked for making a decision, even though he/she is not able to formulate it based on the available knowledge. To address this issue, rule-based systems should support a form of hypothetical reasoning, where, first, one or more assumptions are made on missing information, then they are processed to draw a set of outcomes, and, finally, these latter are evaluated with respect to their possible impacts in order to support the user in his/her final choice. To the best of our knowledge, none of the existing approaches has been designed by considering the specific requirements of mobile health and wellness applications and, thus, they may result inadequate or intractable on mobile devices due to their limited resources. Indeed, the generation and evaluation of one or more hypothesis could be computationally intensive to be performed directly on mobile devices, with the risk of exhausting their computing and memorization resources, if not properly optimized.

Starting from these considerations, this paper proposes a mobile hypothetical reasoning system able to evaluate set of hypotheses, with the assumption that they must be alternatives among them, directly on mobile devices. In particular, it offers facilities to: (i) build specific scenarios starting from different initial hypothesis formulated by the user; (ii) optimize them by eliminating common domain-specific elements and avoiding their processing more than once; (iii) efficiently evaluate a set of logic rules over the optimized scenarios on the mobile devices and infer the logical consequences by providing timely responses and limiting the consumption of their resources. A case study has been arranged in order to evaluate the system's effectiveness within a mobile wellness application for managing personal diets according to daily caloric needs.

In the following, Sect. 2 introduces background and related work. In Sect. 3, the mobile hypothetical reasoning system is presented, whereas the case of study is described in Sect. 4. Finally, Sect. 5 concludes the work.

2   Background and Related Work

Hypothetical reasoning is a form of reasoning that considers the possibility of uncertain or incomplete knowledge. A typical hypothetical reasoning system tries to explain an observation by dividing the knowledge base into many possible assumptions, in order to provide evidence against hypotheses by testing their logical consequences [1, 2]. Existing approaches to hypothetical reasoning are mainly designed as Truth Maintenance Systems (TMSs). In detail, given an observation and a set of assumptions, a TMS is able to perform: (i) the evaluation of the coexistence and contradictions of assumptions; (ii) the retraction of not viable assumptions; (iii) the preservation of existing dependencies among the valid assumptions and the inferred beliefs. A pioneer hypothetical reasoning system is presented in [3], which consists into a TMS able to evaluate different assumptions and work as a cache by storing all inferences (justifications) made on the basis of the defined assumptions.

An Assumption-based TMS is proposed in [4, 5], which is able to manipulate both justifications and assumptions, i.e. each belief is labeled with the set of assumptions under which it holds, besides the justifications that support it. Some recent works have been focused on the automatic generation of hypotheses when a piece of knowledge is missing, on the basis of preconfigured admitted assumptions. These approaches typically demand a lot of computational resources spent in combinatorial calculations for evaluating conflicts and overlays in computed scenarios [6, 7].

Summarizing, none of these existing approaches is specifically thought to be executed directly on mobile devices, and even if a desktop-oriented TMS could be adapted for being applied to mobile health and wellness scenarios, it might soon become intractable due to the great amount of information stored and maintained. Moreover, this adaption may represent a useless waste of computational and memorization resources on mobile devices, since the possible hypotheses to be considered in the scenarios of interest are mainly alternative among them, and, thus, the complex management of coexisting hypotheses is not required.

All these considerations represent the rationale for the proposed hypothetical reasoning system, which is diffusely described in the next section.

3   The Proposed Hypothetical Reasoning System

The main components of the proposed hypothetical reasoning system, organized according to a typical layered software architecture, are shown in Fig. 1.

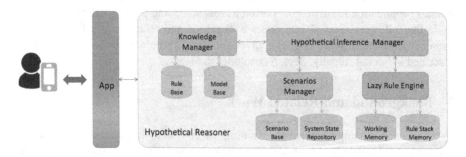

Fig. 1. The main components of the proposed reasoning system.

In detail, the **Knowledge Manager** (KM) and the **Hypothetical Inference Manager** (HIM) are the main interfaces between the reasoning system and other application components. The HIM manages the hypothetical reasoning cycle and it is in charge of invoking other components in order to ensure the correct flow of inference execution, the proper knowledge updating, and the notification of inference outcomes to external components.

The KM is responsible of handling knowledge repositories containing the domain knowledge and the procedural rule set encoding the behavior of the application. In this respect, the **Model Base** (MB) is the repository containing the terminological knowledge, which describes the specific domain in terms of classes and properties. It usually contains the significant assertional knowledge of the domain, i.e. collections of facts, encoded as individuals (instances of concepts) with the corresponding instances of properties. All the information stored in the MB is codified in the N-Triples serialization of OWL language [8], in the form of collections of subject, predicate and object elements. This solution ensures decidability over expressive power and offers a lightweight format for ontologies, which results easier to parse and process in mobile applications [9]. The **Rule Base** (RB) is the repository where production rules are stored. To this aim, a subset of the Jena rule language [10] is used, since it is suitable for being parsed on resource-limited settings, and its predicates include classes and properties encoded as N-Triples. The **Scenarios Manager** (SM) is in charge of defining and evaluating the hypotheses created by the user. In detail, given the ontology O describing domain-specific knowledge, and denoted with R the set of production rules built on top of the ontology O, the couple $K = (O, R)$ can be referred as the knowledge base of the system. When a reasoning process is performed on K, the set $Th(K)$ of logical consequences generated on the basis of K can be eventually used for updating the ontology O according to the executed rules. Given the set C of concepts defined in O, and the set I of possible instances of C, a hypothesis h built on the basis of I is an unordered list of n elements of I, where n is a positive integer, such that $h \cup O$ is semantically consistent.

Note that, given n hypotheses $h_1, \ldots, h_n$ defined by the user, they represent alternative actions that he/she wants to evaluate for determining the best one to choose according to the possible inference outcomes produced by the system. Starting from them, a set of n hypothetical scenarios $S(h_1), \ldots, S(h_n)$ are built on the basis of the domain knowledge and must be submitted to the HIM for evaluating their logical consequences. However, since the hypothetical scenarios can be determined as $S(h_1) = (h_1 \cup O, R) \ldots S(h_n) = (h_n \cup O, R)$, they can often share common domain knowledge that will be evaluated repeatedly when more scenarios are submitted to the HIM. To face this issue, the SM is also in charge of modifying these scenarios, before submitting them to the HIM, with the goal of reducing the amount of information to be processed during their evaluation. In detail, all the knowledge characterizing the hypothetical scenarios are processed for determining the common elements, which can be defined as follows:

$$O_c[S(h_1), \ldots, S(h_n)] = \bigcap_{i=1}^n [h_i \cup O] = O \cup \left[\bigcap_{i=1}^n h_i\right]$$

In this way, a hypothetical "base scenario" $Sc(h_1, \ldots, h_n) = [O_c(h_1, \ldots, h_n), R]$ is automatically determined, representing the common knowledge elements shared among the n hypotheses $h_1, \ldots, h_n$ defined by the user. Such a knowledge will produce the same consequences in all the hypotheses and, thus, should be processed only once for reducing the computational and memorization resources involved during the evaluation of the hypothetical scenarios. In fact, the distinctive knowledge drawn by the scenarios can be determined by re-using the results of the $\mathbf{Th}[Sc(h_1, \ldots, h_n)]$:

$$\mathbf{Th}[S(h_1)] = \mathbf{Th}[Sc(h_1, \ldots, h_n)] \cup \mathbf{Th}[S'(h_1)] \ldots$$
$$\mathbf{Th}[S(h_n)] = \mathbf{Th}[Sc(h_1, \ldots, h_n)] \cup \mathbf{Th}[S'(h_n)]$$

where the sets $S'(h_1), \ldots, S'(h_n)$ are composed as follows:

$$S'(h_1) = [h_1 \bigcup O - O_c(h_1, \ldots, h_n), R] \ldots$$
$$S'(h_n) = [h_n \bigcup O - O_c(h_1, \ldots, h_n), R]$$

Finally, the $n + 1$ scenarios $[Sc(h_1, \ldots, h_n), S'(h_1), \ldots, S'(h_n)]$ are stored in the repository named **Scenario Base** (SB) and, successively, submitted to the HIM for their evaluation. In this respect, the HIM repeatedly configures and invokes the **Lazy Rule Engine** (LRE), which is based on a lazy pattern matching algorithm, proposed by the authors in [9] and specifically designed and implemented as a light-weight solution suitable for resource-limited mobile devices. By exploiting this algorithm, the LRE is able to provide timely responses without maintaining complex memory structures for processing all the rules contained in the RB. In detail, the LRE evaluates all the rules stored in the RB with respect to the domain knowledge elements characterizing each hypothetical scenario, which are maintained and updated into the **Working Memory** (WM). The current state of this rule evaluation process is maintained into the **Rule Stack Memory** (RSM), in order to enable the possibility of pausing and resuming the search for rule instances that have to be still assessed and eventually executed. At each reasoning cycle, the content of both WM and RSM represents the system's state and is stored into the **System State Repository** (SSR). In particular, when the common scenario $Sc(h_1, \ldots, h_n)$ is evaluated, the LRE generates the logical consequences drawn from it, i.e. Output($Sc(h_1, \ldots, h_n)$), and stores it into the SSR. Successively, when the other n scenarios $[S'(h_1), \ldots, S'(h_n)]$ are considered, Output($Sc(h_1, \ldots, h_n)$) is resumed from SSR, without being recalculated, and is used to incrementally generate the Output $(S'(h_1)), \ldots,$ Output($S'(h_n)$).

Finally, at the end of the scenarios' evaluation, the outcomes generated are returned to the application and presented to the user, with the goal of enabling the user to select the single hypothesis h_{best} to make all its outcomes persistent in the MB.

Summarizing, the global reasoning scheme is the following:

```
Load Sc(h₁,..,hₙ);
Reason;
Output(Sc(h₁,..,hₙ)) = SystemState;
For i=1..n do
    SystemState = Output(Sc(h₁,..,hₙ));
    SystemState = SystemState + S'(hᵢ);
    Reason;
    Output(S'(hᵢ)) = SystemState;
End;
Input(h_best)
SystemState = Output(S'(h_best))
```

4   Case of Study

As a proof of concept, the presented reasoning system has been implemented for mobile devices equipped with the Android platform and embedded within a mobile application for monitoring and managing the personal diet according to daily caloric needs. In detail, the application supports users to monitor the food portions consumed during a meal, over a week of observation and alert him/her when potential abnormal situations are detected (e.g. inadequate or excessive consumption of aliments, with respect to the caloric need of the user). For each aliment, a set of diet recommendations has been formulated describing the right portion of food for a meal, for a day, and for a week. Right portions are distilled in terms of minimum and maximum quantities that are recommended and, respectively, forbidden to consume for a given period.

The domain knowledge describing the health status of the user and stored in the MB has been formalized by means of the ontology model outlined in Fig. 2.

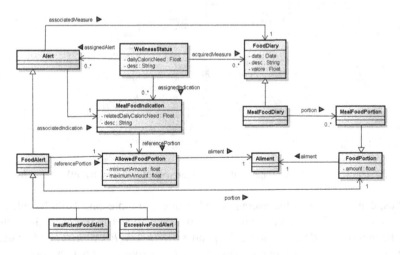

Fig. 2. The ontology model arranged for the case of study considered.

On top of this ontology model, which is diffusely described in [11], a collection of logic rules has been formulated and inserted into the RB of the system. Such rules are aimed at: (i) evaluating the user's daily caloric needs in order to determine the most pertaining diet recommendations; (ii) comparing the selected recommendations with the health status of the user for detecting abnormal food portions; (iii) generating alerts in accordance with the abnormal consumptions detected.

The case of study here considered for this application foresees three possible hypotheses of meals with respect to a personal diet, that are formulated by the user. The hypothesis h_1 consists into a wellness state s composed of 2600 calories as daily caloric needs, and a meal food diary m containing a portion $p1$ of 100 g of fresh cheese, and a portion $p2$ of 350 g of fish. The hypothesis h_2 consists into a wellness state s composed of 2600 calories as daily caloric needs, and a meal food diary m containing a portion $p1$ of 200 g of fresh legumes, and a portion $p2$ of 80 g of meat. Finally, the hypothesis h_3 consists into a wellness state s composed of 2600 calories as daily caloric needs, and a meal food diary m containing a portion $p1$ of 100 g of fresh cheese, and a portion $p2$ of 200 g of fresh legumes.

These hypotheses are submitted to the HIM that interacts with the SM to build three hypothetical scenarios $S(h_1)$, $S(h_2)$, $S(h_3)$ on the top of them by exploiting the ontology model above mentioned. Successively, the SM determines the common knowledge $O_c[S(h_1), S(h_2), S(h_3)]$ among them by calculating the intersection among the scenarios $S(h_1)$, $S(h_2)$, $S(h_3)$ previously computed. In particular, it is worth noting that these hypotheses differ for the type of aliment consumed, and for the number of grams consumed, while the knowledge about the caloric need, and the structure of the objects containing the food portions, is mainly unchanged among them. In detail, with respect to a set of 22 total assertions formulated for encoding the hypotheses h_1, h_2, h_3, a set of 12 assertions has resulted to be shared among them, as reported in Fig. 3.

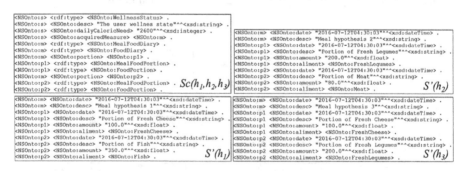

Fig. 3. The scenarios for evaluating the consequences of the meal hypotheses h_1, h_2, h_3.

Thus, denoted with N_c the average number of condition elements in the rules, and denoted with $card(S(h_i))$ the cardinality of the ontology model associated to the scenario $S(h_i)$, the numbers $KB[S(h_1), S(h_2), S(h_3)]$ and $KB[S'(h_1), S'(h_2), S'(h_3)]$ of comparisons required for evaluating the hypotheses h_1, h_2, h_3, before and after the optimization performed by the SM, can be approximately estimated as follows:

$\text{KB}\big[S(h_1), \ldots, S(h_3)\big] = n * \text{card}(O) * \big[\text{card}\big(S(h_1)\big) + \ldots + \text{card}\big(S(h_n)\big)\big]$
$* \text{card}(R) * N_c = 95 * 10^6$

$\text{KB}\big[S'(h_1), \ldots, S'(h_3)\big] = \big[\text{card}(O) + \text{card}(O_c) + \text{card}\big(S'(h_1)\big) + \ldots + \text{card}\big(S'(h_n)\big)\big]$
$* \text{card}(R) * N_c = 490 * 10^3$

where

$n = 3, \text{card}(O) = 2000, \text{card}\big(S(h_i)\big) = 22, \text{card}\big(O_c\big) = 12, \text{card}\big(S'(h_i)\big) = 10, \text{card}(R) = 20, N_c = 12$

As a consequence, the proposed approach enables to drastically reduce the amount of comparisons that are required for comparing rules with the ontology assertions, since all the shared information are computed only once, and properly re-used during the evaluation of each hypothetical scenario. Successively, after the elaboration performed by the SM, the actual scenarios are submitted to the HIM, which repeatedly configures and invokes the LRE for collecting the inference outcomes drawn on the basis of them. In particular, two of the submitted hypotheses generate an excessive food alert, whereas the last one generates no alarm. Thus, the application reports this result to the user, who is enabled to choose the third hypothesis as actual meal to consume.

5 Conclusions

This paper proposes a mobile hypothetical reasoning system able to evaluate set of hypotheses, made on missing information and with the assumption that they must be alternatives among them, infer their outcomes and assess the possible impacts in order to support the user in choosing the best one. Differently from existing solutions, the proposed system is not aimed at automatically generating hypotheses to be validated with respect to specific scenarios and detecting eventual conflicts and overlays. Indeed, the novelty of this system mainly consists into its facilities to: (i) build specific scenarios starting from different initial hypothesis formulated by the user; (ii) optimize them by eliminating common domain-specific elements and avoiding their processing more than once; (iii) efficiently evaluate a set of logic rules over the optimized scenarios directly on the mobile devices and infer the logical consequences by providing timely responses and limiting the consumption of their resources.

A case study has been arranged in order to evaluate the system's effectiveness within a mobile wellness application for managing personal diets according to daily caloric needs, showing its capability of efficiently evaluating scenarios determined on the basis of the hypotheses formulated from the user, as well as reducing the amount of data to process singularly, with respect to the number of comparisons required.

Next step of the research activities will be, on the one hand, to define a more formal and mathematical background to describe the proposed hypothetical reasoning scheme and, on the other hand, to minutely evaluate the performance of the proposed system in terms of computation and memorization resources required when executed in several scenarios and subjected to different load situations.

Acknowledgment. This work has been partially supported by the Italian project "eHealthnet" funded by the Italian Ministry of Education, University, and Research.

References

1. Poole, D., Goebel, R., Aleliunas, R.: Theorist: a logical reasoning system for defaults and diagnosis. In: Cercone, N., McCalla, G. (eds.) Knowledge Frontier: Essays in the Representation of Knowledge, pp. 331–352, Springer, New York (1987)
2. Poole, D.: A logical framework for default reasoning. Artif. Intell. **36**(1), 27–47 (1988)
3. Doyle, J.: A truth maintenance system. Artif. Intell. **12**(3), 231–272 (1979)
4. de Kleer, J.: An assumption-based TMS. Artif. Intell. **28**(2), 127–162 (1986)
5. de Kleer, J.: Extending the ATMS. Artif. Intell. **28**(2), 163–196 (1986)
6. Giannikis, G.K., Daskalopulu, A.: Assumption-based reasoning in dynamic normative agent systems. Web Intell. Agent Syst. **8**(4), 343–362 (2010)
7. Tahara, I.: Computing scenario from knowledge with preferentially ordered hypotheses. Syst. Comput. Jpn. **35**(4), 19–26 (2004)
8. Patel-Schneider, P., Hayes, P., Horrocks, I., et al.: OWL web ontology language semantics and abstract syntax. W3C Recommendation, 10 (2004). http://www.w3.org/TR/owl-semantics/
9. Minutolo, A., Esposito, E., De Pietro, G.: Design and validation of a light-weight reasoning system to support remote health monitoring applications. Eng. Appl. Artif. Intell. **41**, 232–248 (2015)
10. Carroll, J.J., Dickinson, I., Dollin, C., Reynolds, D., Seaborne, A., Wilkinson, K.: Jena: implementing the semantic web recommendations. In: Proceedings of the 13th International World Wide Web Conference on Alternate Track, New York, USA, pp. 74–83 (2004)
11. Minutolo, A., Esposito, M., Pietro, G.: An ontology-based approach for representing medical recommendations in mHealth applications. In: Chen, Y.-W., Tanaka, S., Howlett, Robert J., Jain, Lakhmi C. (eds.) Innovation in Medicine and Healthcare 2016. SIST, vol. 60, pp. 171–182. Springer, Cham (2016). doi:10.1007/978-3-319-39687-3_17

Systems and Apps for Movement Analysis and Detection

Accuracy of the Microsoft Kinect System in the Identification of the Body Posture

Paolo Abbondanza, Silvio Giancola, Remo Sala, and Marco Tarabini[✉]

Department of Mechanical Engineering, Politecnico di Milano, Via La Masa 1, Milan, Italy
{paolo.abbondanza,silvio.giancola,remo.sala,
marco.tarabini}@polimi.it

Abstract. Markerless motion capture systems have been developed in an effort to evaluate human movements in a natural setting. However, the accuracy and reliability of these systems remain nowadays understudied. This paper describes a study performed to evaluate the accuracy and repeatability of the identification of posture using the Microsoft Kinect V2 markerless motion capture system. The measurement repeatability has been studied by observing a mannequin from different positions, with different light conditions, with obstacles partially hiding the lower limbs and with different clothes. The metrics for the evaluation of repeatability were the length of forearms, arms, thighs, legs and spine and the angle of the elbows and knees. Results showed the preferential positions of measuring in terms of distance and angular position between the sensor and the target. The presence of occluded or hidden limbs and close subject represent the most critical problems of body detection returning misleading results.

Keywords: Kinect V2 · Body posture · Uncertainty estimation

1 Introduction

Motion capture techniques are used in several applications, starting from digital animation for entertainment to biomechanics analysis for clinical, sport applications and rehabilitation. There are different human body tracking systems available on the market and their performances mainly depends on the adopted measurement principle. According to the literature review on the human motion tracking for rehabilitation [1], there are three main categories of tracking systems, i.e. the visual-based, non-visual based and the robot-aided methods.

Then visual-based methods use one or more cameras to identify the different body segments, using markers placed in known position or recognizing the body posture using proper algorithms. The non-visual based methods use inertial sensors (accelerometers [2] and gyroscopes), magnetometers or acoustic sensors [3, 4] to detect the relative position of the sensors with respect to fixed elements located in known positions. The robot-aided techniques basically identify the position of the limbs starting from the geometrical configuration of the exoskeleton that is assisting the patient movements.

The Kinect V2 is a Time of Flight camera manufactured by Microsoft; it is available in the market since 2014. The device was originally built for the Xbox console and

© ICST Institute for Computer Sciences, Social Informatics and Telecommunications Engineering 2017
P. Perego et al. (Eds.): MobiHealth 2016, LNICST 192, pp. 289–296, 2017.
DOI: 10.1007/978-3-319-58877-3_37

allowed the video games to be controlled by voice recognition and body movements. The Kinect is based on a continuous wave time of flight camera, that uses an array of 3 lasers and a monochrome camera with a resolution of 512×424 pixels; the field of view is $70° \times 60°$ and the measurement ranges between 0.5 and 4.5 m. The device also integrates an RGB camera and an array of 4 microphones for the voice command interpretation. The SDK allows to visualize in real-time and to acquire color images, infrared images, depth images and audio streams. The most useful feature for our purposes is the identification, performed with a machine vision algorithm, of the position and orientation of the 25 joints of the human body (Fig. 1).

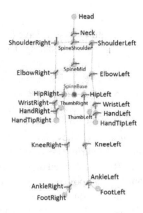

Fig. 1. Name and position of the 25 points detected by the Kinect V2.

The metrological performances of the first version of Kinect were studied in several works. The most comprehensive study of the posture was performed by Plantard, Auvinet et al. [5]. Asteryadis studied the motion of subjects using different Kinect sensors [6] while Lun and Zhao reviewed the possible application in the human motion recognition with the Kinect [7]. The Kinect was also used for the fall detection of older adults in houses [8].

The number of studies focused on the Kinect V2 is more limited [9]. The performances of the Kinect V2 were compared to those of the first version by Zennaro, Munaro et al. [10]. Authors studied the accuracy in the identification of common objects (a ball, a book, a bear puppy). Results showed that Kinect V2 is approximately two times more accurate in the near range; the gap increased at large distances. The new sensor was also more robust versus the artificial illumination and the sunlight. The metrological performances of the Kinect V2 in the reconstruction of geometrical features were analysed in [11]; results evidenced that the temperature of the Kinect V2 has an influence in the distance measurement, that uncertainty increases with the depth and the radial coordinate and that the measurement error usually depend on the material and other surface characterisitics. The performance of the Kinect V2 in 3D reconstruction and people tracking also improved significantly with respect to the Kinect V1. Recently, performances of the open source software for multi-camera people tracking OpenPTrack has been studied by Munaro, Basso and Menegatti [12]. OpenPTrack is an open source project for people tracking and uses a network of heterogeneous 3D sensors all to track people in colour, infrared and disparity images. Results evidenced the supremacy of Microsoft Kinect V2 over the other sensors in people tracking and the benefits deriving from the calibration procedure.

In this paper we describe the accuracy of the Kinect V2 system in the identification of the human body posture. The Kinect V2 can be used in several fields where the Kinect V1 showed some limitations as, for instance, in the monitoring of workers' posture or for the identification of elders' falls in dwellings. Our work is divided in two parts: in the first we analyse the accuracy in the identification of the posture of a mannequin. The mannequin position was fixed and its position was measured by the Kinect V2 placed in 39 positions inside the room. For each Kinect position the posture was measured with and without clothes, in two sensors heights and in two different light conditions. The paper is structured as follows: Sect. 2 describes the experiments and the data processing techniques; experimental results are presented in Sect. 3. The discussion and the conclusions were grouped in Sect. 4.

2   Method

The Kinect V2 SDK was used to identify the position and the orientation of the 25 joints shown in Fig. 1 with a sampling rate of 30 Hz. Data are stored in an ASCII file and afterwards processed with Matlab.

The dummy used in our tests is shown in Fig. 2. The two elbows have angles of approximately 90 and 160° while the legs are straight and the feet are in contact with the ground. The dummy is located at approximately 0.5 m from a room wall.

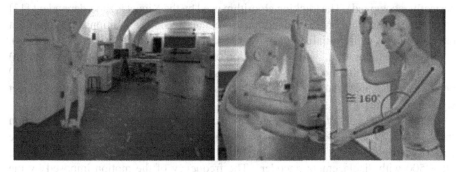

Fig. 2. Positions from where the subject was observed.

Two series of tests were performed. In the first one the mannequin was fixed and the Kinect was moved to the positions shown in Fig. 2. The dummy is always observed from the left side (see Fig. 3): this consideration is driven by the necessity of assessing the performances of the Kinect when the subject is not observing the sensor and by the fact that the mannequin trunk is symmetrical with respect to the sagittal plane. The sensor was located on circumferences with radii of 2, 3 and 4 m each 15°. The mannequin posture was observed in different conditions:

- Naked/Dressed mannequin
- Lights on/off
- Horizontal sensor (sensor height 1.45 m)/Tilted sensor (Sensor height 1.80 m, 15° tilted downward)
- Mannequin partially hidden by a table.

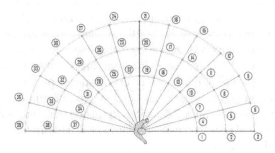

Fig. 3. Positions from where the subject was observed.

In static tests the dummy position was observed for around 30 s. Globally, more than 200 observations were performed. The metrics used to evaluate the measurement repeatability were:

- The length of specific body segments (arms, forearms, legs, trunk)
- The left and right elbow extension

The median value was chosen instead of the mean for the error estimation because of the presence of different outliers (points in which the mannequin position was not correctly recognized). The tracking algorithm used by the Kinect is time-dependent [13] and takes into account previous depth measurement. In static conditions, the algorithm have difficulties in the initialization and can return erroneous joint position (i.e. outliers).

In each configuration, the actual position of the limb (or the actual segment length) was estimated by the median of all the measures (900 frames for each position, 39 positions of the naked dummy in best light conditions, both horizontal and tilted Kinect sensor, no obstacles).

In the second series of tests the mannequin oscillated around its equilibrium position thanks to the force generated by an electrodynamic shaker. The motion measured by the Kinect was compared to the motion measured by a laser Doppler vibrometer (Polytec OFV 500 with displacement decoder). The frequency of the motion imposed by the shaker ranged between 1 and 10 Hz with steps of 0.5 Hz. The displacement varied with the frequencies and with the observed body part (head, torso, wrist). The dynamic tests last 10 s per frequency, in best light conditions.

3 Results

Experimental results of the static tests showed that, when the upper limb is not hidden by the body, the measurement error (the median of the measurements performed in a specific condition minus the reference value) is lower than 2 cm. Figure 4 show the measurement errors (in m) for the left (top figure) and right (bottom figure) forearms.

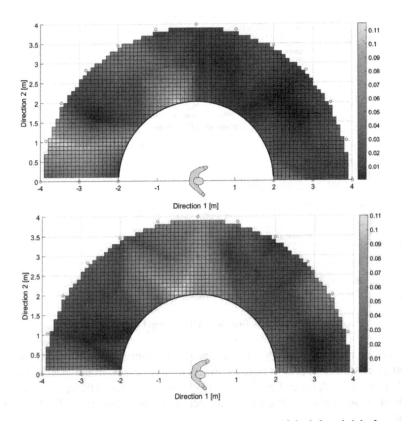

Fig. 4. Errors (median in m) for the estimation of the length of the left and right forearm

Results showed that the lightning conditions do not influence the skeleton measurement and that results obtained with the dressed dummy are more reliable than those obtained with the naked dummy. Larger errors occur from angles between 90° and 135° for both the right and left forearm. In these positions, the arms are not completely visible, and the machine vision algorithm fails in the identification of the upper body posture. The same analyses were performed on the arms, on the upper and lower part of the leg and on the trunk. Errors were always lower than 2 cm when the observed parts were clearly visible. The analysis on the elbow angle are shown in Fig. 5.

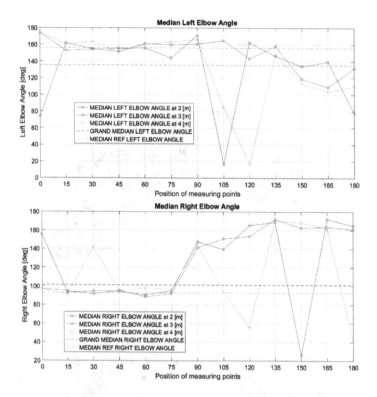

Fig. 5. Positions from where the subject was observed.

Errors are usually lower when the mannequin is observed from angles between 15° and 90°, where errors are lower than 10° except for three cases (frontal position, distance 2 m, left and right elbow and 30°, 3 m, right elbow angle) where the error is larger than 45°. In all these condition there are partial occlusions preventing from clearly observing the elbow.

The dynamic tests evidenced that, in general, the amplitude of the motion is estimated better when the motion occurs in planes orthogonal to the optical axis, although the behaviour is unpredictable and not related to the excitation frequencies. The next figures show three examples obtained with a lateral excitation; when the motion occurs along the Kinect optical axis, the amplitude of the motion is usually underestimated. Three examples are shown in Fig. 6; one can notice that at the frequency of 1 Hz the motion is underestimated both in lateral and fore-and-aft direction; conversely, at 2 Hz, the motion of the forehead is perfectly estimated in lateral direction. The limitations arose above 5 Hz, where a systematic underestimation occurred independently from the measurement direction.

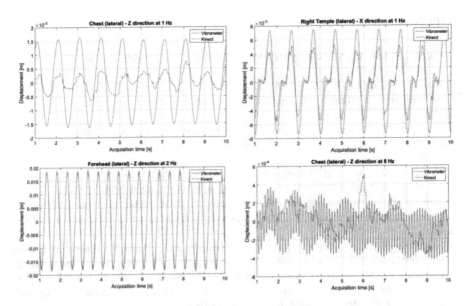

Fig. 6. Comparison between the signals measured by the Kinect (orange) and the ones measured by a vibrometer (blue). Lateral motion imposed by a shaker; Z direction is aligned with the Kinect axis, X direction is the direction connecting the mannequin shoulders. (Color figure online)

4 Discussion and Conclusions

In this work, we described the analyses performed to identify the accuracy and repeatability in the identification of posture of single subject in dwellings using the Microsoft Kinect V2. The first series of tests was performed observing a mannequin from different positions and in different experimental conditions. Results evidenced that, in general, the measurement error does not depend from the light condition nor from the presence of clothes. The main source of errors are the occlusions, that basically prevent from detecting the position of subjects in a room using a unique Kinect; in general, when one of the limbs is not perfectly visible, the posture is not correctly recognized and the error magnitude is often so large that the arithmetic average between measurements performed in different frames does not reduce the measurement uncertainty.

Dynamic measurements evidenced that below 5 Hz the main limit arises as the consequence of the resolution of the instrument; if the displacement is larger than 5 mm the motion reconstruction is usually correct. On the contrary, when the displacement is lower and/or the frequency is larger, the amplitude of the motion is not estimated correctly. This may represent a limitation in case of reconstruction of very fast movements of subjects, preventing from instance the adoption of the Kinect to track the motion of athletes in sports. Given the adoption of the machine learning algorithm to reconstruct the skeleton starting from the measured cloud of points, this limitation should be endorsed to the algorithm itself and not to the limited dynamic performances of the sensor.

References

1. Zhou, H., Hu, H.: Human motion tracking for rehabilitation—a survey. Biomed. Sig. Process. Control **3**, 1–18 (2008)
2. Tarabini, M., Saggin, B., Scaccabarozzi, D., Moschioni, G.: The potential of micro-electro-mechanical accelerometers in human vibration measurements. J. Sound Vibrat. **331**, 487 (2012)
3. Moschioni, G., Saggin, B., Tarabini, M.: 3-D sound intensity measurements: accuracy enhancements with virtual-instrument-based technology. IEEE Trans. Instrum. Meas. **57**, 1820–1829 (2008)
4. Moschioni, G., Saggin, B., Tarabini, M., Hald, J., Morkholt, J.: Uncertainty of array-based measurement of radiated and absorbed sound intensity. Appl. Acoust. **78**, 51–58 (2014)
5. Plantard, P., Auvinet, E., Pierres, A.L., Multon, F.: Pose estimation with a kinect for ergonomic studies: evaluation of the accuracy using a virtual mannequin. Sensors **15**, 1785–1803 (2015)
6. Asteriadis, S., Chatzitofis, A., Zarpalas, D., Alexiadis, D.S., Daras, P.: Estimating human motion from multiple kinect sensors. In: Proceedings of the 6th International Conference on Computer Vision/Computer Graphics Collaboration Techniques and Applications, p. 3 (2013)
7. Lun, R., Zhao, W.: A survey of applications and human motion recognition with microsoft kinect. Int. J. Pat. Recognit. Artif. Intell. **29**, 1555008 (2015)
8. Stone, E.E., Skubic, M.: Fall detection in homes of older adults using the microsoft kinect. IEEE J. Biomed. Health Inform. **19**, 290–301 (2015)
9. Giancola, S., Giberti, H., Sala, R., Tarabini, M., Cheli, F., Garozzo, M.: A non-contact optical technique for vehicle tracking along bounded trajectories. J. Phys. Conf. Ser. **658**, 1–13 (2015)
10. Zennaro, S., Munaro, M., Milani, S., Zanuttigh, P., Bernardi, A., Ghidoni, S., Menegatti, E.: Performance evaluation of the 1st and 2nd generation kinect for multimedia applications. In: 2015 IEEE International Conference on Multimedia and Expo (ICME), pp. 1–6 (2015)
11. Corti, A., Giancola, S., Mainetti, G., Sala, R.: A metrological characterization of the kinect V2 time-of-flight camera. Robot. Auton. Syst. **75**(Part B), 584–594 (2016)
12. Munaro, M., Basso, F., Menegatti, E.: OpenPTrack: open source multi-camera calibration and people tracking for RGB-D camera networks. Robot. Auton. Syst. **75**, 525–538 (2016)
13. Shotton, J., Sharp, T., Kipman, A., Fitzgibbon, A., Finocchio, M., Blake, A., Cook, M., Moore, R.: Real-time human pose recognition in parts from single depth images. Commun. ACM **56**, 116–124 (2013)

A Web Based Version of the Cervical Joint Position Error Test: Reliability of Measurements from Face Tracking Software

Angelo Basteris[1(✉)], Luke Hickey[2], Ebony Burgess-Gallop[2], Ashley Pedler[2], and Michele Sterling[2]

[1] School of Mechanical and Aerospace Engineering, Nanyang Technological University, Singapore, Singapore
angelobasteris@gmail.com
[2] Recover Injury Research Center, Griffith University, Parklands Drive, Gold Coast, QLD 4222, Australia

Abstract. The cervical joint position error test is a method to assess proprioception. This test is particularly relevant for people with neck pain and whiplash associated disorder, and it is of potential interest for people with neurological disorders. In clinical practice, patients are asked to move their head and match the original position while wearing a laser pointer on their head. The error is measured manually as the distance between the projection of the laser on a target before and after neck movement. We developed a web page which delivers this test while measuring the position of the head with a head tracking software. We tested the reliability of our application, using our software simultaneously to the laser method on 14 healthy volunteers. Our results show good correlation ($r = 0.83$, 0.69 and 0.68 after extension, right and left rotation, respectively, all with, $p < 0.001$) and limits of agreement (± 2.64 cm) between the two methods, suggesting that our application can be used for measuring the joint position sense error.

Keywords: Neck · Proprioception · Movement analysis · Face tracking

1 Introduction

The cervical joint position error test is a method to assess cervical spine proprioception in people with neck pain. In clinical practice, patients are asked to move their head in a desired position (neutral or rotated with respect to the trunk). They are then instructed to move the head away from this pose and match the original position as accurately as possible. Error from the original starting position is measured using a laser pointer mounted on the head. Although simple and inexpensive, this test is time intensive, requires special equipment, and relies on repositioning of the head by the therapist between trials. This makes the test potentially prone to error, as witnessed by its poor inter- and intra-rater reliability [1].

Movement analysis, and specifically head tracking software, may provide more accurate results while making the test simpler. For this work, we used a free head tracking

© ICST Institute for Computer Sciences, Social Informatics and Telecommunications Engineering 2017
P. Perego et al. (Eds.): MobiHealth 2016, LNICST 192, pp. 297–301, 2017.
DOI: 10.1007/978-3-319-58877-3_38

software publicly available for download (xLabs, Australia). This software tracks head motion using the Active Shape Model algorithm via a video acquired from a webcam and it provides a 2D projection of the head position on the screen [2]. We developed a web version of the test which makes the test potentially self-delivered and ready for home use. In a pilot study for testing the viability of this method, we found values comparable to normative values from literature in a population of 22 healthy volunteers [3]. In this work, we test the reliability of our software by comparing the results from our method with those measured using the standard method, i.e. the laser pointer.

2   Methods

2.1   Setup

Figure 1 shows the experimental setup. Participants sat in front of a laptop, lifted on a support so that the embedded camera was in front of their face. The same height was maintained for all subjects.

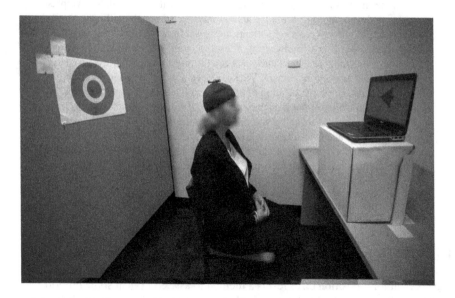

Fig. 1. Experimental setup

We used our application based on the head tracking software simultaneously to the traditional method – i.e. using a laser pointer mounted on a headband.

Traditionally, the target is positioned in front of the subjects. Because of the presence of the laptop, we mounted a panel with an A3 sized target for measuring the repositioning error behind the participant.

Both the camera and the target were positioned at an approximate distance of 90 cm from the subject's head. The positioning of the target panel, the chair and the laptop stand was controlled for by placing markers on the floor and on the table.

2.2 Task

The task consisted of an active head repositioning task to the neutral position with eyes closed. The experiment consisted of eight repetitions of each of three movement directions (extension, left and right rotation) in pseudo-randomized order. The first two trials in each direction were considered as familiarization and not included in subsequent analyses.

The initial position after the familiarization phase was marked by one experimenter as the initial position (neutral head position). The error was measured with respect to this position for all subsequent trials.

After each trial, the participant confirmed verbally the final position, and one tester marked the position of the laser pointer with a sticker on the target, while another tester clicked so that the software acquired the 2D position of the face (on the frontal plane) as measured by the head tracking software.

After this, the participant was instructed to move the head and then open the eyes, so that there was no feedback about the error in the previous trial.

With the eyes open, the subject moved the head back to the initial position for a new trial, using the feedback provided by a cursor representing the 2D position of the face.

2.3 Subjects

Fourteen healthy subjects (12M, 2F, age 24 ± 4) participated in this study. Subjects were volunteers, with no previous history of injury or surgery to the cervical spine, who had not received or sought treatment for neck pain within the past 6 months. This study was approved by the Griffith University Human Research Ethics Committee.

2.4 Data Analysis

Task performance can be measured by several metrics, with different meaning and implications [4]. For this study, we measured the error in the primary direction of movement only.

For each trial, we measured one value of error on the target (difference between marker and initial position, in cm) and one with the software. Because the software provides dimensionless output, we used a LSE for fitting it to the errors measured with the laser output. For both the camera and the laser method, positive errors indicate overshooting.

The most frequently used test outcome is the average absolute error. We averaged this for each direction and subject, for both the laser-based measure and the software estimate.

We considered as indicators of reliability the root mean squared error and the Pearson correlation coefficient between the laser measurement and the software estimate. We also considered the limits of agreement between the two methods using the Bland-Altman method [5].

3 Results

Figure 2 shows the correlation between all the values measured with the two methods. For all the three directions we observed a significant ($p < 0.001$) Pearson correlation coefficient, substantially higher for the vertical error after extension than for horizontal error after rotation.

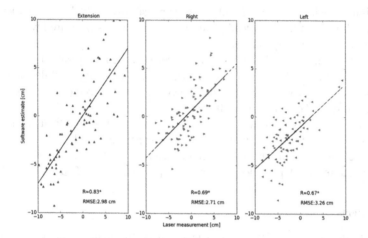

Fig. 2. Correlation for laser measurement in primary direction only and estimate based on software for all trials, all subjects, for different movement directions.

Figure 3 shows the level of agreement between the two methods for the mean value (across repetitions) for all subjects. The bias of 0.93 cm indicates that the software tends to underestimate the error in comparison to the laser, while the 95% limit of agreement is at ±2.64 cm.

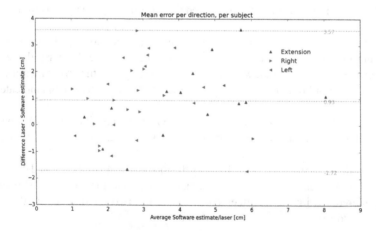

Fig. 3. Level of agreement for the mean value of absolute error across direction for all subjects.

4 Discussion and Conclusions

Our results show the viability of our application for measuring the joint position sense error. We found good correlations between the software and laser methods across all directions, and our results suggest that the face tracking software is more reliable in measuring the error after extension than after rotation. This is in contrast with our previous experience, where lateral movements appeared to be tracked more accurately than vertical movements.

When considering the mean value of absolute error for each direction, which is the standard measurement of task performance, we observed that the software tends to underestimate the error measured with the laser procedure. It is noteworthy that using the laser involves the tester's intervention for placing the marker in the final position and measuring the distance between final and initial position. Movement of the headband that is used to mount the laser on the subject's head may also affect the measurement.

The measured 95% level of agreement between the two methods corresponds to an angular error of 1.68° (at a distance of 90 cm from the target), well within the suggested cut-off scores for "normal" cervical proprioception (4.5°, [6]).

Our system is web-based and uses a Google Chrome browser extension for measuring the position and orientation of the head. While at this stage extensions are not supported for the smartphone version of the browser, once this becomes possible our tool will be available on smartphones and tablets too, regardless of their operating system. Future work will aim at overcoming the limitations of this work, namely the small population and the use of a calibration matrix for transforming the dimensionless camera coordinates in absolute values.

Acknowledgments. MS receives a fellowship from the National Medical and Research Council of Australia. AB and AP salaries are funded from an unrestricted grant from the Motor Accident Insurance Commission of Queensland.

References

1. Strimpakos, N., Sakellari, V., Gioftsos, G., Kapreli, E., Oldham, J.: Cervical joint position sense: an intra- and inter-examiner reliability study. Gait Posture **23**, 22–31 (2006). doi: 10.1016/j.gaitpost.2004.11.019
2. Cootes, T.F., Taylor, C.J., Cooper, D.H., Graham, J.: Active Shape Models-Their Training and Application. Comput. Vis. Image Underst. **61**, 38–59 (1995). doi:10.1006/cviu.1995.1004
3. Basteris, A., Pedler, A., Sterling, M.: Evaluating the neck joint position sense error with a standard computer and a webcam. Manual Ther. **26**, 231–234 (2016). doi:10.1016/j.math.2016.04.008
4. Lee, H.-Y., Teng, C.-C., Chai, H.-M., Wang, S.-F.: Test-retest reliability of cervicocephalic kinesthetic sensibility in three cardinal planes. Manual Ther. **11**, 61–68 (2006). doi:10.1016/j.math.2005.03.008
5. Bland, J.M., Altman, D.G.: Statistical methods for assessing agreement between two methods of clinical measurement. Lancet **1**, 307–310 (1986)
6. Revel, M., Andre-Deshays, C., Minguet, M.: Cervicocephalic kinesthetic sensibility in patients with cervical pain. Arch. Phys. Med. Rehabil. **72**, 288–291 (1991)

Motion Capture: An Evaluation of Kinect V2 Body Tracking for Upper Limb Motion Analysis

Silvio Giancola[1]([✉]), Andrea Corti[1], Franco Molteni[2], and Remo Sala[1]

[1] Vision Bricks Laboratory, Dipartimento di Meccanica,
Politecnico di Milano, Via La Masa, 1, 20156 Milan, Italy
{silvio.giancola,remo.sala}@polimi.it, andreacorti@outlook.it
[2] Movement Analysis Lab of Valduce Hospital, "Villa Beretta" Rehabilitation
Centre, Via Nazario Sauro, 17, 23845 Costa Masnaga, LC, Italy
franco56molteni@gmail.com

Abstract. In this study, we evaluate the performances of the body tracking algorithm of the Kinect V2 low-cost time-of-flight camera for medical rehabilitation purposes. Kinect V2 is an affordable motion capture system, capable to monitor patients ability to perform the exercise programs at home after a training period inside the hospital, which is more convenient and comfortable for them. In order to verify the reliability of the body tracking algorithm of the Kinect V2, it has been compared with an actual stereophotogrammetric optoelectronic 3D motion capture system, routinely used in a Motion Analysis Laboratory in a Rehabilitation Centre, focusing on the upper limb rehabilitation process. The results obtained from the analysis reveal that the device is suitable for the rehabilitation application and, more generally, for all the applications in which the required accuracy related to the joint position does not exceed a couple of centimetres.

Keywords: Motion capture · Kinect V2 · Stereoscopic system

1 Introduction

Due to nervous, muscle's or skeletal system lesions, people may lose a part of their motor control with an impairment of abilities and performances. In order to try to restore those functions, intensive, complex and long term rehabilitation procedures are necessary.

Depending on the distance from the onset of the disability and the level of impairment, the rehabilitation team plans short-medium-long term rehab program that the patients start to perform as in or out-patient. The rehabilitation team have to maintain under control the training session and to perform regular follow up. They need to monitor functional changes of the ability of the patients in order to select the best exercise programs that fit the level of difficulty depending on the patient abilities. For neurorehabilitation, the duration of the treatment can last several months.

© ICST Institute for Computer Sciences, Social Informatics and Telecommunications Engineering 2017
P. Perego et al. (Eds.): MobiHealth 2016, LNICST 192, pp. 302–309, 2017.
DOI: 10.1007/978-3-319-58877-3_39

Regarding upper limb rehabilitation, task and goal-directed exercises are planned to involve arms, forearms, shoulders and backbone, executing activity of daily life. Patients are asked to control upper limb to manipulate small objects and/or to explore peripersonal and personal space using an echological approach to increase the engagement of the patient. Serious game [1], with the support of Virtual Reality (VR), helps patients to project themselves in a virtual world where they can naturally interact and the surrounding environment will not interfere with the neutrality of their movements.

Motion analysis focuses on the biomechanical study of the human body. The skeleton can be interpreted as a complex multi-body system composed of bones, linked together in joints and actuated by muscles. Shippen [2–4] presents a complex model composed of 31 rigid body and 35 joints actuated by 539 muscles for human motion analyses in sports and dance.

Direct and inverse kinematics and dynamics study analyses the body capability to perform a defined movement. Muscle activity are generally tracked with electromyography (EMG) that transforms contractions in an interpretable signal [5]. Regarding motion tracking, different techniques already exist [6].

In the late 1970's, Bajd et al. [7] developed electrogoniometers based on potentiometers able to record joint angles and to realise online gait analysis of the lower limb. This technique was improved in the 1980's with the use of triaxial goniometers, with a complex setup. In the same period, Furnee et al. [8] and successively Jarret et al. [9] were starting to use computer vision system to register human motion. They were using markers on people and animal body in order to tracking their motion in 2D and 3D spaces. Vision-based systems are contact-less methods, that does not introduce any load for the patient, more suitable for rehabilitation since patients keep their movement's freedom.

Our study compare two vision-based systems for human body tracking. The ground truth one is a Multi-View Stereoscopy (MVS) system that tracks markers in space. The position of those markers approximates selected joints that represent the articulation of a partial skeleton. Since it is the most widely used system for human body tracking, due to its maturity and its 0.1 mm accuracy, it will be used for reference data. The second system is a 3D Time-of-Flight (TOF) camera that evaluate the human body position in space from a measured point cloud. Similar comparison with MVS systems has been done with structured light depth camera in [10], providing interesting results. Since TOF technology provides better results in depth measurement [11], we are expecting improvements for body tracking precision.

In a first part we will present both techniques. Then, we will analyse the Kinect V2 TOF performances for absolute position and relative orientation estimation respect to a BTS Smart-DX 7000 MVS system. Finally, uncertainty in position tracking will be estimated for the Kinect V2 system.

2   Vision System for Gait Analysis

Vision systems are non-contact optical measurement techniques that do not introduce any loading effects like IMUs or goniometers do and that could lead in changing the mechanical properties of the multi-body system and impede the patient natural movement.

2.1   Multi-view Stereoscopy: BTS Smart-DX 7000

The multi-view stereoscopy is an active vision technique that use 2 or more cameras for tracking markers in space. They are typically composed of infrared (IR) emitters that enlighten the camera field of view and IR filters that permeate other light wavelength than the one emitted. Reflective objects, typically spheres, are emphasised and tracked from multiple points of view. Using epipolar geometry between the cameras, single points are reconstructed in 3D.

In order to evaluate the performance of the Kinect V2 body tracking algorithm, we use the BTS multi-view stereo system as ground truth measurement provided by the Movement Analysis Lab of Valduce Hospital "Villa Beretta" Rehabilitation Centre in Costa Masnaga, Lecco, Italy. It is a multi-view stereo system composed of 8 cameras, with a resolution of 2048 * 2048 pixel each and a maximum frame rate of 250 fps. The lightening system strobe a 850 nm wavelength light on spherical markers fixed on the patient body. The setup provides marker position measurement in a 6 * 6 * 3 m working space with an uncertainty of 0.1 mm. The cameras are beforehand calibrated in order to correct eventual lens distortion and register the cameras respect to a common reference system.

In order to get the joint position in space, markers have to be placed astutely on he patient body in order to measure the actual articulation. Many marker placement exists: Body Segment CM, Plug-in-gait (Vycon), Helen Hayes (Davis), Cleveland Clinic and Golfer Full-Body are the more common. They typically use multiple markers for a single joint in order to return a better identification of the articulation position. In most rehabilitation cases, simpler marker placement are preferred, using a single marker per joint in order to reduce preparation time. A limited number of markers does not reconstruct the exact position of the centre of a joint, but guaranty an acceptable similarity with the real movement, with a satisfying repeatability. Also, the expected performances are usually not reached for the articulation measurements since markers are fixed on soft tissues that are not rigidly fixed with the skeleton.

2.2   Time-of-Flight Camera: Microsoft Kinect V2

Time-of-Flight cameras are depth sensors that return dense point clouds. A TOF camera is composed of a pulsed cIR lightening system and an IR matrix sensor that measures the phase between the codified light sent and the received one for every single pixel. The phase between emitted and received signals is actually proportional to the distance covered by the light back-and-forth. Every single pixel measure the distance of the first obstacle it sense; put together it returns a 2.5D representation of a scene.

The second version of the Microsoft Kinect (Kinect V2) is an RGB-D camera based on the TOF technology. The Kinect V2 is composed of a 512 * 424 pixel TOF IR camera and a 1080 * 1920 pixel RGB camera. They are registered and

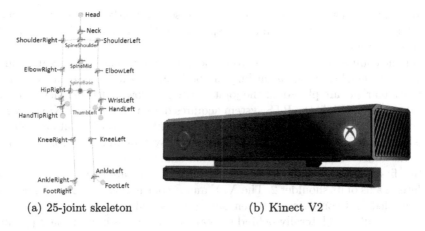

(a) 25-joint skeleton   (b) Kinect V2

Fig. 1. Human body skeleton tracking with Kinect V2 according to Shotton et al. [12]

return a 217.088 organised coloured point cloud at a 30 Hz frequency. The depth goes from 0.5 to 4.5 m and previous study claimed a best-case precision of 1.5 mm for the point cloud reconstruction [11].

The Kinect V2 has an integrated SDK function for markerless human-motion capture based on Shotton et al. [12] algorithm based on SVMs and Randomized Decision Forests. This markerless human-motion tracking method can fully track up to 6 human body simultaneously, defined with 25 joints as shown in Fig. 1, respect to the reference system defined by the TOF sensor.

3 Experimental Setup and Preliminary Results

The Kinect V2 system seems to be a cheap alternative to the expensive MVS technology. Since the 2 vision-based devices have different reference systems, it is necessary to register one system with another, in order to compare both upper limb trajectories in a common reference system.

We define the BTS reference system as the main one since it provides ground truth data. The (X, Y) plane is horizontal and the Z axis is vertical, centred in the room and directed versus top. The Kinect V2 is fixed on a tripod that frames the pedestal where the patient will be tracked.

For the registration, a set of markers composed of a thin black 80 mm-diameter disk and a 15 mm semi-sphere are disposed casually on the scene, in order to measure the position of those custom markers with both systems. The Kinect V2 IR camera identify the black disk and its barycentre is measured through a blob analysis with sub-pixel precision, which is then reprojected into the point cloud in order to obtain the 3D points in the Kinect V2 reference system. The BTS system directly returns the 3D position of semi-sphere in its own reference system. The 2 set of points are then aligned through the solving of the Procrustes problem [13] with an SVD-based algorithm [14] that minimise the root mean squared distances between the sets of markers. The transformation that align the 2 sets of point corresponds to the registration between the 2 reference systems.

For the comparison, the person to track sit down on a chair placed at around 2.5 m of the TOF camera. Regarding the body motion measurement, spherical reflective markers are placed on the joint to track, following the classical routine for the patients. While the BTS system acquires data at 250 Hz, the Kinect V2 is limited at 30 Hz. We have interpolated and re-sampled Kinect V2 data at 250 Hz, transformed the trajectory in the BTS reference system and synchronises times with the time-stamps and a cross-correlation analyses.

In a first motion recording, the patient is asked to rotate its right arm around the lateral axis of its shoulder 2. The X, Y and Z coordinates of the wrist position are recorded and compared between our systems. Different posture have been tested, frontally and laterally behind the camera, as well as intermediate posture of the body. The Kinect V2 body tracking system seems more accurate when the body is placed in front of the sensor oriented at 45° along the medial axis.

4   Neuro-Rehabilitation Motion Analysis

The following study will focus on comparing performances in motion tracking between the 2 techniques during neuro-rehabilitation exercises.

Exercises for an upper limb rehabilitation program [15] were performed in the "Villa Beretta" rehabilitation centre, the which require the use of 5 reflective markers for the analysis of a single upper limb as shown in Fig. 2. The exercises are 3, during which he performs 10 times the same simple daily life movement in a seated position.

The first exercise is called *"abduction"*, the patient needs to rigidly stand its arm along the lateral axis inside the coronal plane, starting from a relaxed caudal direction. In the second exercise, called *"reaching"*, the patient needs to extend its arm in front of him along the sagittal plan anterior direction, starting from

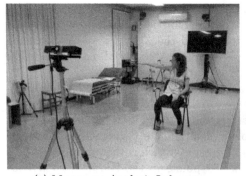
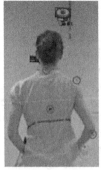
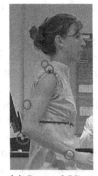
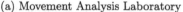

(a) Movement Analysis Laboratory   (b) Back View   (c) Lateral View

Fig. 2. Experimental setup and marker placement

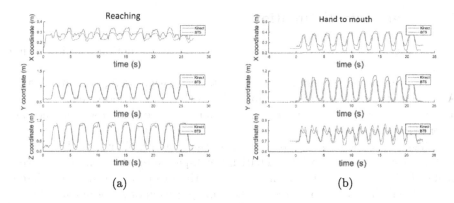

Fig. 3. X, Y and Z coordinates of the wrist position during Reaching and Hand-to-mouth exercises

the same relaxed position than in the previous exercise. In the third exercise, called *"hand-to-mouth"*, the patient is asked to reach his mouth with his hand, starting with his hand on his thigh.

During the exercise, the position in space and time of the wrist, elbow, shoulder, cervical C7 and thoracic T5 vertebrae. The last 2 correspond to the SpineShoulder and SpineMid joints in the Kinect V2 skeleton representation (see Fig. 1a).

Some of the plots of the wrist trajectory during the exercise are shown in Fig. 3. Note that a 5 Hz 2nd order low-pass Butterworth filter has been applied in order to remove high frequency noise in the trajectories.

Even if the trajectories shape look similar, they are not perfectly superimposed. First of all, the position of the marker introduce an offset in the measurement, as seen previously. As long as the markers are placed in the same position on the body, the process can be considered as repeatable. Also, a limb position close to the body is challenging to distinguish in the point cloud, which result in more erroneous full body reconstruction. Finally, a frontal position for the camera produce an occlusion of the torso with the limb, especially in the reaching and the hand-to-mouth exercises.

We can actually denote that the trajectory have a maximum deviation of 20 mm, especially shown in the range of motion extrema, when switching direction occurs. We can assume that the body tracking algorithm takes into consideration both speed and previous positions [12] to estimate the current position of the joint, since it returns worse results when switching direction. Also we can note a systematic error in the trajectories, which has been assigned to the inaccurate marker placement on the ulnar styloid, and not on the centre of the wrist. Nevertheless, the system actually provides a repeatable measurement for the position.

5   Uncertainty Estimation

In this section we estimate the uncertainty for the wrist motion tracking with a Kinect V2 device.

The arm of the patient is kept in a static position along the lateral axis. A metallic structure ensures the immobility of the limb for more than a minute. The position of the wrist is measured at 30 Hz, more than 1800 samples are recorded.

Then, the same 5 Hz 2nd order low-pass Butterworth filter is used to remove high frequency noises, as well as a 0.01 Hz high-pass filter that removes an eventual drift due to the patient strain in staying still during 60 s. Test with different limb attitude has been done, return the same precision order of magnitude.

Precision is defined as the standard deviation of the static measurement, and the root mean square of the standard deviation along the 3 main axis, which has been estimated around 1 mm for the wrist position measurement. Accuracy is not provided since it is impossible to estimate the wrist as a single point, nevertheless an offset of around 20 mm has been estimated in the previous exercises.

Similar test has been carried on the elbow angle, which return a 0.25° precision. We believe the accuracy of the Kinect V2 algorithm for angle measurement is better than the multi-view stereo system with single marker placement at the joints, since a completely extended arm return 180° with the Kinect V2 but only 160° with the BTS system.

6   Conclusion

In this paper the Kinect V2 motion tracking algorithm has been evaluated to analyse movement of the upper limb. It has been applied in a rehabilitation exercise program and compared in terms of precision of detection of the movement with a state-of-the-art MVS marker tracking system already used in medical field.

We found that the Kinect V2 body tracking system has a good 1 mm precision. On the other side, the accuracy is larger but hard to improve due to the difficulty to define the position of the wrist as a single point. In any case, the Kinect V2 accuracy is better than a single marker placement per joint with the multi-view stereo marker tracking system analysis.

Kinect V2 is a markerless technique that reduces preparation time for medical staff. We have shown that this low-cost system is user-friendly, by not being invasive to the patient. We believe patients will be able to use it at home during custom training sessions, associated with serious game frameworks.

Microsoft initially reveals the possibility to contemporary use multiple Kinect V2 systems. Combining information from different system, it is possible to solve the occlusion problem as well as improving the human body tracking performances by meaning information.

Future exploitation of this work will be extended with complete body tracking and real-time inverse dynamics evaluation.

References

1. Abt, C.C.: Serious Games. University Press of America, Lanham (1987)
2. Shippen, J., May, B.: Teaching Biomechanical Analysis Using the Bob Matlab/Simulink Model
3. Shippen, J.M., May, B.: Calculation of muscle loading and joint contact forces during the rock step in irish dance. J. Dance Med. Sci. **14**(1), 11–18 (2010)
4. Wagner, D.W., Stepanyan, V., Shippen, J.M., DeMers, M.S., Gibbons, R.S., Andrews, B.J., Creasey, G.H., Beaupre, G.S.: Consistency among musculoskeletal models: caveat utilitor. Ann. Biomed. Eng. **41**(8), 1787–1799 (2013)
5. Sutherland, D.H.: The evolution of clinical gait analysis part l: kinesiological EMG. Gait Posture **14**(1), 61–70 (2001)
6. Sutherland, D.H.: The evolution of clinical gait analysis: part II kinematics. Gait Posture **16**(2), 159–179 (2002)
7. Bajd, T., Stanič, U., Kljajić, M., Trnkoczy, A.: On-line electrogoniometric gait analysis. Comput. Biomed. Res. **9**(5), 439–444 (1976)
8. Furnée, E., Halbertsma, J., Klunder, G., Miller, S., Nieukerke, K., Van der Burg, J., van der Meché, F.: Proceedings: Automatic analysis of stepping movements in cats by means of a television system and a digital computer. The Journal of Physiology **240**(2), 3P (1974)
9. Jarrett, M., Andrews, B., Paul, J.: A television/computer system for the analysis of human locomotion. In: IERE Golden Jubilee Conference, An exhibition on Application of Electronics in Medicine, Southampton University, Southampton, England (1976)
10. Galna, B., Barry, G., Jackson, D., Mhiripiri, D., Olivier, P., Rochester, L.: Accuracy of the microsoft kinect sensor for measuring movement in people with Parkinson's disease. Gait Posture **39**(4), 1062–1068 (2014)
11. Corti, A., Giancola, S., Mainetti, G., Sala, R.: A metrological characterization of the kinect v2 time-of-flight camera. Robot. Auton. Syst. **75**, 584–594 (2016)
12. Shotton, J., Sharp, T., Kipman, A., Fitzgibbon, A., Finocchio, M., Blake, A., Cook, M., Moore, R.: Real-time human pose recognition in parts from single depth images. Commun. ACM **56**(1), 116–124 (2013)
13. Schönemann, P.H.: A generalized solution of the orthogonal procrustes problem. Psychometrika **31**(1), 1–10 (1966)
14. Besl, P.J., McKay, N.D.: Method for registration of 3-D shapes. In: Robotics-DL tentative, International Society for Optics and Photonics, pp. 586–606 (1992)
15. Caimmi, M., Carda, S., Giovanzana, C., Maini, E.S., Sabatini, A.M., Smania, N., Molteni, F.: Using kinematic analysis to evaluate constraint-induced movement therapy in chronic stroke patients. Neurorehabilitation Neural Repair **22**(1), 31–39 (2008)

Use of Wearable Inertial Sensor in the Assessment of Timed-Up-and-Go Test: Influence of Device Placement on Temporal Variable Estimation

Stefano Negrini[1,2], Mauro Serpelloni[3], Cinzia Amici[4], Massimiliano Gobbo[1],
Clara Silvestro[5], Riccardo Buraschi[2], Alberto Borboni[4], Diego Crovato[5],
and Nicola Francesco Lopomo[3(✉)]

[1] Dipartimento di Scienze Cliniche e Sperimentali, Università degli Studi di Brescia,
Viale Europa 11, Brescia, BS, Italy
{stefano.negrini,massimiliano.gobbo}@unibs.it

[2] IRCCS Fondazione Don Carlo Gnocchi ONLUS, Piazzale Morandi 6, Milano, MI, Italy
rburaschi@dongnocchi.it

[3] Dipartimento di Ingegneria dell'Informazione, Università degli Studi di Brescia,
Via Branze 38, Brescia, BS, Italy
{mauro.serpelloni,nicola.lopomo}@unibs.it

[4] Dipartimento di Ingegneria Meccanica e Industriale, Università degli Studi di Brescia,
Via Branze 38, Brescia, BS, Italy
{cinzia.amici,alberto.borboni}@unibs.it

[5] BTS S.p.A., Viale Forlanini 40, Garbagnate Milanese, MI, Italy
{clara.silvestro,diego.crovato}@btsbioengineering.com

Abstract. The "Timed Up and Go" (TUG) test is widely used in various disorders to evaluate subject's mobility, usually evaluating only time execution. TUG test specificity could be improved by using instrumented assessment based on inertial sensors. Position of the sensor is critical. This study aimed to assess the reliability and validity of an inertial sensor placed in three different positions to correctly segment the different phases in the TUG test. Finding demonstrated good reliability of the proposed methodology compared to the gold standard motion analysis approach based on surface markers and an optoelectronic system. Placing the sensor just beneath the lumbar-sacral joint reported the lower values of deviation with respect to the gold standard. Optimized position can extend the proposed methodology from the clinical context towards ubiquitous solutions in an ecological approach.

Keywords: Inertial sensor · Sensor position · Timed-Up and Go test · Optoelectronic system · Phases durations

1 Introduction

The "Timed Up and Go" (TUG) test is one of the most widely used criteria to assess subject's mobility and balance. TUG test is specifically composed of several distinct subtasks that aim to mimic in a clinical context several elements of normal daily life

© ICST Institute for Computer Sciences, Social Informatics and Telecommunications Engineering 2017
P. Perego et al. (Eds.): MobiHealth 2016, LNICST 192, pp. 310–317, 2017.
DOI: 10.1007/978-3-319-58877-3_40

activities. In particular, TUG test requires that the subject is observed and timed while he/she rises from a chair, walks for a defined distance (usually short range, such as 3 meters), turns, walks back, turns and sits down again [1]. TUG test was reported to have good correlation with subject's performance in activities of daily living, gait speed and static and dynamic balance abilities, and patient's capacity to safely walk around [2]. TUG test is, for instance, classified as "recommended" for the assessment of gait and balance in Parkinson's disease (PD) [3] and plays a fundamental role in the prediction of falls in frail older patients [4] and post-stroke subjects [5], it can be used to assess also musculoskeletal disease, such as spine impairments and degenerative conditions [6, 7] and hip fracture [8]. In TUG test temporal information about subtasks duration and transitions are fundamental to assess subject's cognitive and motor performance and define precise constraints able to support clinicians in the diagnosis of specific diseases [9, 10].

The necessity to increase the specificity and sensitivity of the test for the quantification of age-related performance in mobility, balance and overall function - led to the introduction of instrumented assessment [11–17]. In particular, wearable and mobile technologies have been providing optimal configurations and good results in the assessment of balancing [18], elderly frailty [19], fall risk [20–22], in the classification of PD patients [23] and early-stage multiple sclerosis [24] detection of freezing of gait (FOG) [17] - providing feedbacks to both subjects and clinicians [16, 25–27], in the evaluation of cognitive impairments including day-long acquisitions [13] and their relationship with motor function [28] and ageing [29]. Furthermore, instrumented TUG can provide also information about the kinematics of the functional tasks, including accelerations, and angular velocities [30, 31]. However, there are several issues, scientific literature only partially dealt with. Timing and transitions between different phases could in fact drive important clinical information from both diagnostic and prognostic point of view [9]. Correct estimation of times are therefore fundamental.

Following the state-of-the-art and scientific literature, we hypothesized to be able to correctly estimate the TUG phases in terms of temporal information by using a single inertial sensor placed on the lower back of the subject. In this perspective, it was worth to analyze how the placement of this sensor could specifically influence the estimation of TUG timing and phases. Therefore, the main objective of this study was to evaluate the reliability and validity of using acceleration and angular velocity data during the performance assessment associated in a TUG test, with respect to a gait analysis system used as "gold standard".

2   Materials and Methods

2.1   Study Design and Subjects Selection

An observational transversal analytical study with repeated measurements was designed to test intra-subject variability and validity of the proposed method with respect to the gold standard. Exclusion criteria were the presence of musculoskeletal disorders, any malignancy, pain or prior surgeries to limbs and spine.

2.2 Instrumentations

G-Sensor device (BTS Bioengineering, Italy) was the inertial sensor used in this study. This module integrated 4 triaxial accelerometer (16 bit/axes with multiple sensitivity ±2, ±4, ±8, ±16 g), 4 triaxial magnetometer (13 bit, ±1200 uT), 4 triaxial gyroscope (16 bit/axes, with multiple sensitivity ±250, ±500, ±1000, ±2000 °/s) and a GPS receiver (with a position accuracy of 2.5 m up to 5 Hz, or 3.0 m up to 10 Hz), within a volume of $70.0 \times 40.0 \times 18.0$ mm. The inertial unit could thus provide both accelerations and angular rates (up to 200 fps). The sensors fusion technology could provide also information about sensor orientation and position. For the acquisitions performed in this study accelerometer range was set to ±2 g, gyroscope range to ±2000 °/s, acquisition frequency to 100 Hz. Connectivity to laptop for acquisition was ensured via Bluetooth 3.0 (class 1.5, range up to 60 m LOS). In order to set the gold standard reference, an 8-cameras optoelectronic motion analysis system (Smart DX, BTS Bioengineering, Italy) with passive retroreflective spherical surface markers (15 mm diameter) was used to acquire kinematic data (100 fps). Specifically designed markers protocol is hereinafter reported, whereas a specific kinematic model was develop to allow for correct tracking and parameters identification. After the proper procedure, a calibrated area of about $4000 \times 3000 \times 3000$ mm, with an error on marker position identification <1 mm, was obtained.

2.3 Acquisition Protocol

The participants wore the inertial sensor attached in a semi-elastic neoprene belt on the lower back. Three different placement of the inertial sensor were used. In particular, the device was placed [**POS 1**] just over the iliac alae (i.e. above the iliac crests), [**POS 2**] just beneath the lumbar-sacral joint (i.e. under the line connecting the two posterior superior iliac spines - PSIS) and [**POS 3**] just over the lumbar-sacral joint. Subjects were also marked with retroreflective hemispherical markers on specific landmarks, including head of the 5th metatarsal bones, most posterior part of the calcaneus, left and right PSIS, sacral spine (S2) and thoracic-lumbar spine (T12-L1). Trajectories of the markers on the feet were specifically used to define the stance phases, whereas the two markers on the spine were used to estimate trunk flexion-extension. Markers placement procedure was performed by a single operator in order to reduce the variability in the definition of the reference setting. Once placed sensor and markers, the subjects were instructed to rise from a chair (without armrests), walk on a straight line for 3 m (turning point was identified on the floor with the tape), turn 180°, walk back, turn 180° and sit down again (Fig. 1).

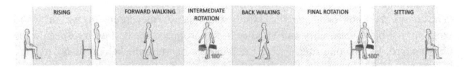

Fig. 1. Analyzed phases of the Timed-Up and Go (TUG) test.

The subjects performed the movement three times. Acceleration and angular rate data were acquired by using a dedicated software (G-Studio, BTS Bioengineering, Italy). Three-dimensional trajectories of each marker was also acquired by a dedicated software (SMART Capture, BTS Bioengineering, Italy). Synchronization between inertial sensor and optoelectronic system was performed by manually introducing an external shared trigger.

2.4 Data Analysis

Three-dimensional data from the optoelectronic system and inertial data (i.e. three-dimensional acceleration and angular rate), were processed using a software for multi-purpose biomechanical analysis (SMART Analyzer, BTS Bioengineering, Italy). After the definition a proper kinematic model, the different phases in TUG test were manually estimated as follows:

- **Chair Rising Start:** it corresponded to the beginning of the trunk flexion (estimated for both the systems on the first increase in the trunk flexion-extension velocity);
- **Chair Rising End:** it corresponded to the maximal trunk extension or, when it occurred before, to the first foot strike (estimated for both the systems on the first decrease in the trunk flexion-extension velocity or on the lowest value in the vertical component of the trajectories of the markers on the posterior calcaneus bones for the optoelectronic system and on the lowest value of antero-posterior acceleration for the inertial sensor);
- **Forward Walking Start:** it corresponds to the first foot strike after the chair rising (estimated on the lowest value in the vertical component of the trajectories of the markers on the posterior calcaneus bones for the optoelectronic system and on the lowest value of antero-posterior acceleration for the inertial sensor);
- **Forward Walking End = Intermediate Rotation Start:** it corresponds to the beginning of the rotation movement (estimated by using the angle between the pelvis and the global reference for the optoelectronic system and on the vertical component of the angular rate for the inertial sensor);
- **Intermediate Rotation End = Back Walking Start:** it corresponds to the conclusion of the rotational movement and to the beginning of the back walking phase (estimated between the pelvis and the global reference for the optoelectronic system and on the vertical component of the angular rate for the inertial sensor);
- **Back Walking End = Final Rotation Start:** it corresponds to the beginning of the rotational movement (estimated between the pelvis and the global reference for the optoelectronic system and on the vertical component of the angular rate for the inertial sensor);
- **Final Rotation End:** it correspond to the conclusion of the rotational movement (estimated between the pelvis and the global reference for the optoelectronic system and on the vertical component of the angular rate for the inertial sensor);
- **Chair Sitting Start:** it corresponded to the beginning of the trunk flexion (estimated for both the systems on the first increase in the trunk flexion-extension velocity).
- **Chair Sitting End:** it correspond to the complete trunk extension (estimated for both the systems on the first decrease in the trunk flexion-extension velocity).

Data analysis included the identification of the times of start/end and duration of each phase for both the systems. Values of shift in time and variations in duration for each phase were used to evaluate the RMS deviation between the measurements performed with the inertial sensor – considering the three different placements – and the values obtained by using the optoelectronic system. Furthermore, bias, lower and upper limits from Bland-Altman test were used also to investigate statistical agreement between the two methodologies.

3   Results

Figure 2 reports an example of the data acquired during the test including accelerations and rotations for the inertial sensor and trunk flexion-extension for the optoelectronic system.

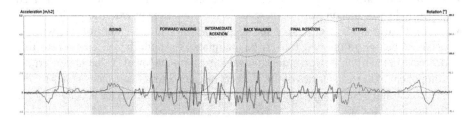

Fig. 2. Example of inertial data and phases segmentation. Antero-posterior acceleration (blue line) and rotation around vertical axis (red line) are reported. (Color figure online)

RMS deviation in start/end events and phase durations are reported in Fig. 3.

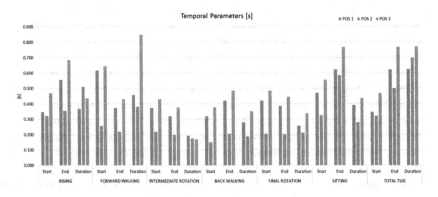

Fig. 3. Root Mean Square (RMS) deviation in start/end events and phase durations.

Average RMS deviations were 0.367 ± 0.144 s, 0.349 ± 0.196 s and 0.479 ± 0.245 s, for POS 1, POS 2 and POS 3, respectively. Average bias [with lower and upper limits] for phase durations were 0.112 ± 0.244 $[-0.478 \pm 0.372; 0.702 \pm 0.252]$ s, 0.183 ± 0.212

[−0.372 ± 0.252; 0.738 ± 0.375] s and 0.202 ± 0.307 [-0.561 ± 0.388; 0.965 ± 0.530] s for POS 1, POS 2 and POS 3, respectively.

4   Discussion

In this study, we investigated the reliability of using an inertial sensor to identify the different phases present in the standard TUG test, considering three different placements on the lower-back part of healthy subjects and comparing the start/end events and durations with the values identified by using a validated motion analysis methodology. RMS deviations for the duration of the overall TUG test and for the rising phase - which is one of the most important parameter used in diagnosis - reported values that are low, even if higher with respect to the findings identified in literature [11, 32]. Furthermore, Bland-Altman analysis reported good level of agreement with low value of bias. In general, the durations of each phase are almost identical for the two methodologies with negligible differences even if the methodology based on the inertial sensor was inclined to underestimate them. From the point of view of sensor placement, we found that POS 2 (i.e. just beneath the lumbar-sacral joint) reported the lower values of RMS deviation with respect to the optoelectronic system for all the analyzed parameters with the exception of the overall TUG duration which, as previously reported, was more influenced by the last phase. This finding could be due to the specific performed motion, which affected more the lower part of the subject's back, corresponding to POS 2. Anyhow, considering overall duration POS 1 was the most reliable. Considering also the Bland-Altman analysis, POS 2 reported the narrowest range concerning limits of agreement averaged for all the phases, whereas POS 1 reported the lowest bias values. Considering the importance of estimating also kinematic parameters, unlike POS 2, POS 1 - being not influenced by the pelvic tilt - could allow to easily identify also flexion-extension movement of the lumbar part, which is fundamental in TUG test, especially during rising/sitting phases.

5   Conclusion

This study sought to shed a light on the reliability of using an inertial sensor during TUG test, with respect to the placement of the sensor itself. This issue is fundamental whenever clinical data about mobility and balance in elderly are required both in a clinical context and during domiciliary assessment. Furthermore, the use of a wireless wearable sensor can be thus optimized to be extended towards the possibility to use ubiquitous solutions with different kinds of data acquisitions, sharing and available information, including subject's kinematics.

Acknowledgments. All the authors would like to thank Francesco Tirapelle for his huge contribution to the study. SN, MG and NFL acknowledge also the "Laboratorio di Fisiologia Clinica Integrativa" (FCI Lab) of the "Università degli Studi di Brescia" for the support.

References

1. Mathias, S., Nayak, U.S., Isaacs, B.: Balance in elderly patients: the "get-up and go" test. Arch. Phys. Med. Rehabil. **67**, 387–389 (1986)
2. Podsiadlo, D., Richardson, S.: The timed "Up & Go": a test of basic functional mobility for frail elderly persons. J. Am. Geriatr. Soc. **39**, 142–148 (1991)
3. Bloem, B.R., Marinus, J., Almeida, Q., Dibble, L., Nieuwboer, A., Post, B., Ruzicka, E., Goetz, C., Stebbins, G., Martinez-Martin, P., Schrag, A.: Movement disorders society rating scales committee: measurement instruments to assess posture, gait, and balance in Parkinson's disease: critique and recommendations. Mov. Disord. **31**(9), 1342–1355 (2016)
4. Cardon-Verbecq, C., Loustau, M., Guitard, E., Bonduelle, M., Delahaye, E., Koskas, P., Raynaud-Simon, A.: Predicting falls with the cognitive timed up-and-go dual task in frail older patients. Ann. Phys. Rehabil. Med. **60**, 83–86 (2016)
5. Timmermans, C., Roerdink, M., van Ooijen, M.W., Meskers, C.G., Janssen, T.W., Beek, P.J.: Walking adaptability therapy after stroke: study protocol for a randomized controlled trial. Trials **17**, 425 (2016)
6. Gautschi, O.P., Joswig, H., Corniola, M.V., Smoll, N.R., Schaller, K., Hildebrandt, G., Stienen, M.N.: Pre-and postoperative correlation of patient-reported outcome measures with standardized Timed Up and Go (TUG) test results in lumbar degenerative disc disease. Acta Neurochir. (Wien) **158**, 1875–1881 (2016)
7. Gautschi, O.P., Corniola, M.V., Joswig, H., Smoll, N.R., Chau, I., Jucker, D., Stienen, M.N.: The timed up and go test for lumbar degenerative disc disease. J. Clin. Neurosci. **22**, 1943–1948 (2015)
8. Kristensen, M.T., Bandholm, T., Holm, B., Ekdahl, C., Kehlet, H.: Timed Up & Go test score in patients with hip fracture is related to the type of walking aid. Arch. Phys. Med. Rehabil. **90**, 1760–1765 (2009)
9. Weiss, A., Mirelman, A., Giladi, N., Barnes, L.L., Bennett, D.A., Buchman, A.S., Hausdorff, J.M.: Transition between the timed up and go turn to sit subtasks: is timing everything? J. Am. Med. Dir. Assoc. **17**, 864.e9–864.e15 (2016)
10. Reinfelder, S., Hauer, R., Barth, J., Klucken, J., Eskofier, B.M.: Timed Up-and-Go phase segmentation in Parkinson's disease patients using unobtrusive inertial sensors. Proc. Conf. IEEE Eng. Med. Biol. Soc. EMBS, 5171–5174 (2015)
11. Mellone, S., Tacconi, C., Chiari, L.: Validity of a smartphone-based instrumented Timed Up and Go. Gait Posture **36**, 163–165 (2012)
12. Salarian, A., Horak, F.B., Zampieri, C., Carlson-Kuhta, P., Nutt, J.G., Aminian, K.: iTUG, a sensitive and reliable measure of mobility. IEEE Trans. Neural Syst. Rehabil. Eng. **18**, 303–310 (2010)
13. Smith, E., Walsh, L., Doyle, J., Greene, B., Blake, C.: The reliability of the quantitative timed up and go test (QTUG) measured over five consecutive days under single and dual-task conditions in community dwelling older adults. Gait Posture **43**, 239–244 (2016)
14. Van Lummel, R.C., Walgaard, S., Hobert, M.A., Maetzler, W., Van Dieën, J.H., Galindo-Garre, F., Terwee, C.B.: Intra-rater, inter-rater and test-retest reliability of an instrumented Timed Up and Go (iTUG) test in patients with Parkinson's disease. PLoS One **11**, 1–11 (2016)
15. Coulthard, J.T., Treen, T.T., Oates, A.R., Lanovaz, J.L.: Evaluation of an inertial sensor system for analysis of Timed-Up-and-Go under dual-task demands. Gait Posture **41**, 882–887 (2015)
16. Zampieri, C., Salarian, A., Carlson-Kuhta, P., Aminian, K., Nutt, J.G., Horak, F.B.: The instrumented timed up and go test: potential outcome measure for disease modifying therapies in Parkinson's disease. J. Neurol. Neurosurg. Psychiatry **81**, 171–176 (2010)

17. Mancini, M., Priest, K.C., Nutt, J.G., Horak, F.B.: Quantifying freezing of gait in Parkinson's disease during the instrumented timed up and go test. Conf. Proc. Annu. Int. Conf. IEEE Eng. Med. Biol. Soc., 1198–201 (2012)
18. Sheehan, K.J., Greene, B.R., Cunningham, C., Crosby, L., Kenny, R.A.: Early identification of declining balance in higher functioning older adults, an inertial sensor based method. Gait Posture **39**, 1034–1039 (2014)
19. Greene, B.R., Doheny, E.P., O'Halloran, A., Kenny, R.A.: Frailty status can be accurately assessed using inertial sensors and the TUG test. Age Ageing **43**, 406–411 (2014)
20. Lockhart, T.E., Yeoh, H.T., Soangra, R., Jongprasithporn, M., Zhang, J., Wu, X., Ghosh, A.: Non-invasive fall risk assessment in community dwelling elderly with wireless inertial measurement units. Biomed. Sci. Instrum. **48**, 260–267 (2012)
21. Zakaria, N.A., Kuwae, Y., Tamura, T., Minato, K., Kanaya, S.: Quantitative analysis of fall risk using TUG test. Comput. Methods Biomech. Biomed. Engin. **5842**, 37–41 (2013)
22. Greene, B.R., Redmond, S.J., Caulfield, B.: Fall risk assessment through automatic combination of clinical fall risk factors and body-worn sensor data. IEEE J. Biomed. Health Informat. PP, 1 (2016). Epub ahead of print
23. Palmerini, L., Mellone, S., Rocchi, L., Chiari, L.: Dimensionality reduction for the quantitative evaluation of a smartphone-based Timed Up and Go test. Proc. Annu. Int. Conf. IEEE Eng. Med. Biol. Soc. EMBS, 7179–7182 (2011)
24. Greene, B.R., Rutledge, S., McGurgan, I., McGuigan, C., O'Connell, K., Caulfield, B., Tubridy, N.: Assessment and classification of early-stage multiple sclerosis with inertial sensors: comparison against clinical measures of disease state. IEEE J. Biomed. Heal. Informat. **19**, 1356–1361 (2015)
25. Coste, C.A., Sijobert, B., Pissard-Gibollet, R., Pasquier, M., Espiau, B., Geny, C.: Detection of freezing of gait in Parkinson disease: preliminary results. Sensors (Switzerland) **14**, 6819–6827 (2014)
26. Capecci, M., Pepa, L., Verdini, F., Ceravolo, M.G.: A smartphone-based architecture to detect and quantify freezing of gait in Parkinson's disease. Gait Posture **50**, 28–33 (2016)
27. Zampieri, C., Salarian, A., Carlson-Kuhta, P., Nutt, J.G., Horak, F.B.: Assessing mobility at home in people with early Parkinson's disease using an instrumented Timed Up and Go test. Parkinsonism Relat. Disord. **17**, 277–280 (2011)
28. Mirelman, A., Weiss, A., Buchman, A.S., Bennett, D.A., Giladi, N., Hausdorff, J.M.: Association between performance on Timed Up and Go subtasks and mild cognitive impairment: further insights into the links between cognitive and motor function. J. Am. Geriatr. Soc. **62**, 673–678 (2014)
29. Vervoort, D., Vuillerme, N., Kosse, N., Hortobágyi, T., Lamoth, C.J.C.: Multivariate analyses and classification of inertial sensor data to identify aging effects on the Timed-Up-and-Go test. PLoS One **11**, e0155984 (2016)
30. Galán-Mercant, A., Cuesta-Vargas, A.I.: Differences in trunk accelerometry between frail and non-frail elderly persons in functional tasks. BMC Res. Notes **7**, 100 (2014)
31. Galán-Mercant, A., Cuesta-Vargas, A.I.: Clinical frailty syndrome assessment using inertial sensors embedded in smartphones. Physiol. Meas. **36**, 1929–1942 (2015)
32. Weiss, A., Herman, T., Plotnik, M., Brozgol, M., Maidan, I., Giladi, N., Gurevich, T., Hausdorff, J.M.: Can an accelerometer enhance the utility of the Timed Up & Go Test when evaluating patients with Parkinson's disease? Med. Eng. Phys. **32**, 119–125 (2010)

Advances in Soft Wearable Technology
for Mobile-Health

Development of a Sustainable and Ergonomic Interface for the EMG Control of Prosthetic Hands

Emanuele Lindo Secco[✉], Cedric Moutschen, Andualem Tadesse Maereg, Mark Barrett-Baxendale, David Reid, and Atulya Kumar Nagar

Robotic Laboratory, Department of Mathematics and Computer Science, Liverpool Hope University, Hope Park, Liverpool L16 9JD, UK
{seccoe,maerega,barretm,Reidd,nagara}@hope.ac.uk, cedric.moutschen@imaxpro.be

Abstract. Most of the interfaces of the current upper limb prosthetic device are rigid. However, human limbs and body are a combination of rigid and soft parts. Such a combination inherently suggests to implement soft ergonomic interfaces between the human body and such prosthetic devices. To this aim we have developed a novel set of wearable solutions, including a textile sleeve embedding EMG electrodes for the control of hand prosthesis. This interface has been integrated and preliminary tested in order to control a 5 d.o.f. low cost robotic hand.

Keywords: Textile wearable human-machine interface · EMG textile electrodes · Upper limb prostheses

1 Introduction

In 2008, about 3 million people in the world were affected by arm amputation, due to congenital, tumors and other diseases. The occurrence of traumatic event is the main cause of these amputation with a percentage rate of 77%. According to the National Center for Health Statistics, every year in the only USA, there are about 50,000 new amputations. Focusing on upper limb amputation in humans, it should be noticed that the human hands are certainly one of the most dexterous and versatile parts of the human's body. Performing daily life tasks without the hands is really demanding and it causes a lot of deficiencies. Therefore, it is mandatory to perform new strategies in order to recover such loss of motor capacities [1, 2].

In this paper we deal with a novel designed interface for the control of a robotic prosthetic hand to help people who have lost their own limbs. There are already plenty of different prosthetic hands and interfaces on the market. Nevertheless, these systems do not always offer good wear-ability as well as proper anthropomorphic design and sustainability. The development of an affordable system for prosthetic hand that will adapt to the amputees with an improved ergonomic is the main purpose of this work.

© ICST Institute for Computer Sciences, Social Informatics and Telecommunications Engineering 2017
P. Perego et al. (Eds.): MobiHealth 2016, LNICST 192, pp. 321–327, 2017.
DOI: 10.1007/978-3-319-58877-3_41

2 Architecture

In this work we will focus on the interface between the end-user and the prosthetic device. Nevertheless, the overall project behind this work has required the development of a new robotic hand and of the aforementioned interface. Therefore, for a better understanding of this approach, it is more useful to briefly present the overall architecture and different components of the project architecture. An overview of the proposed approach is reported in the next figure (Fig. 1).

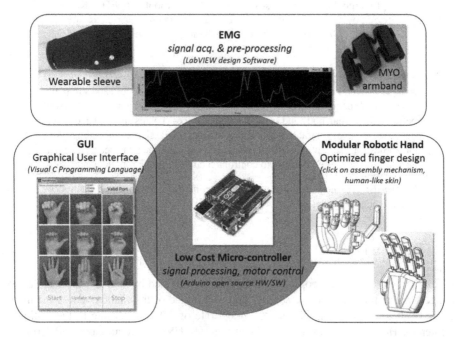

Fig. 1. Overview of the project architecture: design of the robotic and prosthetic hand, of its Graphical User Interface (GUI), EMG signal processing and microcontroller programming.

The first element regards the processing of the EMG signals in order to control a robotic hand. This approach quite mimics the natural way of controlling the hand of a healthy subject. In a second element the design of the hardware is considered, namely the development of a novel prosthetic hand. Within this contribution, an important aspect of the design concerns the implementation and the optimization of the fingertips. As soon as the EMG command signals are available, a proper set of functions in order to manipulate and use the signals has to be designed: this role is played from an open source and low cost microcontroller, which commands the motors of the prosthetic hand and read some information from a set of sensors embedded within the hand. Finally, a Graphical User Interface (GUI) is implemented to allow the end-user learning how to use and control the prosthetic hand. The GUI has been designed to display the EMG signals and different grasping configuration that the user can achieve with the robotic hand.

3   The EMG Wearable Interface

In terms of EMG signal strategy, the project has been focusing on two approaches, namely two different set of signals which may be used to control the hand.

Project 1 - In order to contain the cost of the prototype, we assume to be able to control the robotic hand with a 2-dimensional EMG input, according to previous literature where it has been shown that most of the daily grasping activity can be detailed with two PCs (Principal Components) of the finger angular displacements of human grasping. That means a less number of EMG electrodes may be used to control the hand which will benefit in terms of simplicity of the use, irrespective of the hand dexterity [3–5].

Project 2 - In a second stage of the project, we face the possibility of using more electrodes to control the robotic hand. This approach was based on the usage of a pack of electrodes which offers more possibilities in terms of signal classification and future developments.

These two approaches required the design of specific and different software, even if some common elements have been preserved within both the setup. Therefore, within each of the following paragraph, specific requirements related to each approach wil be distinguished.

3.1   Optimization of the EMG Electrodes Position vs. Muscles Sites

Generally speaking, the control of a prosthetic hand may be performed by contracting any muscle of the body. However, controlling a prosthetic hand by improper muscles is not really practical. According large literature, the best choice to control hand prosthesis is to focus on the muscles of the subject forearm. According to the number of the used electrodes, the following muscles were recruited through these electrodes.

Project 1 - in order to select two muscles or groups of muscles which have to be controllable independently, the locus of the *abductor pollicis longus*, *extensor pollicis brevis* and *extensor pollicis longus* was chosen for the first electrode, since this group of muscle is only activating with the thumb movement [6]. The second locus was chosen in correspondence of the *flexor carpi*: this area refers to muscles that are only contracting when the other fingers are moving (i.e. all fingers except the thumb) [7].

According to the level of the amputation, some of these muscles may be not available. If this is the case, we should clearly refer to another muscular strategy.

Project 2 - in this application we will used six electrodes of a commercial product, namely the Myo Armband bracelet that will mainly collect the signals of all the flexor muscles of the forearm [8]. Interestingly, all muscle activities will be captured and transmitted in six different cluster of signals, according to the design of the interface.

3.2   The EMG Wearable Interfaces

Different surface electrodes were used, since the needle electrodes are quite invasive, may cause some pain and safety issue.

Project 1 - The first type of used electrodes was the H124SG [9], which are really useful because they are easy to place and allows us to make some tests to better know where is the most appropriate place to place the electrodes. Moreover, the signal from these electrodes is quite clean from movement artefacts. Unfortunately, these devices have a limited lifetime and are not reusable. Therefore, a novel EMG sleeve interface was conceived and designed in order to make the electrodes reusable. The sleeve is made of an elastic fabric combined with a DIY "Conductive Fabric Electrodes" which are sewed on the sleeve. Thanks to this manufacturing process the sleeve is reusable and easily wearable. Figure 2 show the inner and outer surface of the sleeve after the preparation on the left and right panels, respectively.

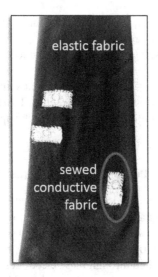 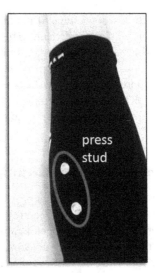

Fig. 2. On the left and right panels, the inner and outer layer surface of the homemade & reusable conductive electrodes.

The operational functioning of the device is simple: by sewing the conductive tissue on an appropriate place, we are able to detect the EMG signal. These tissues play the role of the electrodes. The armband is elastic and allows to have a great contact between the skin and the conductive. Some press studs have been attached to the centre of the electrode to perform a click-on mechanism and allow to snap the cables to the electrodes in order to externally transmit the EMG signals out of the wearable sleeve (Fig. 3).

A customized acquisition system based on open source hardware was developed in order to test the system, as well as a dedicated software interface was designed to visualize the signals. The Fig. 4 shows the EMG data output as it was obtained from the reusable electrodes. This visualization was developed under the Labview Design Software (from National Instruments) [10].

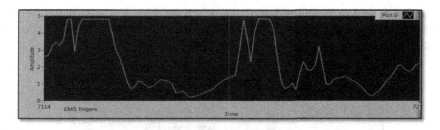

Fig. 3. Rectified and amplified signal from preliminary trial with the homemade reusable electrodes

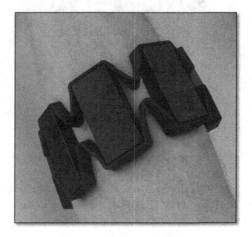

Fig. 4. The Myo Armband bracelet

Project 2 - As it was mentioned before, another integrated device was used to acquire the EMG signals and control the robotic hand, namely a Myo Armband bracelet embedding multiple electrodes.

This device works with Bluetooth that makes it really portable and design. Moreover, it can recognize different limb gestures which allows to easily interface with the prosthetic hand.

4   Data Acquisition System

To be contracted a muscle needs to receive an electrical information from the motor neurons. Such a signal has to be amplified and filtered in order to be used. The Myo Armband already integrates its own amplifier and rectifier electronic board. Therefore, this board will not be discussed here, rather we will detail the prototyping of the amplifier and filter which has been used for the Project 1.

Design of self-prototyping board - A data acquisition hardware prototype was designed and realized according to instructions reported on [11]. The final manufacturing is reported in Fig. 5.

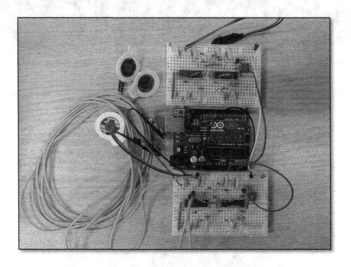

Fig. 5. The self-developed data acquisition system

This electronic set-up was finally working properly and it allowed to read two amplified and rectified EMG signals. However, a smaller device would be desirable to be easily integrated within our application.

5   Discussion and Conclusion

There are plenty of systems and products, which allow to capture and process the human EMG body signals. However, some of these solutions are currently quite expensive or not really functional. Here we suggest a set of more ergonomic and low cost solutions for better comfort of use in prosthetic applications.

The proposed wearable textile sleeve is an attempt to conjugate a low cost device with good ergonomic optimization. This solution may be combined with open source hardware implementing the signal processing and communication. On the other side, the Myo Armband is a commercial product which allow to control a large number of grasping positions. This product is not so much more expensive than the other solution and offers a lot of possibilities.

Acknowledgments. We thank all the staff of the Department of Mathematics and Computer Science for their valuable support and in particular: Mrs. S. Benson, Ms J. Burnett and Mr. M. Butler.

This work was presented in thesis form in fulfilment of the requirements for the MSC in Engineering for the student C. Moutschen under the supervision of E.L. Secco from the Robotics Laboratory, Department of Mathematics & Computer Science, Liverpool Hope University.

References

1. LeBlanc, M.: Estimated of Amputee Population (2008). https://web.stanford.edu/class/engr110/2011/LeBlanc-03a.pdf. Accessed 5 May 2016
2. ISHN. Statistics on hand and arm loss (2014). http://www.ishn.com/articles/97844-statistics-on-hand-and-arm-loss. Accessed 5 May 2016
3. Matrone, G., Cipriani, C., Secco, E.L., Carrozza, M.C., Magenes, G.: Bio-inspired controller for a dexterous prosthetic hand based on principal component analysis. In: 31st Annual International Conference of the IEEE Engineering in Medicine and Biology Society – EMBC, pp. 5022–5025 (2009)
4. Matrone, G., Cipriani, C., Secco, E.L., Magenes, G., Carrozza, M.C.: Principal components analysis based control of a multi-DoF underactuated prosthetic hand. J. NeuroEng. Rehabil. **7**, 16 (2010)
5. Matrone, G., Cipriani, C., Secco, E.L., Carrozza, M.C., Magenes, G.: A biomimetic approach based on principal components analysis for multi-DoF prosthetic hand control. In: Workshop CORNER Genova – IIT, 14–15 December 2009
6. U4 L41 Forearm Muscles. https://www.studyblue.com/notes/note/n/u4-l41-forearm-muscles-digits-2-5/deck/3109440. Accessed 1 Sep 2016
7. http://www.danasoidb.top/anterior-forearm-muscles/. Accessed May 2016
8. The MYO Armband https://www.myo.com. Accessed 1 Sep 2016
9. The H124SG electrodes Data Sheet. https://www.adafruit.com/product/2773. Accessed 1 Sep 2016
10. LabVIEW Design Instrument. www.ni.com/labview. Accessed 1 Sep 2016
11. EMG Circuit for a Microcontroller. http://www.instructables.com/id/Muscle-EMG-Sensor-for-a-Microcontroller/. Accessed 1 Sep 2016

Synergy-Driven Performance Enhancement of Vision-Based 3D Hand Pose Reconstruction

Simone Ciotti[1,2(✉)], Edoardo Battaglia[1], Iason Oikonomidis[3],
Alexandros Makris[3], Aggeliki Tsoli[3], Antonio Bicchi[1,2],
Antonis A. Argyros[3], and Matteo Bianchi[1]

[1] Research Center E. Piaggio, University of Pisa,
Largo L. Lazzarino 1, 56126 Pisa, Italy
{simone.ciotti,e.battaglia,bicchi,matteo.bianchi}@centropiaggio.unipi.it
[2] Department of Advanced Robotics (ADVR), Istituto Italiano di Tecnologia (IIT),
via Morego 30, 16163 Genova, Italy
[3] Institute of Computer Science, Foundation for Research and Technology, Hellas,
Heraklion, Greece
{oikonom,amakris,aggeliki,argyros}@ics.forth.gr

Abstract. In this work we propose, for the first time, to improve the performance of a Hand Pose Reconstruction (HPR) technique from RGBD camera data, which is affected by self-occlusions, leveraging upon *postural synergy information*, i.e., *a priori* information on how human most commonly use and shape their hands in everyday life tasks. More specifically, in our approach, we ignore joint angle values estimated with low confidence through a vision-based HPR technique and fuse synergistic information with such incomplete measures. Preliminary experiments are reported showing the effectiveness of the proposed integration.

1 Introduction

In recent years, the need for accurate 3D Hand Pose Reconstruction (HPR) has gained an increasing attention in many application fields such as virtual reality, ambulatory human motion/activity monitoring, biomechanics, rehabilitation and human robot interaction [1]. Different methods proposed for HPR can be classified as glove-based HPR (e.g., [2–4]) and vision-based HPR (e.g., [5]). The first type of approaches relies on the usage of wearable resistive, inertial or piezoelectric sensors [1,6,7] to measure quantities related to joint angles. Vision-based methods employ data acquired from cameras (typically RGBD) to reconstruct hand kinematics information. However, both these approaches can be affected by constraints that arise from the complexity in modeling the biomechanics of the human hand, measurement noise, sensor resolution and visual occlusion, among others [4]. To improve HPR performance, an important asset is the work laid out in [1,4,8–12], where the existence of postural synergies was exploited to enhance kinematic and joint angle reconstruction performance and to design optimized gloves with a limited number of sensing elements. The basic idea was to interpret *postural synergies*, that is, goal-directed kinematic

© ICST Institute for Computer Sciences, Social Informatics and Telecommunications Engineering 2017
P. Perego et al. (Eds.): MobiHealth 2016, LNICST 192, pp. 328–336, 2017.
DOI: 10.1007/978-3-319-58877-3_42

activation or inter-joint covariation patterns [13,14], in terms of statistical *a priori* information on the probabilistic distribution of human poses in common tasks like grasping. This information can be fused with incomplete and possibly inaccurate measurements provided by an HPR to increase its performance [4] and can be used for optimal placement of sensors on a glove for HPR in order to reconstruct hand posture, especially with a limited number of sensors [10].[1] In this work, we push forward our investigation and apply, for the first time, synergy-inspired performance enhancement to a vision-based HPR method [5]. This vision-based technique proposes to recover and track in real-time 3D position, orientation and full articulation of a human hand from marker-less visual observations obtained by the commercial RGBD camera Xtion PRO[2] following the optimization approach described in [5,17]. Despite its simplicity and effectiveness, such a reconstruction procedure is affected by some intrinsic limitations. For example, no-matter how the camera is placed w.r.t the hand, there are always self-occlusions that limit the reconstruction accuracy. In this paper we propose to discard joints estimated with low confidence and to complete HPR through synergistic information, integrating techniques reported in [4,5].

2   Synergy-Based Hand Pose Reconstruction

For the sake of clarity, let us summarize the definitions and results from [4,8]. Let us consider an n degrees of freedom kinematic hand model, with $y \in \mathbb{R}^m$ measures provided by an HPR system. In this case, the joint variables $x \in \mathbb{R}^n$ and measurements y are related by the equation $y = Hx + \nu$, with $H \in \mathbb{R}^{m \times n}$ ($m < n$) the full row rank matrix and $\nu \in \mathbb{R}^m$ the vector of measurement noise, with a zero mean and Gaussian distribution with covariance matrix R. Our objective is to determine hand posture, which can be represented by joint angles x in a hand model (Fig. 1), from a reduced set of measures y. This objective can be achieved by using postural synergy information. Hand synergies are goal-directed, combining muscle and kinematic activation, leading to a reduction of the dimensionality of the motor and sensory space. Furthermore, in robotics, hand synergies have represented a highly effective solution for the fast and simplified design and control of artificial systems (see [14] for a comprehensive review on hand synergies and their applications). From a kinematic point of view, hand synergies can be defined in terms of inter-joint covariation patterns, which were observed both in free hand motion and object manipulation [14]. In [4], following the approach introduced in [13], we embedded synergy information in an *a priori* set of imagined grasped object poses N, defining a $X \in \mathbb{R}^{n \times N}$ matrix. This information can be summarized in a covariance matrix $P_o \in \mathbb{R}^{n \times n}$, i.e., $P_o = \frac{(X-\bar{x})(X-\bar{x})^T}{N-1}$, where $\bar{x}$ is a matrix $n \times N$ whose columns contain the mean

---

[1] It is worth to mention that robotics research has leveraged upon neuroscientific insights on synergies to inform the design and control of artificial hands, see e.g. [14–16].

[2] Images and depth maps are captured at $640 \times 480@24$ bit and $640 \times 480@16$ bit, respectively.

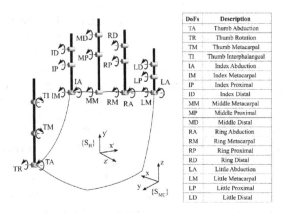

DoFs	Description
TA	Thumb Abduction
TR	Thumb Rotation
TM	Thumb Metacarpal
TI	Thumb Interphalangeal
IA	Index Abduction
IM	Index Metacarpal
IP	Index Proximal
ID	Index Distal
MM	Middle Metacarpal
MP	Middle Proximal
MD	Middle Distal
RA	Ring Abduction
RM	Ring Metacarpal
RP	Ring Proximal
RD	Ring Distal
LA	Little Abduction
LM	Little Metacarpal
LP	Little Proximal
LD	Little Distal

Fig. 1. Hand Model used for the synergy-based Hand Pose Reconstruction.

values for each joint angle arranged in vector $\mu_o \in \mathbb{R}^n$. According to [4], the hand pose reconstruction can be obtained through the minimum variance estimation (MVE) technique as:

$$\hat{x} = \mu_o - P_o H^T (H P_o H^T + R)^{-1} (H \mu_o - y). \tag{1}$$

3   Visual Tracking of Hand Posture

The visual tracking of hand posture described in this paper relies on the technique described in [5][3]. Within the vision-based HPR methods, a distinction can be made between discriminative and generative: the former rely on large datasets of hand poses to learn a mapping from the visual input to the hand pose space [18,19], while the latter rely on 3D models of the kinematics and appearance of a human hand, and try to match these models to the visual input by rendering the 3D hand model and comparing it to the visual observations. This explicit handling of a 3D hand model allows the calculation of the occluded parts of the hand and, indirectly, the level of estimation confidence. The approach presented in [5] falls in the second category. We use as input to our method the Xtion PRO, a camera that captures RGBD data, and the appearance of the hand model is approximated by appropriately transformed and positioned cylinders and spheres as shown in the left panel of Fig. 2, while the kinematics is illustrated in the right panel of the same figure. To perform tracking-based HPR for each input frame, we begin from an initial hand pose, which is used to start a search using our own variant of Particle Swarm Optimization (PSO) [17], as described in [5]. During tracking, a hand pose x is sought that matches the observations $O = (o_s, o_d)$, respectively the silhouette and the depth map of the observed hand. The core of optimization involves

---

[3] Implementation available online at: http://cvrlcode.ics.forth.gr/handtracking/.

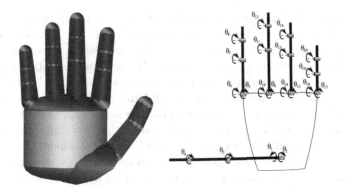

Fig. 2. Appearance (left) and kinematics (right) model of the hand used for tracking-based HPR. The hand appearance is built out of appropriately positioned cylinders and spheres. Colors encode different types of geometric primitives.

the comparison of a candidate hand pose x against O, with a matching error computed from per-pixel depth differences. Specifically, a hand pose hypothesis x, given the camera calibration information C yields a rendered depth map $r_d(x, C)$. We compare this map with the respective observation o_d, computing a "matched depths" binary map $r_m(x, C)$. This map in turn is compared to the observed silhouette, so that the objective function exhibits an optimum when the hypothesized and observed silhouettes match. Overall, the D is computed as:
$D(O, x, C) = \frac{\sum min(|o_d - r_d|, d_M)}{\sum (o_s \vee r_m) + \epsilon} + \lambda \left(1 - \frac{2 \sum (o_s \wedge r_m)}{\sum (o_s \wedge r_m) + \sum (o_s \vee r_m)} \right)$, where D_M serves
as a maximum penalty in depth difference, used to smooth out the behavior of the objective function around the optimum and λ is an experimentally determined weight factor. We formulate the final objective function by adding to the quantity D an appropriately weighted penalty term to prevent configurations in which hand parts (e.g., palm, fingers) occupy the same physical space. Based on the values of this objective function, PSO improves the candidate hand poses, eventually coming up with a hand pose that matches the input data. For more details on the employed tracking-based HPR method, the reader is referred to [5].

4 Assessing the Confidence of Vision-Based Joint Angles Estimation

Obtained a hand pose, in order to select the most trusted joints to be used in the synergy-based HPR stage (Sect. 2), an estimation of the confidence for each of them is required. We determine this confidence by capitalizing on occlusion information. Intuitively, the confidence of each estimated joint angle is at least partly determined by the level of occlusion of the two parts on either side of the joint. Therefore, we first compute the occlusion for each rigid part of the hand. Then, the confidence for each joint is computed as the product of the occlusion levels of the two rigid hand parts linked by that joint. More specifically, given a hand pose x we can count the number of pixels that are drawn using each geometric primitive of the hand model shown in Fig. 2, left. In order to provide a normalized estimate of the visibility for each hand part, a reference pose x_r is used, in which all the hand parts are visible. In our implementation this pose is an open hand with the palm facing the camera (see Fig. 3, left). The reference pose is rendered offline and the area of each hand part is calculated (in pixels). Assuming this information, we then compute the percentage of each part within the reference pose as the ratio of its rendered pixels over the total number of rendered pixels. Specifically, let a be the area in pixels of a hand part. Then the i-th hand part in the reference pose x_r has an area $a_i(x_r)$ and respective ratio $r_i(x_r) = \frac{a_i(x_r)}{\sum_{k \in P} a_k(x_r)}$, where P denotes the set of all part indices. The vector of precomputed ratios for all the hand parts $r_i(x_r), i \in P$ is stored for use during the visibility check of arbitrary hand poses. Provided an arbitrary hand pose x, a similar computation is carried out. We first count the number of pixels $a_i(x)$ per hand part in that pose. An area percentage $r_i(x)$ is again computed as the ratio of hand part pixels over total occupied. The final visibility score per part $v_i(x)$ is obtained as the ratio of its two percentages, the one computed using the target pose over the precomputed one on the reference pose $v_i(x) = \frac{r_i(x)}{r_i(x_r)}$. Computed the visibility score for each hand part, the final decision per DoF is taken by checking the two hand parts corresponding to it. If the product of its visibility ratios is over a given threshold then we retain the estimation for this DoF, otherwise we discard it. Figure 3 illustrates this process. The posture is then completed with the synergy-based techniques described in Sect. 2. Note that the visual tracking HPR method has negligible measurement noise ($< 0.2°$) and hence we have not considered it within the synergy-based reconstruction, which was proven to be robust to noise [8].

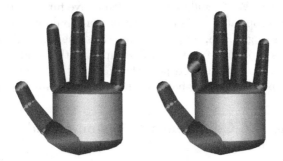

Fig. 3. Illustration of the main idea for assessing the confidence of joint angles estimation. The proximal interphalangeal joint of the index finger connects the proximal phalanx to the intermediate one (highlighted in purple). The areas of the highlighted phalanges in the reference pose (left) are computed offline and stored. Assuming an arbitrary hand pose (right), we perform the same computation and compare the visibility ratios v_i for each of the two phalanges. In this example, the intermediate phalanx is almost completely occluded, lowering the confidence in the estimation for the examined joint. (Color figure online)

5   Integration

As detailed in the previous sections, the tracking-based HPR and the synergy-based HPR rely on two different hand models. The model used in tracking-based HPR is naturally induced by the parametrization of the fingers as a succession of 3D points clusters, while the model used in synergy-based HPR was derived from a biomechanical model of the hand [13]. For this reason, the two models, while being fairly similar overall, differ substantially in the description of the thumb. In order to provide a rough mapping to feed thumb angle joints from the tracking-based HPR model to the synergy-based HPR model, a sparse sampling of direct kinematics for the tracking-based HPR model was performed, for a large number K of values of joint angles. For each of these instances, inverse kinematics was performed in the model used for synergy-based HPR, imposing a minimal distance between the position of joint centers with a least-squares approach, assuming the same length for each phalanx. At the end of this process we obtained a matrix of joint angles $\Theta_S \in \mathbb{R}^{4 \times K}$ in the synergy-based HPR, for which each column corresponds to joint angles in the tracking-based HPR hand model $\Theta_V \in \mathbb{R}^{4 \times K}$. From these values a matrix $Q = \Theta_S((\Theta_V^T)^{-1})^T$ can be obtained which gives an approximate mapping of joint angles for the thumb from one model to the other, and an estimate of joint values in the synergy-based HPR model can be obtained from values in the tracking-based HPR model as $\theta_S = Q\theta_V$. For the other fingers this conversion is straightforward, as it is simply a change in sign. Figure 4 shows a block-diagram with the different phases of integration of the tracking-based HPR system with the synergy-based HPR algorithm. The tracking-based HPR is implemented with a python script, while the synergy-based HPR is implemented in C++. This, together with the fact that it is a closed form formula, ensures that the additional computational cost introduced by the synergy-based HPR is negligible. Python script, C++ code, and hand pose visualization all run from the same PC through UDP. The whole loop is executed with a frequency of 2 Hz (± 0.1 Hz). Both input (from the tracking-based HPR) and output (from synergy-based HPR) joint angles are filtered with a smoothing filter.

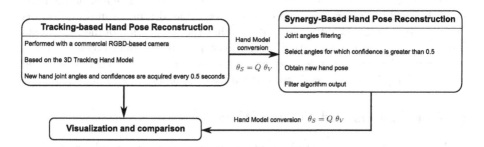

Fig. 4. Integration of visual-based HPR system and synergy-based HPR algorithm.

6   Preliminary Results

Preliminary experiments were performed with one 28 years old male subject and 3 objects (bag, book, and key). In the experiments the subject was provided a picture of the object to grasp, and asked to perform a grasp action for the target object (similarly to what was done in [13]). The subject was asked to maintain the hand posture for 5 s. In Fig. 5 we show results of the hand pose reconstruction from different points of view.

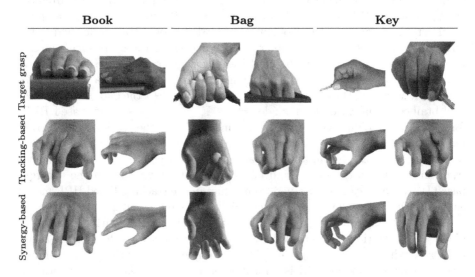

Fig. 5. Hand Pose Reconstruction results.

Referring to Fig. 1, we chose to use as input to the synergy-based HPR algorithm the following angles from the visual tracking outcomes: TA and MP for the bag; TA, IA, IM, IP, RA, RM, LA, and LM for the book; TA, MM, MP, RA, RM, RP, LA and LM for the key. We selected these angles since their confidence (whose assessment is detailed in Sect. 4) is greater than 0.5. The rest of kinematics is obtained by fusing these data with synergy-based a priori information (as described in Sect. 2). What is noticeable is that the integration of measurements and postural synergy information on the most probable human poses enables a more human-like and reliable posture reconstruction, in cases where the visual tracking of hand posture needs to deal with low-confidence estimated angles.

7   Conclusions and Future Work

In this work we have presented an integrated approach that combines optimal HPR based on *a priori* synergistic information on probabilistic distribution of human hands, and an optimization procedure to accurately track and reconstruct hand pose from visual data provided by a commercial RGBD camera.

More specifically, hand joint values estimated through such an optimization procedure are discarded if the confidence in their estimation is low. Hand posture is then completed by fusing synergy information with the remaining estimates in a Bayesian optimal fashion. Preliminary qualitative results show that the integrated approach provides more realistic and accurate 3D hand tracking than the original optimization techniques. This is particularly true in those conditions where occlusions of parts of the tracked hands can be observed. While the performed experiments considered human grasping, there is no inherent limitation that prevents the applicability of our approach to other types of hand activities. Future works will further develop the integration of different sensing modalities as done e.g. in [12]. The idea is to push forward under-sensing approach for wearable sensors [1] and synergy-based performance enhancement, taking advantage from both visual (unobtrusive, usable) and non-visual (wearable) HPR to increase performance in ambulatory monitoring, virtual reality and human-robot interaction. Finally, we will perform a more quantitative evaluation of the results in real-time hand tracking tasks, investigation how synergy information can be used to reduce the search space for the methods described in [5].

Acknowledgment. This work is supported in part by the European Research Council under the Advanced Grant SoftHands (No. ERC-291166), by the EU H2020 projects SoftPro (No. 688857) and SOMA (No. 645599), and by the EU FP7 project WEARHAP (No. 601165).

References

1. Ciotti, S., et al.: A synergy-based optimally designed sensing glove for functional grasp recognition. Sensors **16**(6), 811 (2016)
2. Sturman, D.J., et al.: A survey of glove-based input. IEEE Comput. Graphics Appl. **14**(1), 30–39 (1994)
3. Dipietro, L., et al.: A survey of glove-based systems and their applications. IEEE Trans. Syst. Man Cybern. Part C Appl. Rev. **38**(4), 461–482 (2008)
4. Bianchi, M., et al.: Synergy-based hand pose sensing: Reconstruction enhancement. Int. J. Robot. Res. **32**(4), 396–406 (2013)
5. Oikonomidis, I., et al.: Efficient model-based 3D tracking of hand articulations using kinect. In: British Machine Vision Conference (BMVC 2011), vol. 1, no. 2, pp. 1–11. BMVA, Dundee (2011)
6. Muth, J.T., et al.: Embedded 3D printing of strain sensors within highly stretchable elastomers. Adv. Mater. **26**(36), 6307–6312 (2014)
7. Hsiao, P.-C., et al.: Data glove embedded with 9-axis imu and force sensing sensors for evaluation of hand function. In: 2015 37th Annual International Conference of the IEEE Engineering in Medicine and Biology Society (EMBC), pp. 4631–4634. IEEE (2015)
8. Bianchi, M., et al.: On the use of postural synergies to improve human hand pose reconstruction. In: 2012 IEEE Haptics Symposium (HAPTICS), pp. 91–98. IEEE (2012)
9. Bianchi, M., et al.: Synergy-based optimal design of hand pose sensing. In: 2012 IEEE/RSJ International Conference on Intelligent Robots and Systems (IROS), pp. 3929–3935, October 2012

10. Bianchi, M., et al.: Synergy-based hand pose sensing: optimal glove design. Int. J. Robot. Res. **32**(4), 407–424 (2013)
11. Bianchi, M., et al.: Exploiting hand kinematic synergies and wearable under-sensing for hand functional grasp recognition. In: 2014 EAI 4th International Conference on Wireless Mobile Communication and Healthcare (Mobihealth), pp. 168–171, November 2014
12. Bianchi, M., et al.: A multi-modal sensing glove for human manual-interaction studies. Electronics **5**(3), 42 (2016)
13. Santello, M., et al.: Postural hand synergies for tool use. J. Neurosci. **18**(23), 10 105–10 115 (1998)
14. Santello, M., et al.: Hand synergies: integration of robotics and neuroscience for understanding the control of biological and artificial hands. Phys. Life Rev. **17**, 1–23 (2016)
15. Catalano, M.G., et al.: Adaptive synergies for the design and control of the Pisa/IIT softhand. Int. J. Robot. Res. **33**(5), 768–782 (2014)
16. Matrone, G.C., et al.: Principal components analysis based control of a multi-dof underactuated prosthetic hand. J. Neuroeng. Rehabil. **7**(1), 1 (2010)
17. Kennedy, J., et al.: Particle swarm optimization. In: International Conference on Neural Networks, vol. 4, no. 3, pp. 1942–1948. IEEE, January 1995
18. Sun, X., et al.: Cascaded hand pose regression. In: Proceedings of the IEEE Conference on Computer Vision and Pattern Recognition, pp. 824–832 (2015)
19. Keskin, C., Kıraç, F., Kara, Y.E., Akarun, L.: Hand pose estimation and hand shape classification using multi-layered randomized decision forests. In: Fitzgibbon, A., Lazebnik, S., Perona, P., Sato, Y., Schmid, C. (eds.) ECCV 2012. LNCS, vol. 7577, pp. 852–863. Springer, Heidelberg (2012). doi:10.1007/978-3-642-33783-3_61

A Quantitative Evaluation of Drive Patterns in Electrical Impedance Tomography

Stefania Russo[1(✉)], Nicola Carbonaro[2], Alessandro Tognetti[2,3], and Samia Nefti-Meziani[1]

[1] Autonomous System and Robotics Research Centre, University of Salford, Manchester, UK
{s.russo1,s.nefti-meziani}@salford.ac.uk
[2] Research Centre E. Piaggio, University of Pisa, Pisa, Italy
{nicola.carbonaro,a.tognetti}@centropiaggio.unipi.it
[3] Department of Information Engineering, University of Pisa, Pisa, Italy

Abstract. Electrical Impedance Tomography (EIT) is a method used to display, through an image, the conductivity distribution inside a domain by using measurements taken from electrodes placed at its periphery. This paper presents our prototype of a stretchable touch sensor, which is based on the EIT method. We then test its performance by comparing voltage data acquired from testing with two different materials, using the performance parameters Signal-to-Noise Ratio (SNR), Boundary Voltage Changes (BVC) and Singular Value Decomposition (SVD). The paper contributes to the literature by demonstrating that, depending on the present stimuli position over the conductive domain, the selection of electrodes on which current injection and voltage reading are performed, can be chosen dynamically resulting in an improved quality of the reconstructed image and system performance.

Keywords: Electrical Impedance Tomography · EIT · Drive patterns · Stretchable sensors

1 Introduction

EIT is a method that utilises electrodes placed at the periphery of a conductive body for both injecting a small current inside the conductive domain, and measuring the consequently induced potentials. The EIT method is mostly applied in clinical applications [1], but it can be used to create artificial sensitive skins by using thin, conductive and flexible fabric materials that respond to a mechanical solicitation by changing their internal resistance. The main advantage of such EIT systems is the possibility to achieve a stretchable sensor without internal wires, which can be easily mounted over 3D and deformable surfaces showing multi-touch sensing capabilities [2]. In literature, some other EIT applications are for damage detection [3] and pressure sore prevention [4].

The main issue with EIT is its low resolution, being an inverse ill-posed problem [5] where the aim is to reconstruct the internal conductivity based on the voltages which are measured at the boundary. For this reason, recent studies [6–8] have focused on developing different drive patterns for current excitation and voltage reading in order to

© ICST Institute for Computer Sciences, Social Informatics and Telecommunications Engineering 2017
P. Perego et al. (Eds.): MobiHealth 2016, LNICST 192, pp. 337–344, 2017.
DOI: 10.1007/978-3-319-58877-3_43

improve the image resolution and object distinguishability. Being a drive pattern a strategy that selects the electrodes pairs on which current injection and voltage reading are performed, it affects system performance as different current injections result in different current density distribution across the transducer, and different voltage readings influence how big of a portion of the material is been read. However, these studies have not considered the correlation between drive patterns and the contact position of the input stimuli.

This work describes a comparison of different performance parameters of three drive patterns for EIT. The results are compared according to the location of the input stimuli.

2   Materials and Methods

2.1   EIT for Artificial Sensitive Skin

EIT works by minimising the difference between the voltages measured at the periphery of a conductive body, and a model called forward operator which predicts these values [3]. In the EIT method, measurements are conducted initially without any load in order to get a set of baseline potentials V_0 and a difference imaging technique is then performed by comparing V_0 and measurements taken once a load is applied. Then, the forward operator is linearized around an initial known conductivity σ_0, giving the solution:

$$\partial V \approx J \partial \sigma + w. \tag{1}$$

Where ∂V represents the difference between the measured voltages, w represents the noise, and J is the Jacobian matrix that relates the voltage across the electrodes to the changes in electrical conductivity within the medium when a known current is applied.

The Jacobian matrix has many entries which are close to zero, and they create numerical sensitivity when reconstructing the conductivity σ. This is solved by approximating the solution through regularisation [9], assuming that the conductivity inside the medium is changing smoothly. A common regularization method is the Tikhonov regularization, which provides the following solution:

$$\delta \sigma = (J^T J + \alpha^2 Q)^{-1} (J^T \partial V). \tag{2}$$

Here, α is a hyper-parameter that controls the extent of regularisation, and Q is a combination of regularisation matrices controlling the "smoothness" of the solution. The calculation for the forward model and the Jacobian along with setting parameters α and Q is done only once at the start, while the reconstruction of the internal conductivity is performed on-line each time a voltage data set is acquired.

2.2   EIT Fabric Sensor and Hardware System

Two sample materials have been tested. Sample #1 is a Medtex 130 conductive knit fabric, silver-plated highly conductive and stretchable in both directions; this material is light-weight, low cost, and has a homogeneous conductivity distribution. Sample #2 is an EEONTEX™ conductive stretchable fabric from Eeonyx Corporation; it is a knitted nylon coated with doped polypyrrole (PPY) which is an inherently conducting polymer.

Both sample materials were cut into a circular shape of 10 cm diameter, where 8 stainless steel electrodes were pierced equidistantly. The materials were then placed in a fixture presenting a soft foam support at the bottom in order to reduce the sensitivity to stretching in the vertical axis when a load is applied. The two sensors are shown in Fig. 1.

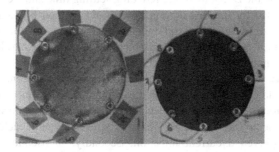

Fig. 1. On the left, conductive Medtex fabric and on the right EEONTEX™ conductive fabric.

A typical EIT hardware is made of a constant current generator, a switching mechanism for current injection and a data acquisition (DAQ) unit for voltage measurements.

The schematics of our hardware design are shown in Fig. 2. We developed a constant current source supplied with 5 V. The output of the circuit is connected to the multiplexer stage used for current injection switching. A National Instruments USB-6353 DAQ card

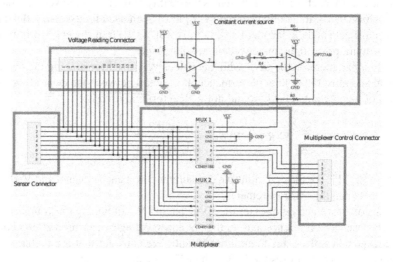

Fig. 2. Circuit schematics of the injection and measurement setup. On the top right the constant current generator, on the bottom right the two multiplexers with the connector to the DAQ and, on the left, the connection to the electrodes and the voltage reading block to the DAQ card.

was used for power supply, differential voltage readings and controlling multiplexers. Our hardware design guarantees a straightforward switch between drive patterns and change between different current amplitudes.

Being the calculated surface resistance of the sensors approximately 30 Ω for sensor #1 and 30 KΩ for sensor #2, current amplitudes of 0.9 mA and 0.9 μA were applied respectively.

In contrast to previous works [10, 11] where 4 multiplexers were used, we only used 2 for controlling the current injection pattern, while voltage readings were acquired in differential mode by the DAQ, therefore reducing settling time and electrical noise. The multiplexers are used for limiting current flow to one of their 8 channels; one of the multiplexers was used as a current sink, while the other one as a current source. Each of the multiplexers is controlled via 3 variables which are set using the DAQ at each injection step, by changing the output voltage on its digital lines.

In our work we will use three drive patterns made out of different combinations of current injection and voltage reading modalities: first, in the adjacent drive (AD) pattern, the current injection is performed between adjacent electrodes, while voltages are read on the remaining electrodes. This is performed progressively until each pair of adjacent electrodes has received a current injection. Secondly, in pseudo-polar (PP) drive patterns, the first injection is performed between a pair of electrodes, where the electrodes are opposite to each other, with one of them shifted one electrode to the side. The voltage readings are taken through pairs of neighbouring electrodes. Lastly, the PP-PP pattern is the one where the current injection and voltage readings have the same distribution of electrodes as when performing PP current injection.

2.3 Theoretical Considerations

One of the main aspects of an EIT system is the quality of the measured voltage changes. Three performance parameters inspired by [6] have been used for assessing the quality of the voltage data and the Jacobian, in order to evaluate the transducer sensitivity to the applied stimuli, prior to the image reconstruction stage.

The first parameter is the SNR which is extensively used for judging the quality of the signal and thus, the system performance. It is a ratio between the desired signal and the level of the unwanted background noise. The formula used is:

$$SNR = -20log_{10}\frac{|E[V_i]|}{\sqrt{Var(V_i)]}} \tag{3}$$

Where $E[V_i]$ is the mean of multiple measurements on each channel and $Var(V_i)$ the variance between these measurements.

The second parameter expresses the BVC, having V_0 containing the voltage data set which was used as a reference and V_1 the boundary voltages measured after a conductivity change takes place due to an input stimuli. We consider that the preferred drive pattern is one that maximises the BVC. The BVC is calculated as:

$$BVC = \|V_1 - V_0\| \tag{4}$$

Lastly, the third parameter is the rank of the Jacobian, accessible through SVD by looking at the singular values of the Jacobian. The rank is expected to be higher for the drive pattern which brings more information, thus showing a better accuracy of the inverse solution.

2.4 Experiments

We carried out 3 experiments on both sample materials, where we applied stimuli in 3 different positions using the presented drive patterns to determine which is optimal.

A 2 cm radius non-conductive load of 400 g is applied during each test in different locations. We will call P1 the experiment conducted with the load close to electrodes 1–2, P2 when the pressure is applied in the centre of the conductive medium and P3 when a two-point contact pressure is applied close to electrodes 1–2 and 5–6.

3 Results and Discussion

3.1 Performance Parameters

In Table 1, the mean SNR for the two sample materials is shown for the three drive patterns. The results indicate that the PP-PP pattern has the best performance in terms of SNR compared to the other patterns, since a current flowing crosswise in almost opposite electrodes presents an increased density, and so improves the SNR to the same extent of noise of the other drive modalities.

Table 1. SNR for sample material #1 and #2. All values are displayed in dB

	Sample #1			Sample #2		
	AD	PP	PP-PP	AD	PP	PP-PP
Mean SNR	30.9	39.4	48.1	35.8	42.5	43.5

The BVC for both sample materials is then calculated when performing three experiments, each with the same three different drive patterns. As shown in Table 2, for both sample materials, across all different drive patterns, the AD produces a higher BVC when compared to the PP in experiment P1, because of the increased density of current flowing near the electrodes. However, the PP-PP pattern presents even better results since, even though the current is more spread out over the conductive medium, the voltages are acquired over a bigger area of material. The PP and PP-PP patterns result in a better performance for experiments P2 and P3 respectively, because of the increased distribution of current flowing in the area of pressure. The decreased resolution in areas far from the electrodes is the main problem of an EIT system so, following our results, a PP pattern is optimal, although a PP-PP pattern could be used when 2 or more contact point locations are applied.

Table 2. BVC for sample material #1 and #2. All values are displayed in mV

Experiment	Sample #1			Sample #2		
	AD	PP	PP-PP	AD	PP	PP-PP
P1	6.8	3.5	7.3	16.3	7.9	14.2
P2	6.7	7.8	6.4	12.8	15.0	5.9
P3	10.8	12.9	15.3	9.2	15.2	15.4

The SVD has been applied to show how different drive patterns influence to what extent the problem can be considered as ill-posed. The plots in Fig. 3 display a sharp decrease in the singular values, evidently showing that the PP pattern for both samples has less sensitivity of solution to small changes in the voltage data. The rank of the Jacobian is equal to the number of non-zero singular values; here, there is a certain amount of singular values that are close to zero, which have no numerical meaning and are indication of noise. For this reason, the rank of the Jacobian is calculated by investigating the singular values spectra, and finding the singular value position where the fastest decrease in value results. The rank of J for the AD, PP and PP-PP patterns are respectively 26, 28, 28 for sample material #1, and 25, 28, 28 for sample material #2, thus confirming that the PP and PP-PP patterns present an inverse solution with better accuracy.

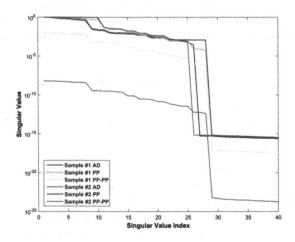

Fig. 3. Normalised SV of the Jacobian on a logarithmic scale for the two samples with AD, PP and PP-PP patterns.

3.2 Image Reconstruction

After performing the experiments, the voltage data were sent to an open source MATLAB toolkit (EIDORS software algorithm [12]), which through the use of the finite element method, reconstructs the image of the conductivity changes inside the transducer. Figure 4 shows a comparison of reconstructed images between drive patterns for the three different experiments, where we see that the drive patterns that perform best at the different loading scenarios are the AD pattern for P1, PP for P2, and PP-PP for P3.

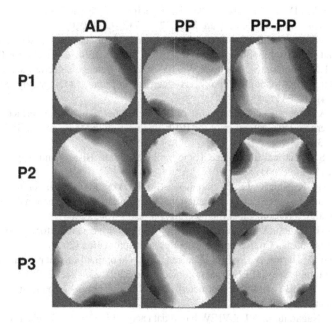

Fig. 4. Reconstructed images for different drive patterns in the case of P1, P2 and P3 load. The area in blue shows a decrease in conductivity due to the applied load. AD pattern shows an improved performance for P1, PP for P2 and PP-PP for P3. The blurred areas in the pictures are due to the high hysteresis of the materials. (Color figure online)

4 Conclusion

In this study, we compared the performance of three drive patters for EIT. Our experimental results indicate that, in order to improve the resolution and quality of the reconstructed image, it is preferable to dynamically change the injection and reading modalities accordingly to the location of the input stimuli. Therefore, the selection of the most appropriate drive pattern will result in more accurate excitations and readings over that specific region of the conductive material, enabling the performance optimisation of an EIT system. Our future work includes developing a 16 electrode system with a further investigation on the optimisation strategies of drive patterns which will lead to more accurate EIT systems.

Acknowledgments. The research leading to these results has received funding from the People Programme (Marie Curie Actions) of the European Union Seventh Framework Programme FP7/2007-2013/under REA grant agreement number 608022.

References

1. Bodenstein, M., David, M., Markstaller, K.: Principles of electrical impedance tomography and its clinical application. Crit. Care Med. **37**(2), 713–724 (2010)
2. Silvera-Tawil, D., Rye, D., Soleimani, M., Velonaki, M.: Electrical impedance tomography for artificial sensitive robotic skin: a review. IEEE Sens. J. **15**(4), 2001–2016 (2015)
3. Tallman, T.N., Gungor, S., Wang, K.W., Bakis, C.E.: Damage detection and conductivity evolution in carbon nanofiber epoxy via electrical impedance tomography. Smart Mater. Struct. **23**(4), 045034 (2014)
4. Knight, R.A., Lipczynski, R.T.: The use of EIT techniques to measure interface pressure. In: Annual International Conference of the IEEE Engineering in Medicine and Biology Society, pp. 2307–2308 (1990)
5. Holder, D.S.: Electrical Impedance Tomography Methods. History and Applications. CRC Press, Boca Raton (2004)
6. Xu, C., Dong, X., Shi, X., Fu, F., Shuai, W., Liu, R., You, F.: Comparison of drive patterns for single current source EIT in computational phantom. In: 2nd International Conference on Bioinformatics and Biomedical Engineering, pp. 1500–1503 (2008)
7. Silvera Tawil, D., Rye, D., Velonaki, M.: Improved EIT drive patterns for a robotics sensitive skin. In: Australasian Conference on Robotics and Automation (2009)
8. Demidenko, E., Hartov, A., Soni, N., Paulsen, K.D.: On optimal current patterns for electrical impedance tomography. IEEE Trans. Biomed. Eng. **52**(2), 238–248 (2005)
9. Lionheart, W.R.B.: EIT reconstruction algorithms: pitfalls, challenges and recent developments. Physiol. Measur. **25**, 125–142 (2004)
10. Bera, T.K., Nagaraju, J.: A LabVIEW based data acquisition system for electrical impedance tomography (EIT). In: Pant, M., Deep, K., Nagar, A., Bansal, J.C. (eds.) Proceedings of the Third International Conference on Soft Computing for Problem Solving. AISC, vol. 259, pp. 377–389. Springer, New Delhi (2014). doi:10.1007/978-81-322-1768-8_34
11. Soleimani, M.: Electrical impedance tomography system: an open access circuit design. Biomed. Eng. Online **5**(28), 28 (2006)
12. Adler, A., Lionheart, W.R.B.: Uses and abuses of EIDORS: an extensible software base for EIT. Physiol. Measur. **27**(5), S25 (2006)

Wearable Augmented Reality Optical See Through Displays Based on Integral Imaging

Emanuele Maria Calabrò[1], Fabrizio Cutolo[1(✉)], Marina Carbone[1], and Vincenzo Ferrari[1,2]

[1] EndoCAS, University of Pisa, Via Paradisa, 2, 56124 Pisa, Italy
{emanuele.calabro,fabrizio.cutolo,marina.carbone,
vincenzo.ferrari}@endocas.unipi.it
[2] Department of Information Engineering, University of Pisa, Via Caruso 15, 56122 Pisa, Italy

Abstract. In the context of Augmented Reality (AR), industrial pioneers and early adopters have considered the wearable optical see-through (OST) displays as proper and effective tools in applications spanning from manufacturing and maintenance up to the entertainment field and the medical area, because they provide the user with an egocentric viewpoint maintaining the quality of the visual perception of the real world.

The common OST displays paradigm entails intrinsic perceptual conflicts owing to mismatched accommodation between real 3D world and virtual 2D images projected over semitransparent surfaces. Such paradigm is suitable for augmenting the reality with simple virtual elements (models, icons or text), but various shortcomings remain in case of complex virtual contents. The major shortcoming is due to the tedious and error prone calibration methods required to obtain geometrical consistency, pivotal in many of the aforementioned fields of application. These shortcomings are due to the intrinsic incompatibility between the nature of the 4D light field, related to the real world, and the nature of the virtual content, rendered as a 2D image.

In this paper we describe a radical rethinking of the wearable OST displays paradigm by generating, through integral imaging technique, the virtual content as a light field, in order to overcome the typical limitations of the traditional approach. This paper describes the hardware components and an innovative rendering strategy in more details in respect to a previous work. Furthermore we report early results with the implementation of the integral imaging display using a lens array instead of a pinhole array.

Keywords: Augmented Reality · Integral imaging · Optical see through · Light fields

1 Introduction

Augmented Reality (AR) based on visual enhancements represents an emerging technology whose growing penetration in the consumer market is nowadays possible both owing to all the frontier research carried out in the past and to the increased availability

© ICST Institute for Computer Sciences, Social Informatics and Telecommunications Engineering 2017
P. Perego et al. (Eds.): MobiHealth 2016, LNICST 192, pp. 345–356, 2017.
DOI: 10.1007/978-3-319-58877-3_44

of hand-held devices with breakthrough hardware capabilities, like smartphones and tablets.

Wearable AR devices, commonly referred to as head-mounted displays (HMDs), provide the user with a natural egocentric viewpoint and allow him/her to work hands free. HMDs can be either binocular or monocular, depending on whether they provide stereovision or not.

As demonstrated by the huge number of publications in the medical area, AR is a promising technology in the field of image-guided surgery since it may constitute a functional and ergonomic integration between navigational surgery and virtual planning [1–13]. In this field of application, wearable devices offer the most ergonomic solution for those medical tasks manually performed under user's direct vision (open surgery, introduction of biopsy needle, palpation, etc.).

As a general rule, the quality of an AR experience depends on how well virtual content is integrated into the real world spatially, photometrically and temporally [14]. The fundamental condition for an AR surgical navigation system is to guarantee the geometric coherence in the augmented scene (i.e. registration) [15]. The HMD AR capability can be accomplished using either an optical or a video see-through method.

With a video see-through HMD, the real-world view is captured with external cameras rigidly fixed in front of the HMD, and the virtual content generated by a virtual camera is electronically combined with the video representation of the real world. An accurate registration between the virtual and the real scene is obtained through different methods [7, 10].

With optical-see-through HMDs, the real world is not mediated by external cameras, but it is generally observed through semi-transparent surface of projections placed in front of the user's eyes where the virtual information is projected. The optical see-through paradigm of HMDs (Google Glass, Microsoft HoloLens, Epson Moverio, Lumus optical) is still the same described by Benton [16]. A straightforward implementation of the optical see-through paradigm comprises the employment of a beam combiner to merge real view and virtual content. The user's own view is herein augmented by rendering the virtual content on a 2D micro display and by sending it to the beam combiner. Lenses can be placed between the beam combiner and the display to focus the virtual 2D image so that it appears at a comfortable viewing distance on a Semitransparent Surface of Projection (SSP) (Fig. 1) [17, 18]. As an alternative, the use of high-precision waveguide technologies allow the removal of the bulky optical engine placed in front of the eyes [19].

The industrial pioneers, as well as the early adopters of wearable AR technology properly considered the camera-mediated view as drastically affecting the quality of the visual perception and experience of the real world [20]. By contrast, optical see-through systems provide the user with a natural view of the real world with full resolution.

Although the optical see-through HMDs were once at the leading edge of the AR research [20], the degree of adoption and diffusion in many applications has slowed down over the years due to technological and in particular perceptual limitations.

In optical see-through HMDs, the user is indeed forced to accommodate his/her eye for focusing all the virtual objects on the SSP placed at a fixed distance. On the other hand, the focus distance of each physical object in the 3D world depends on its relative

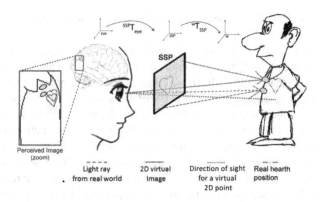

Fig. 1. Schematic of a standard optical see-through HMD display. A semi-transparent surface of projection (SSP) displays the virtual 2D image (heart). The user perceives light rays from the world combined with the 2D virtual image. The perceived image of the 2D virtual image can be misaligned in respect to the real view of the world (see the heart peak) due to user dependent calibrations issues.

distance from the observer and may dynamically vary over time. This means that, even if an accurate geometric registration of virtual objects to the real scene is attained on the 2D SSP plane, the user may not be able to view both elements in focus at the same time.

The second major shortcoming of the standard optical see-through HMDs is related with the geometric registration required to obtain a geometrically consistent augmentation of the reality, which is an essential condition in medical and surgical application. The spatial alignment of the virtual content with the real 3D world needs for: (a) the tracking of the HMD SSP relative to the real world (in Fig. 1); (b) a user-specific calibration for estimating the relative pose between HMD SSP and user's eye, namely the extrinsic calibration (in Fig. 1); (c) the definition of a projective model of the virtual viewpoint which is consistent to the human eye projective model, namely the intrinsic calibration.

State-of-the-art methods for tracking the HMDs (a), yield accurate results in terms of HMD pose estimation, whether they exploit external trackers or not. Differently, the calibration step needed to estimate user's eye pose in relation to the SSP (b) often entails a tedious and error prone method [21–24]. Further, this process should be repeated each time the HMD moves causing a change in the relative position between SSP and user's eye, and it should be autonomous and real-time. Current and more advanced calibration methods [25], albeit they work in real-time, do not incorporate the user-specific and real-time estimation of the eye projective model (c), which can change over time with the focus distance due to the accommodation process.

In real world, under the simplifying assumptions of geometrical optics, each point emits, transmits or reflects light rays in all directions. The light rays flowing in every direction along every point in space can be described as a light field (LF). Light rays directions in a 3D environment can be parameterized with a 5D (plenoptic) function [26], whereas light rays directions crossing a surface are parameterized with a 4D function (e.g. 2 dimensions for defining the position on the surface and 2 dimensions for defining the zenith and the azimuth angles).

A user wearing a traditional optical see-through display perceives the chromatic information of some of the light rays coming from the real world and crossing the semi-transparent surface SSP of the HMD. If we consider the real light field crossing the SSP, the rays perceived by the user through the SSP are a function of the pose of the real world in relation to the SSP, the pose of the SSP in relation to the eye, and of the actual projective model of the eye. The user perceives the virtual information as coherently aligned with the real world if the following condition is met for all the pixels on the SSP. A light ray along the direction passing through a point in the 3D real world and the eye's center, intersects the SSP in a display pixel, and the virtual information rendered in that pixel must match with said point in the 3D real world (Fig. 1). In this regard, the goal of the calibration routine is hence to determine where to render the 2D virtual image so to match the 4D light field perceived.

The major shortcomings of the standard optical see-through HMDs are due to the incompatibility between the nature of the 4D light field, related to the real world, and the nature of the virtual content, rendered as a 2D image on the SSP.

A recent feasibility study demonstrated that an optical see-through HMD based on light field displays potentially solves the perceptual conflict due to mismatched accommodations intrinsic to standard optical see-through HMDs [27]. The efficacy of the proposed method was demonstrated in conjunction with a proof-of-concept monocular prototype, which combined emerging freeform optical technology and microscopic integral imaging.

In a recent feasibility study by our group [28], unlike the work by Hua et al. [27], our focus was not only aimed at solving the perceptual conflict due to mismatched accommodation, but also at dealing with the geometric registration problem affecting the standard implementations of the wearable optical see-through paradigm. Our hardware implementation is a scaled version of the one described in [29], including an innovative rendering strategy that will allow the implementation of small, thus wearable, devices.

This new paper describes the hardware components and the rendering strategy in more details in respect to the previous work. Furthermore we report early results with the implementation of the integral imaging display using a lens array instead of a pinhole array.

2   Methods

2.1   Integral Imaging

Integral Imaging (or integral photography) is a technique dating back to 1908 allowing the acquisition and reproduction of a light field [30, 31]. There is a growing interest in light field acquisition, processing and display nowadays, based on the availability of plenoptic cameras and the growing up of the know-how on the matter.

An integral imaging (II) display is able to optically reproduce a full-parallax view of the scene. An integral imaging based display is composed by the coupling of a 2D

Display Panel (DP) (for example an LCD based display) with a 2D Parallax Array (PA) consisting in a lens array or a pinhole array. The PA is positioned ahead the DP at a fixed distance. The light rays emitted by DP pixels are forced to pass through the Center Of Projections (COP) (Fig. 2). The DP is populated by a 2D array of sub-images that are defined elemental images (EIs). Each EI is coupled with a corresponding COP. Each pixel of each EI describes the chromatic information for the light ray passing through the coupled COP and the pixel itself. Therefore, each couple of EI/COP can be described as a projecting element of light rays passing through the COP. The integration of all the EI/COP couples simulates the light field LF passing through the whole array of COPs.

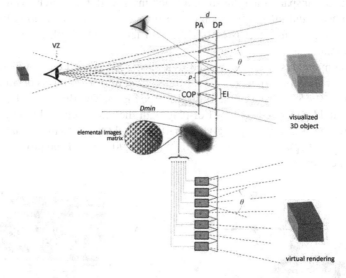

Fig. 2. (Up) Integral Imaging display and (Down) Elemental Images virtual rendering. PA is the parallax array that forces the light rays to pass through the center of projections COPs. Light rays are emitted by each pixel of each elemental image EI on the display panel DP. An array of virtual cameras are placed in a virtual scene to look the EIs virtual content. Each virtual camera acquires the chromatic information coming from different directions and passing through its center of projection. The result is that the user that looks at the integral imaging display will perceive the simulated light field corresponding to the virtual scene. Note that when the point of view is beyond the viewing zone VZ, the user view is double or distorted as some perceived light rays contain correspond to adjacent EIs (wrong).

The array of EIs can be generated by a direct grabbing from the world employing dedicated cameras (LF or plenoptic cameras) or deploying virtual rendering [30]. In the latter case, EIs can be generated simulating a bidimensional array of virtual cameras observing a virtual 3D scene. Each virtual camera acquires the chromatic information of virtual scene light rays crossing the camera center of projection. The virtual cameras array acquire the information for each EI/COP couple of the LF display. If the virtual cameras position, orientation and angle of view exactly replicates the COPs position, display orientation and aperture angle θ of the LF display, the system allow for the visualization of the virtual content in a natural fashion as the elemental images EIs acquired by the virtual cameras are naturally coherent with the LF display.

2.2 Hardware Description

The selected hardware components are: an HAIER w970 6′ Smartphone used as display panel DP (1280 × 720 resolution and 0.1038 mm pixel size); a 3 mm Plexiglas panel covered with a semi-transparent film as beam combiner and a parallax array PA. Two different kind of parallax array were employed. The first is a pinhole array realized printing over a transparent acrylic sheet a black mask with transparent white holes of 0.1 mm diameter and pitch 0.9339 mm. The second one is a lenses array by Fresnel Technologies microlens sheet (item #630), with lens focal length 3.3 mm and lens spacing 1.0 mm.

All the components where embodied in a plastic 3D printed case implementing a display as described in [29], where a semi-transparent mirror, acting as beam combiner (BC), is posed at 45° in front of the II display, see Fig. 3. The BC allows fusion of the virtual light field generated by the II display with the real world light field. The half mirror allows the user's eye to perceive both the real light field and the virtual light field emitted by the II display since the virtual light field is 90° rotated and projected directly in front of the user.

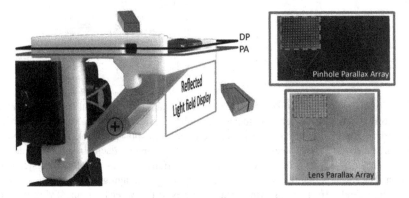

Fig. 3. The experimental integral imaging display: a smartphone display is used as DP and a lenslet array or a pinhole array as PB, (placed below the DP). The beam combiner BC "+" consisting in a half mirror rotates the light field in front of the user's eye. A camera is placed at the user's eye position to acquire the AR results.

If the virtual LF generated by the II display matches with the real LF, the real world and the virtual one are both perceived by the user as consistent from any viewing angle, hence regardless of the eye's projection model and independently from its pose relative to the HMD, all without performing any calibration. We confirmed this hypothesis with an experiment. On a wooden parallelepiped the borders of a virtual colored ones was marked. A mechanical calibration allowed placing the wooden parallelepiped in the correct position and orientation. A real camera was placed in correspondence of the user eye to acquire the scene. We acquired three pictures sliding horizontally the real camera approximately 2 cm left and right in respect to the central position (Fig. 4). The coherence between virtual and real content is clearly reached and maintained despite the point of view movements confirming that no calibration is needed.

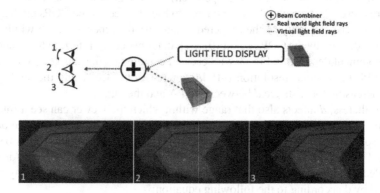

Fig. 4. Both a real object and the display were hold steady to acquire the images. A real camera placed in correspondence of the user's eye was sided in three horizontal position (with 2 cm acquisition steps) to demonstrate that without any eye-display calibration the coherence is naturally achieved.

Since in this experiment we employed as parallax array a pinhole array, the images has to be acquired in reduced light conditions in order to perceive the virtual reality. Using the lens array allowed us to work with normal lighting conditions (Fig. 5).

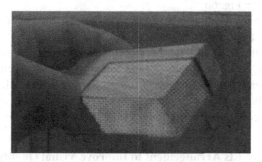

Fig. 5. The AR scene using the lens array: the improved brightness is clearly visible and the scene is comfortably visible in normal lighting conditions.

2.3 EIs Rendering and Limits of the Traditional EIs Arrangement

An off-line rendering of the elemental images EIs was achieved through a Python routine integrated in Blender 2.75a (www.blender.org), and generating a perspective image of the virtual 3D scenario for each EI. The perspective images were obtained by using an array of virtual cameras whose number, spacing, field of view, orientation, and frustum shape, were all opportunely fixed to match the specific LF display hardware parameters (Fig. 2). A 73 × 33 × 28 mm virtual parallelepiped with colored faces is rendered with an orientation of 45° along the X and Y axes (Fig. 2).

Theoretically, high visual quality could be achieved increasing the density of the COPs and/or the number of PPI (pixels per inch) for the EIs. Nonetheless, technological limits are present. As a general rule, referring to Fig. 2, once set the COPs pitch and the EIs PPI, the visual quality of the rendered image strictly depends on the width of the solid angle defined by the COP/EI pair (θ) [32]. In more details, referring to the standard EIs arrangement depicted in Fig. 2, with each EI centered on the coupled COP, given a certain PPI, the angular resolution (~PPI/θ) increases by decreasing the angle θ that means increasing the distance d between the PA and the DP.

Nevertheless, d affects also that range within which the viewer can see a full resolution image, defined as Viewing Zone (VZ) [30]. If the point of view is moved beyond the VZ, some of the perceived rays contain chromatic information which refer to wrong elemental images pixels (Fig. 2), thus the resulting perceived image appears distorted or doubled. VZ lower boundary (Dmin) is directly defined by L (longest display panel), by p, and by d according to the following equation:

$$Dmin = \frac{Ld}{p} \qquad (1)$$

In our setup, if we set d = 7 mm a Dmin of about 100 cm is imposed, indeed: Fig. 6a, showing a good result, was grabbed by a real camera 100 cm away from the LF display, which is clearly a uncomfortable viewing distance in the direction of a wearable implementation. On the other hand, the same image acquired with the same hardware setting from about 15 cm produces a distorted image as the viewpoint is outside the VZ lower boundary as visible in Fig. 6b.

If we reduce d to see the display at distance 15 cm without distortions, we obviously reduce the visual quality as demonstrated in Fig. 6c.

The distance of the viewing zone is proportional to d and so a too large d determines a bulkiness display. With the traditional elemental images arrangement, the designer should have to increase d to obtain high visual quality, but there is a limit due to the fact that increasing d the minimum distance between the eye and the display Dmin also increases, with the consequent need to implement a cumbersome display.

2.4   The Innovative EIs Arrangement to Improve Visual Quality

An innovative strategy that partially allows separating the visual quality output (angular resolution as a function of d) from Dmin, has been proposed by the authors and first presented in the previous work [28].

The key idea behind the proposed new modality consists in a new arrangement of the EIs taking into account the ideal eye position in respect to the display. It is reasonable to force the eye position approximately in the center of the display at a certain distance D.

In particular, as shown in Fig. 7, each EI is centered with the direction pinpointed by the center of the eye in its ideal position and by the corresponding COP. The rendering

Traditional EIs arrangement

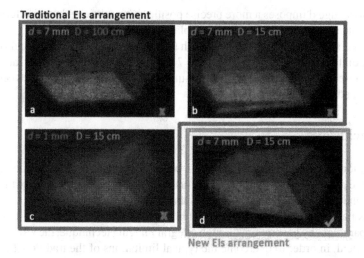

New EIs arrangement

Fig. 6. Different renderings varying d and D with traditional EI arrangement (a, b, c), and an example of the results obtained with the new EI arrangement (d). A black screen was placed behind the reflected LF display so only virtual reality is visible in the picture.

of the EIs is obtained adapting the frustum of the virtual cameras to the new geometries. In this way, a higher value of d is permitted, thus allowing a higher visual quality and guarantee a VZ, around the ideal eye position, in which the eye can be placed to still rightly see the rendered images. In this case a large d reduces the VZ and vice-versa

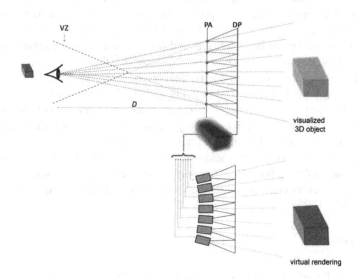

Fig. 7. Improving visual quality with the optimized EIs arrangement. In the new arrangement the EI is centered with the direction crossing the coupled COP and the eye. Virtual cameras position, angle of view and frustum shape are consequently coherently set.

(Fig. 7), so a huge d imposes a more precise positioning of the eye, but no inferior limit in the distance between the eye and the display (Dmin) are imposed.

Figure 6d shows the image rendered with the strategy described above and acquired at a viewpoint distance D = 15 cm with d = 7 mm. According to the figure, the efficacy of the proposed method ensures good image quality also at low distances between user's viewpoint and display.

3   Conclusions

The common optical see-through displays paradigm entails intrinsic incompatibility between the nature of the 4D light field, related to the reality and the nature of the virtual content, rendered as a 2D image on the display.

In this paper we describe a radical rethinking of the wearable optical see-through displays paradigm by generating, through integral imaging technique, the virtual content as a light field, in order to overcome the typical limitations of the traditional approach based on 2D images projected over semitransparent surfaces. Our hardware implementation, consisting in a semi-transparent mirror positioned at 45° in front of an Integral Imaging display, is a scaled version of the one described in [29].

The Integral Imaging displays visual quality relies on: parallax barrier pitch, display PPI, and by the distance d between display and parallax barrier. To obtain high visual quality, large d are required and, with the traditional EIs arrangement, a minimum distance between the eye and the display is forced by an inferior limit proportional to d itself (Eq. 1). For this reason, the miniaturization and the achievement of high visual quality are conflicting objectives.

The proposed rendering strategy based on a new EIs arrangement, which takes into account the ideal eye position in respect to the display, allows increasing the visual quality avoiding inferior limits for the distance between the eye and the display itself (that determine a bulky display). Note that in this EIs arrangement the knowledge of the ideal eye position is required, but the eye can be moved in the VZ maintaining the same visual quality without any distortion in the perceived image.

The presented work is a feasibility study and the implementation of a complete device based on the proposed approach still needs further research and complex technical developments. Two key issues are mandatory to go towards a wearable device: real-time rendering of the light field and real-time tracking of the real scene. In our current implementation we do not implemented tracking of the real scene (the object was mechanically calibrated) and rendering is off-line. Anyway, both issues were previously investigated and there are different possible solutions, which may be integrated with the proposed set-up [29, 33].

References

1. Badiali, G., Ferrari, V., Cutolo, F., Freschi, C., Caramella, D., Bianchi, A., Marchetti, C.: Augmented reality as an aid in maxillofacial surgery: validation of a wearable system allowing maxillary repositioning. J. Craniomaxillofac. Surg. **42**, 1970–1976 (2014)

2. Kersten-Oertel, M., Jannin, P., Collins, D.L.: The state of the art of visualization in mixed reality image guided surgery. Comput. Med. Imaging Graph. **37**, 98–112 (2013)
3. Cutolo, F., Badiali, G., Ferrari, V.: Human-PnP: ergonomic AR interaction paradigm for manual placement of rigid bodies. In: Linte, C.A., Yaniv, Z., Fallavollita, P. (eds.) AE-CAI 2015. LNCS, vol. 9365, pp. 50–60. Springer, Cham (2015). doi: 10.1007/978-3-319-24601-7_6
4. Rankin, T.M., Slepian, M.J., Armstrong, D.G.: Augmented reality in surgery. In: Latifi, R., Rhee, P., Gruessner, W.G.R. (eds.) Technological Advances in Surgery, Trauma and Critical Care, pp. 59–71. Springer, New York (2015)
5. Ferrari, V., Cutolo, F., Calabrò, E.M., Ferrari, M.: HMD video see through AR with unfixed cameras vergence. In: International Symposium on Mixed and Augmented Reality – ISMAR (2014)
6. Cutolo, F., Parchi, P.D., Ferrari, V.: Video see through AR head-mounted display for medical procedures. In: International Symposium on Mixed and Augmented Reality – ISMAR (2014)
7. Ferrari, V., Megali, G., Troia, E., Pietrabissa, A., Mosca, F.: A 3-D mixed-reality system for stereoscopic visualization of medical dataset. IEEE Trans. Biomed. Eng. **56**, 2627–2633 (2009)
8. Meola, A., Cutolo, F., Carbone, M., Cagnazzo, F., Ferrari, M., Ferrari, V.: Augmented reality in neurosurgery: a systematic review. Neurosurg. Rev. 1–12 (2016). doi:10.1007/s10143-016-0732-9 [epub ahead of print]
9. Abe, Y., Sato, S., Kato, K., Hyakumachi, T., Yanagibashi, Y., Ito, M., Abumi, K.: A novel 3D guidance system using augmented reality for percutaneous vertebroplasty. J. Neurosurg. Spine **19**, 492–501 (2013)
10. Ferrari, V., Ferrari, M., Mosca, F.: Video see-through in the clinical practice. In: 1st International Workshop on Engineering Interactive Computing Systems for Medicine and Health Care, EICS4Med, vol. 727, pp. 19–24 (2011)
11. Ferrari, V.: Letter to the editor on "designing a wearable navigation system for image-guided cancer resection surgery". Ann. Biomed. Eng. **42**, 2600–2601 (2014)
12. Cutolo, F., Carbone, M., Parchi, P.D., Ferrari, V., Lisanti, M., Ferrari, M.: Application of a new wearable augmented reality video see-through display to aid percutaneous procedures in spine surgery. In: Paolis, L.T., Mongelli, A. (eds.) AVR 2016. LNCS, vol. 9769, pp. 43–54. Springer, Cham (2016). doi:10.1007/978-3-319-40651-0_4
13. Parrini, S., Cutolo, F., Freschi, C., Ferrari, M., Ferrari, V.: Augmented reality system for freehand guide of magnetic endovascular devices. In: Conference Proceedings of IEEE Engineering in Medicine and Biology Society 2014, pp. 490–493 (2014)
14. Sielhorst, T., Feuerstein, M., Navab, N.: Advanced medical displays: a literature review of augmented reality. J. Disp. Technol. **4**, 451–467 (2008)
15. Holloway, R.L.: Registration error analysis for augmented reality. Presence Teleop. Virt. **6**, 413–432 (1997)
16. Benton, S.A.: Selected Papers on Three-Dimensional Displays. SPIE Optical Engineering Press, Bellingham (2001)
17. Rolland, J.P., Cakmakci, O.: The past, present, and future of head-mounted display designs, pp. 368–377 (2005)
18. Holliman, N.S., Dodgson, N.A., Favalora, G.E., Pockett, L.: Three-dimensional displays: a review and applications analysis. IEEE Trans. Broadcast. **57**, 362–371 (2011)
19. Mukawa, H., Akutsu, K., Matsumura, I., Nakano, S., Yoshida, T., Kuwahara, M., Aiki, K., Ogawa, M.: Distinguished paper: a full color eyewear display using holographic planar waveguides. SID Int. Symp. Dig. Tech. Papers **39**, 89–92 (2008)

20. Rolland, J.P., Holloway, R.L., Fuchs, H.: A comparison of optical and video see-through head-mounted displays. Telemanipulator Telepresence Technol. **2351**, 293–307 (1994)
21. Tuceryan, M., Genc, Y., Navab, N.: Single-point active alignment method (SPAAM) for optical see-through HMD calibration for augmented reality. Presence Teleop. Virt. **11**, 259–276 (2002)
22. Genc, Y., Tuceryan, M., Navab, N.: Practical solutions for calibration of optical see-through devices. In: International Symposium on Mixed and Augmented Reality, Proceedings, pp. 169–175 (2002)
23. Gilson, S.J., Fitzgibbon, A.W., Glennerster, A.: Spatial calibration of an optical see-through head-mounted display. J. Neurosci. Meth. **173**, 140–146 (2008)
24. Kellner, F., Bolte, B., Bruder, G., Rautenberg, U., Steinicke, F., Lappe, M., Koch, R.: Geometric calibration of head-mounted displays and its effects on distance estimation. IEEE Trans. Vis. Comput. Graph. **18**, 589–596 (2012)
25. Plopski, A., Itoh, Y., Nitschke, C., Kiyokawa, K., Klinker, G., Takemura, H.: Corneal-imaging calibration for optical see-through head-mounted displays. IEEE Trans. Vis. Comput. Graph. **21**, 481–490 (2015)
26. Levoy, M.: Light fields and computational imaging. Computer **39**, 46–55 (2006)
27. Hua, H., Javidi, B.: A 3D integral imaging optical see-through head-mounted display. Opt. Express **22**, 13484–13491 (2014)
28. Ferrari, V., Calabrò, E.M.: Wearable light field optical see-through display to avoid user dependent calibrations: a feasibility study. In: SAI Computing Conference (2016)
29. Liao, H., Inomata, T., Sakuma, I., Dohi, T.: 3-D augmented reality for MRI-guided surgery using integral videography autostereoscopic image overlay. IEEE Trans. Biomed. Eng. **57**, 1476–1486 (2010)
30. Stern, A., Javidi, B.: Three-dimensional image sensing, visualization, and processing using integral imaging. Proc. IEEE **94**, 591–607 (2006)
31. Lippmann, G.: Epreuves reversibles donnant la sensation du relief. J. Phys. Theor. Appl. **7**, 821–825 (1908)
32. Park, S.-G., Yeom, J., Jeong, Y., Chen, N., Hong, J.-Y., Lee, B.: Recent issues on integral imaging and its applications. J. Inf. Disp. **15**, 37–46 (2014)
33. Wang, J., Suenaga, H., Liao, H., Hoshi, K., Yang, L., Kobayashi, E., Sakuma, I.: Real-time computer-generated integral imaging and 3D image calibration for augmented reality surgical navigation. Comput. Med. Imaging Graph. **40**, 147–159 (2015)

Emerging Experiences into Receiving and Delivering Healthcare Through Mobile and Embedded Solutions

Interference Between Cognitive and Motor Recovery in Elderly Dementia Patients Through a Holistic Tele-Rehabilitation Platform

Alberto Antonietti[1]([✉]), Marta Gandolla[1], Mauro Rossini[2], Franco Molteni[2], Alessandra Pedrocchi[1], and The ABILITY Consortium

[1] Neuroengineering and Medical Robotics Laboratory, Department of Electronics, Information and Bioengineering, Politecnico di Milano, Milan, Italy
{alberto.antonietti,marta.gandolla,
alessandra.pedrocchi}@polimi.it
[2] Valduce Hospital, Villa Beretta Rehabilitation Center, Costa Masnaga, Italy
{mrossini,fmolteni}@valduce.it

Abstract. To improve the quality of life of elderly subjects affected by dementia, the rehabilitation environment has to translate from the hospital to the patient's home. A holistic tele-rehabilitation system can be successfully used to support and enhance a home-based rehabilitation process. The ABILITY platform foresees mobile and wireless technologies, integrated into a unique environment in which patients can become primary actors in their own care. In this work, we present a Pilot Study (N = 10) about the motor recovery, and in particular the relationship between the motor recovery and the cognitive recovery, in dementia patients. A group of control patients followed the usual care treatment and another group used the ABILITY platform at home. The results of the study suggested that the use of the tele-rehabilitation platform could improve both the motor skills, the cognitive skill and the interaction between them.

Keywords: Tele-rehabilitation · Tele-medicine · Mobile sensors · Dementia · Domotics · Active aging

1 Introduction

In an aging society like ours, the pathologies which affect elderly people represent a large burden for their families and for the national health system(s). Among the population with more than 65 years, dementia is one of the main causes of disability, causing a substantial drop of the self-sufficiency in the everyday life [1, 2]. The 5% and the 30% of the population respectively with more than 65 and 80 years is affected by neurodegenerative diseases and, every year, several millions of these neurological patients are diagnosed as new cases of dementia. One of the characteristics of dementia is a continuous and evolving decline in motor, behavioral and cognitive skills. The loss in motility and in communication and cognitive abilities can contribute not only to social isolation, but also to dangerous behaviors [3]. For these reasons, the treatment of dementia has become a priority for the public health system. Since, at present, pharmacological

© ICST Institute for Computer Sciences, Social Informatics and Telecommunications Engineering 2017
P. Perego et al. (Eds.): MobiHealth 2016, LNICST 192, pp. 359–366, 2017.
DOI: 10.1007/978-3-319-58877-3_45

therapies do not exist, the treatment of dementia patients is devoted to relatives or in-home nurses (caregivers). Since the house of the patient is his/her principal environment, mobile and wireless technologies placed at the patient's home can provide therapeutic aids, direct communication with general practitioner and assistance to the caregivers. Maximizing the home assistance and tele-rehabilitation will cause a reduction of the treatments' cost of the hospitalization and will improve the patient's quality of life [4, 5].

Given the multifaceted aspects of dementia, the ideal tele-rehabilitation system has to deal with both motor and cognitive impairments, and has to improve capabilities for an independent life.

In this context, the goal of the ABILITY project was to design, develop and validate an integrated platform of services, aiming at supporting and enhancing the home-based rehabilitation process for patients with dementia. The namesake platform, representing the core of the project, consisted of a central unit and of mobile and wireless devices (e.g. tablets, RFID sensors, wireless scale and pressure sensors, activity trackers) for motor and cognitive rehabilitation of elderly people with dementia [6–8]. The project was developed through a collaboration of academic (Politecnico di Milano and Università degli Studi Milano - Bicocca), clinical (IRCCS Fondazione Don Carlo Gnocchi and Ospedale Valduce - Centro di Riabilitazione di Villa Beretta) and industrial partners (Telbios Srl, Astir Srl, Teorema Engineering Srl, Secure Network Srl, AB Tremila Srl and Sait Srl).

2 The ABILITY Platform Architecture

The ABILITY platform was designed to be a holistic tele-rehabilitation system for elderly dementia patients following a home-based rehabilitation treatment. The etiology of dementia can vary, ranging from Mild-Cognitive-Impairment (MCI), to post-stroke dementia (vascular) to degenerative dementia (due to Parkinson Disease or Alzheimer syndrome) [8]. The two main characteristic of the platform were the possibility for the clinicians to assign rehabilitation plans to be performed at home, and the holistic approach to rehabilitation, as the plan includes physical, cognitive and behavioral therapies/exercises. The platform was not used by the patients only, but also by the caregivers, by the neurologist in charge of the patient and by other clinical specialists (e.g. by the neuropsychologists and physiotherapists). Each of the users has proper functions: the patient can see the daily therapy, the neurologist can assign, modify or evaluate the therapeutic plans, the caregiver can interact with the medical personnel or can check how the rehabilitation is going.

The interaction of the different users and the logical architecture of the platform are depicted in Fig. 1. The lower part represents the patient's interaction with the platform. The patient (green circle) might be equipped with different devices that can be provided with the platform: a dedicated PC/Tablet, used by the patient to see the daily activity plan, to play serious games and to receive or write messages to the neurologist; an activity tracker (FITIBIT®) to measure the amount of physical activity of the patient and the quantity of his sleep; RFID sensors placed in different rooms of the house, in order to measure the time spent in the different rooms (e.g. how much time the patient spends in the bedroom during the day); wireless telemetry devices, such as a scale and a blood pressure monitor. The platform foresees also other devices, which are used only at the hospital (e.g. an EEG portable helmet to measure variations in the brain activity of the patients during specific cognitive or attentive tests). The "Middleware layer" manages the communications from the mobile devices to the PC and then forwards the information to the platform as structured data. The upper part of the figure represents the platform side, the intermediate part is transparent to the users and contains the databases, medical knowledge, business intelligence and decision support system tools, which facilitate the generation and the personalization of rehabilitation plans, also suggesting modifications when needed (e.g. the level of the exercises is too hard for the patient). The upper part represents the front-end interfaces, providing access to the platform to all the clinical staff (red circles) and to the caregiver (orange circle).

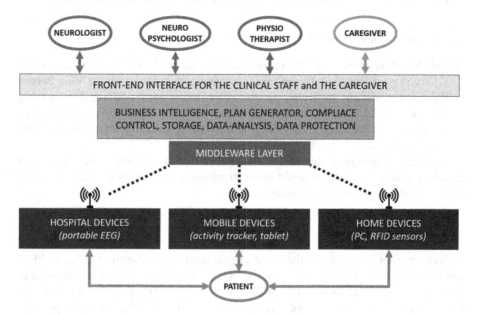

Fig. 1. The ABILITY platform architecture and the interactions of the different users with it. (Color figure online)

3   Pilot Study

3.1   Pilot Study Design

With the aim to investigate the motor aspect of the recovery, and particularly the relationship between the motor recovery and the cognitive recovery, we designed a pilot study. We investigated two small groups of patients: the control group (CTR) that was treated with the standard rehabilitation plan for dementia patients, with both motor and cognitive exercises, and the experimental group (ABIL) that was treated with the support of the ABILITY platform.

3.2   Participants

The participants recruited for the Pilot Study had to satisfy the following criteria. They had to be diagnosed with degenerative dementia: Alzheimer Disease (AD) at mild stage or Mild Cognitive Impairment (MCI) with an high risk to an evolution to AD [9], according to the diagnostic criteria of the DSM-5 [10]. They had to obtain less than 24 points in the Mini-Mental state examination test, they had to have completed at least 3 school years and to be aged between 60 and 85 years. Patients with severe deficits in visual acuity, acoustic perception, communication problems or dysmetria could not take part of the study, because these pathologies could interfere with the activities foresaw by the ABILITY program. The patients were randomly assigned to the ABIL or to the CTR groups. This study and the use of the ABILITY platform was approved by the Ethical Committee of the Valduce Hospital, Villa Beretta Rehabilitation Center.

3.3   Rehabilitation Protocol

The rehabilitation protocol was performed for 6 weeks, bot for CTR and ABIL groups.

CTR group was treated following the usual care protocol in use in the Villa Beretta rehabilitation center. In particular, patients were instructed to perform daily aerobic physical activity, to stimulate cognitive functions with conventional instruments (i.e., crosswords), and to compile a daily diary with physiological variables monitoring (i.e., pressure, weight, etc.).

ABIL group was instructed to use the ABILITY platform daily which allowed to perform cognitive functions rehabilitation with serious games and motor functions rehabilitation with step-by-step instructions.

3.4   Assessment Protocol

Both groups were assessed with the motor-cognitive protocol before the treatment (PRE) and at the end of the 6 weeks of treatments (POST). The proposed protocol consisted of a simple motor test, proposed in two different modalities: (i) classical motor task, and (ii) dual-task, with a cognitive interference in the motor task. The aim of the protocol was to evaluate both the motor performance *per se* and the interaction between the cognitive processes (required during the execution of the motor task), and the execution of the motor exercise itself. The protocol lasted around 20 min and it consisted of two sessions of the 6 min Walking Test (6MWT) [11], separated by a pause of 10 min, to give the possibility to the patient to rest, which was extended upon patient request. The 6MWT, in its classical version (6MWT-S – Simple), was executed with the standard protocol, using an indoor 50 m hallway. The starting and the ending points were marked with adhesive tape on the floor. The participants were informed that the aim of the test was to measure how much they can walk in six minutes. The subjects could decide at which pace take the exercise and also they were allowed to take pauses if they needed. The assisting physiotherapist had to measure the performed distance, the number of the potential pauses and the passed time.

The 6MWT, in the dual-task version (6MWT-DT) [12], was executed in the same way as the 6MWT-S, with the addition of a cognitive task. During the walking, the subjects had to recite the Italian alphabet only every other letter. After 3 min, the assistant changed the starting letter. In the first three minutes, the subjects started with the letter "A" (A-C-E-G-I-M-O-Q-S-U-Z), in the second half of the test the subjects started with the letter "B" (B-D-F-H-L-N-P-R-T-V). In this test, the physiotherapist had also to measure the number of errors made by the subjects.

3.5 Data Analysis

We used the Mann-Whitney U-test to verify if the ages of the subjects in the two groups were significantly different ($p < 0.05$) or not. Afterwards, we computed the average walking speed of the two groups before and after the rehabilitation treatments. We evaluated the walking speeds in both the 6MWT-S and the 6MWT-DT. For the 6MWT-DT we also computed the mean number of errors committed during the task, for both groups (CTR/ABIL) and for both conditions (S/DT). For every measure, we used the Mann-Whitney U-test to verify if there were significant differences ($p < 0.05$) between the groups or between the conditions. In order to verify the interference of the cognitive processes on the motor task, we have defined an ad-hoc index I, which quantify, as a percentage, the improvement (POST-PRE) in the 6MWT-DT versus the improvement in the 6MWT-S task, which was defined as follows (Eq. 1):

$$I = \frac{(Vel_{POST\_DT} - Vel_{POST\_S})}{Vel_{POST\_S}} - \frac{(Vel_{PRE\_DT} - Vel_{PRE\_S})}{Vel_{PRE\_S}} \cdot 100 \tag{1}$$

Where Vel_{POST_S} and Vel_{POST_DT} were the gait velocities in the POST session in the S and in the DT protocols, respectively; Vel_{PRE_S} and Vel_{PRE_DT} were the gait velocities in the PRE session in the S and in the DT protocols, respectively.

4   Results of the Pilot Study

4.1   Participants

6 patients for the control group (CTR), and 4 for the intervention group (ABIL) completed the proposed rehabilitation program. The recruited subjects were all diagnosed with degenerative dementia, with demographics reported in Table 1.

Table 1. Demographic data of the control (CTR) and experimental (ABIL) groups.

	CTR group (N = 6)	ABIL group (N = 4)
Diagnosis	Degenerative dementia	Degenerative dementia
Sex	M = 3, F = 3	M = 1, F = 3
Age (years)	75.0 ± 8.9 (61.1–84.6)	69.8 ± 1.7 (63.0–76.4)
School years	5.0 ± 0.0	6.5 ± 1.7
Mini-mental-state test	19.3 ± 5.8	22 ± 4.7

4.2 Motor and Cognitive Performance and Their Interaction

The subjects of the CTR and ABIL groups could be considered age-matched, since the p-value resulting from the Mann-Whitney test was equal to 0.48 *(>0.05)*. All participants, but one of the CTR group, could be considered as community ambulators, since they had a gait speed higher than the threshold commonly used in literature of 0.8 m/s [13], the mean gait velocities along with their standard deviations of both groups in all the four conditions are reported in Fig. 2 and in Table 2.

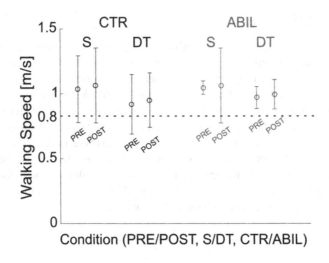

Fig. 2. The gait speeds of the two groups (CTR in black, ABIL in red), in the four conditions (S/DT and PRE/POST). (Color figure online)

Table 2. The gait speeds of the two groups (CTR in black, ABIL in red) in the four conditions (S/DT and PRE/POST) and the number of errors in the DT task are reported as Mean ± Standard Deviation. The *p-values* of the Mann-Whitney test between the CTR and the ABIL group are reported in the last column.

Protocol	Measure	CTR group	ABIL group	p-value
Simple	Vel_{PRE} [m/s]	1.034 ± 0.257	1.046 ± 0.052	1.000
	Vel_{POST} [m/s]	1.063 ± 0.288	1.025 ± 0.091	0.324
Dual task	Vel_{PRE_DT} [m/s]	0.918 ± 0.229	0.970 ± 0.085	0.714
	Vel_{POST_DT} [m/s]	0.951 ± 0.209	0.995 ± 0.113	0.914
	$Errors_{PRE}$	20.6 ± 8.9	6 ± 6.8	0.0381 (*)
	$Errors_{POST}$	17.8 ± 8.5	5.2 ± 4.6	0.0382 (*)

*$p < 0.05$

It is possible to notice that in both CTR and ABIL groups and in both S and DT experiments, there was a general increase of the gait speed induced by the rehabilitation training, which was however not significant, considering the minimally clinical significant change for the gait velocity in the 6MWT of 0.14 m/s [14, 15]. Also, the Mann-Whitney test comparisons performed between the CTR and the ABIL groups showed that in all the four conditions there were no significant differences in the gait speed. Otherwise, the number of errors committed by the ABIL group was significantly lower than the CTR group both in the PRE and in the POST assessments.

About the cognitive interference index I, the improvement of the subjects of the CTR group in the DT with respect to the S task was of the 2.05%, whereas the improvement of the ABIL group was of the 3.98%. However, due to the high variance and the low numerosity of the groups, the Mann-Whitney test did not show a significant variation between the two groups for the index I.

5 Discussion and Conclusions

The results obtained through the designed Pilot Study showed that both the usual care therapy of elderly dementia patients and the use of the ABILITY tele-rehabilitation platform generated an improvement -in a basic motor task- the locomotion. In particular, the gait speed increased from the PRE to the POST of about 0.03 m/s in both groups and in both the Simple (S) and the Dual Task (DT). Focusing on the investigation of the interference of the cognitive processes on the walking task, an interesting result emerged: the improvement in the DT with respect to the improvement in the S task was doubled in the ABIL group. This suggests the hypothesis that the use of a holistic tele-rehabilitation system like the ABILITY platform could help in improving both the motor skills, the cognitive skill and the interaction between them. Since the present is only a pilot study, the statistical significance of the presented results has to be improved by extending the number of the patient's cohorts, and attention might be devoted to differentiate responders and non-responders which has been demonstrated to be an effective approach with post-stroke patients [15, 16]. Moreover, the study might be extended to other motor-cognitive tasks during the rehabilitation of dementia in elderly subjects.

Acknowledgments. Ability is co-funded by Regione Lombardia within the Smart Cities and Smart Communities funding program (MIUR-POR LOMBARDY – ASSE 1 POR FESR 2007–2013).

References

1. Graham, J.E., Rockwood, K., Beattie, B.L., et al.: Prevalence and severity of cognitive impairment with and without dementia in an elderly population. Lancet **349**, 1793–1796 (1997). doi:10.1016/S0140-6736(97)01007-6
2. Lobo, A., Launer, L.J., Fratiglioni, L., et al.: Prevalence of dementia and major subtypes in Europe: a collaborative study of population-based cohorts. Neurologic diseases in the Elderly research group. Neurology **54**, S4–S9 (2000)
3. Young, R., Camic, P.M., Tischler, V.: The impact of community-based arts and health interventions on cognition in people with dementia: a systematic literature review. Aging Ment. Health **20**, 337–351 (2016). doi:10.1080/13607863.2015.1011080

4. McCue, M., Fairman, A., Pramuka, M.: Enhancing quality of life through telerehabilitation. Phy. Med. rehabil. clin. N. Am. **21**, 195–205 (2010). doi:10.1016/j.pmr.2009.07.005

5. Kairy, D., Lehoux, P., Vincent, C., Visintin, M.: A systematic review of clinical outcomes, clinical process, healthcare utilization and costs associated with telerehabilitation. Disabil. Rehabil. **31**, 427–447 (2009). doi:10.1080/09638280802062553

6. Laurin, D., Verreault, R., Lindsay, J., et al.: Physical activity and risk of cognitive impairment and dementia in elderly persons. Arch. Neurol. **58**, 498–504 (2001). doi:10.1001/archneur. 58.3.498

7. Tousignant, M., Boissy, P., Corriveau, H., Moffet, H.: In home telerehabilitation for older adults after discharge from an acute hospital or rehabilitation unit: a proof-of-concept study and costs estimation. Disabil. Rehabil. Assist. Technol. **1**, 209–216 (2006). doi: 10.1080/17483100600776965

8. Antonietti, A., Gandolla, M., Nalin, M., et al.: A telerehabilitation platform for cognitive, physical and behavioral rehabilitation in elderly patients affected by dementia. In: 6° Forum Ital. dell'Ambient Assist. Living. Lecco, pp. 29–35 (2015)

9. Albert, M.S., DeKosky, S.T., Dickson, D., et al.: The diagnosis of mild cognitive impairment due to Alzheimer's disease: recommendations from the national institute on Aging-Alzheimer's association workgroups on diagnostic guidelines for Alzheimer's disease. Alzheimer's Dement. **7**, 270–279 (2011). doi:10.1016/j.jalz.2011.03.008

10. DSM-5 Diagnostic classification. Diagnostic and Statistical Manual of Mental Disorders. (2013). doi:10.1176/appi.books.9780890425596.x00DiagnosticClassification

11. Enright, P.L., McBurnie, M.A., Bittner, V., et al.: The 6-min walk test: a quick measure of functional status in elderly adults. Chest **123**, 387–398 (2003). doi:10.1378/chest.123.2.387

12. Verghese, J., Mahoney, J., Ambrose, A.F., et al.: Effect of cognitive remediation on gait in sedentary seniors. J. Gerontol. A Biol. Sci. Med. Sci. **65**, 1338–1343 (2010). doi:10.1093/gerona/glq127

13. Bowden, M.G., Balasubramanian, C.K., Behrman, A.L., Kautz, S.A.: Validation of a speed-based classification system using quantitative measures of walking performance poststroke. Neurorehabil. Neural Repair **22**, 672–675 (2008). doi:10.1177/1545968308318837

14. Perera, S., Mody, S.H., Woodman, R.C., Studenski, S.A.: Meaningful change and responsiveness in common physical performance measures in older adults. J. Am. Geriatr. Soc. **54**, 743–749 (2006). doi:10.1111/j.1532-5415.2006.00701.x

15. Gandolla, M., Molteni, F., Ward, N.S., et al.: Validation of a quantitative single-subject based evaluation for rehabilitation-induced improvement assessment. Ann. Biomed. Eng. **43**, 2686–2698 (2015). doi:10.1007/s10439-015-1317-4

16. Gandolla, M., Ward, N.S., Molteni, F., et al.: The neural correlates of long-term carryover following functional electrical stimulation for stroke. Neural Plast. **2016**, 1–13 (2016). doi: 10.1155/2016/4192718. Article no. 4192718

Supporting Physical and Cognitive Training for Preventing the Occurrence of Dementia Using an Integrated System: A Pilot Study

Mauro Marzorati[1(✉)], Simona Gabriella Di Santo[2], Simona Mrakic-Sposta[1],
Sarah Moretti[1], Nithiya Jesuthasan[3], Andrea Caroppo[4], Andrea Zangiacomi[5],
Alessandro Leone[4], Marco Sacco[5], and Alessandra Vezzoli[1]

[1] Istituto di Bioimmagini e Fisiologia Molecolare, CNR, Milan, Italy
mauro.marzorati@ibfm.cnr.it
[2] IRCCS Fondazione Santa Lucia, Rome, Italy
[3] Istituto di Tecnologie Biomediche, CNR, Milan, Italy
[4] Istituto per la Microelettronica e Microsistemi, CNR, Lecce, Italy
[5] Istituto di Tecnologie Industriali e Automazione, CNR, Milan, Italy

Abstract. The project proposes a comprehensive preventive program of dementia in elderlies with minor cognitive disorders due to neurodegenerative diseases. The program combines physical and cognitive training, by means of an integrated technological system composed of a Virtual Environment, simulating daily activities, a smart garment measuring physiological parameters, a bicycle ergometer and tailoring the system to the specific patient's status. Preliminary results confirm the feasibility of this intervention and appear promising in order to contrast age-related cognitive neurodegeneration.

Keywords: Physical and cognitive training · MCI · Oxidative stress · Virtual environment · Smart garment

1 Introduction

Age-related cognitive changes may progress from mild cognitive impairment (MCI) to dementia, a condition in which memory, behavior and cognition are impaired due to neurodegeneration in the brain. Different neurodegenerative disorders causing dementias are observed in elderly but Alzheimer's disease (AD) is the most frequent accounting for 60–70% of all the forms. The pathological process of AD precedes of decades the clinical severe manifestations of dementia, suggesting the possibility of early interventions in asymptomatic or early mild symptomatic individuals. Among many possible procedures, exercise training and cognitive stimulation have demonstrated some preventive efficacy. Cross-sectional studies in humans suggest that more active individuals may have reduced risk of impairment and dementia [1]. Furthermore, improvements in cognitive function in older subjects have also been reported from supervised aerobic training interventions [1]. On the other side, it has been recently reported that even

© ICST Institute for Computer Sciences, Social Informatics and Telecommunications Engineering 2017
P. Perego et al. (Eds.): MobiHealth 2016, LNICST 192, pp. 367–374, 2017.
DOI: 10.1007/978-3-319-58877-3_46

simple computer-based virtual environments were effective in enhancing cognition of older adults [2].

Patients with AD and even individuals with MCI [3], often exhibit disorders in Visuospatial (VSP) abilities, such as difficulties with reading, discriminating forms and colors or perceive contrasts, failures to identify objects (agnosia) or to locate them into the environment, deficits of spatial orientation and motion detection, difficulties in developing visual strategies (i.e. to avoid obstacles, point to or grasp objects). Individuals with MCI show preserved brain plasticity and indication exists that cognitive rehabilitation can be a potential efficient method to enhance their cognitive and functional abilities.

Starting from these considerations, this project (GOJI) aimed to develop a comprehensive preventive program tailored on the individual and group characteristics of the cohort (elderly people with minor cognitive disorders) based on the use of a virtual environment and a smart garment, with the purpose of providing an effective and easy accessible technological tool for physical and cognitive stimulation.

2   The Physical and Cognitive Training System

The training system is composed of two main subsystems: a virtual environment simulating daily activities and a smart garment which controls the physiological parameters and regulates the physical exercise intensity properly in order to maintain patient's heart rate at the chosen value.

2.1   Virtual Environment for Supporting Physical and Cognitive Training

The designed virtual environment is composed of two main scenarios, which replicate daily activities: cycling in the park/city and shopping at market.

Both the virtual cycling environment as well as the virtual market one are composed of two steps. The user has to cycle in a park first (purely physical activity) and then in a city, taking care of approaching cars before crossing the streets (jointly physical and cognitive activities). Once in the market, two different tasks, structured according to five different difficulty levels, have to be performed (purely cognitive activity).

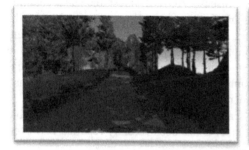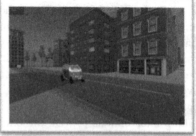

Fig. 1. Screenshots of the virtual cycling scenario

The street scenario, in which the user has to cycle on a cycle-ergometer, is designed according to a subjective point of view. During the route for reaching the market the user has to cross some roads stopping and checking that both sides are clear of traffic before proceeding through the intersection. The user uses a joystick for looking at both sides of the road (Fig. 1).

In the market scenario, the user is provided with a shopping-list and has to select accordingly first the appropriate lane containing the products to be purchased as in a real supermarket. Then he/she is asked to detect and select the correct product from the shelf. The number of products in the list, the number of lanes, the amount of items on the shelf and also the position of the target item increase according to the difficulty level selected. Automatic helps (verbal/visive indications) are provided to users if errors occur (Fig. 2).

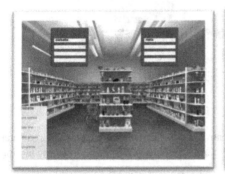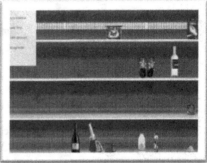

Fig. 2. Screenshots of the virtual market: lane and shelf

Both the street and market scenarios are built in Unity 3D. A cycle-ergometer is integrated into the system (see next paragraph) and a touch-enabled interactive projector is used. The system is thus able to track the gesture of the users and to reveal the point and click activities performed in order to select the proper lane and the requested products on the shelf [4].

2.2 Smart Garment for Heart Rate Monitoring in Virtual Environment Navigation

The navigation of the Virtual Environment for the physical training is carried out by means of a cycle-ergometer (Fig. 3a) and a smart garment (Wearable Wellness System - WWS) (Fig. 3b). The WWS integrates an electronic device for the acquisition, the storage and the wireless transmission of the data. The WWS is designed to be suitable and comfortable, reducing the well-known usability problems of the wearable devices. It integrates two textile electrodes and one textile piezoresistive sensor placed in a pocket at the chest level. It has been designed to monitor continuously the most important vital parameters (as ECG, heart rate and breathe rate) and the movements of the end-user (according to the data of the tri-axial MEMS accelerometer integrated inside). The WWS can operate in streaming mode via Bluetooth up to 20 m in free space or in off-line mode, storing the data on the onboard micro-SD card. Data acquired are sampled with different rates (breath-rate@25 Hz, heart-rate@0.2 Hz, 1-derived ECG channel@250 Hz) and transmitted to the PC on which the Virtual Environment is running.

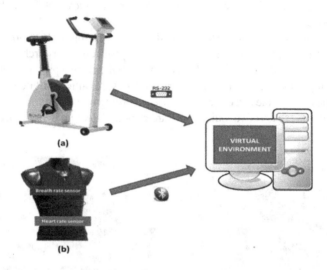

Fig. 3. Overall architecture for fatigue level control at constant HR: (a) the bicycle ergometer used for navigation of VE and (b) the Wearable Wellness System (WWS) used for HR monitoring during the training exercise

An ad-hoc software library manages the user's interaction with the Virtual Environment, integrating functionalities for (a) heart-rate acquisition by the smart garment (via Bluetooth protocol), (b) cycle-ergometer speed acquisition (via RS232 protocol) and (c) setting of the workload of the cycle-ergometer (via RS232 protocol) according to both the cycling speed and the required level of fatigue as defined by the physicians.

The aim of keeping constant the level of effort during training exercise has been reached through the design and the implementation of a digital controller based on a proportional-integral (PI) feedback mechanism.

The control strategy used is inspired from the work of Kawada et al. [5]. In particular, the controller measures the HR provided by the smart garment, compares it with a priori defined HR (heart rate) preset value (about 65% of maximal HR of the subject) and adjusts the workload in order to minimize the difference between them. The difference value is scaled and integrated from the terms of control K_p (proportional gain) and K_i (integral gain). To obtain the correct setting for K_p and K_i a simulation of the overall system was carried out thanks to Simulink Matlab®. The simulation assumes that the controller must stabilize the HR value within specific time constraints. In this work a constraint is that the achievement of the preset HR should be obtained within 3–4 min from the start of the training exercise. From the results obtained, the system is stable in the desired time using the following coefficient: Kp = 0.5, and Ki = 0.04.

3   Description of the Pilot Study

3.1   Experimental Session

This pilot study was performed as a randomized, controlled trial: 10 participants with minor cognitive impairment or mild AD, aged 71 ± 6 years, with 7.6 ± 4.4 years of schooling, were randomly assigned to the experimental group (n = 5), subjected to 3 sessions per week for 6 weeks of Physical and Cognitive Training (Street and Market) for a total of 18 sessions or to a control group (n = 5) that did not receive any kind of stimulation. The duration of training was approximately 40–45 min: 15-20 min of free cycling, about 5 min to perform 5 crossroad passing and 20 min of shopping at the supermarket). The traffic at each intersection (i.e. number and speed of the cars transiting on the road to cross) was determined randomly.

During each session of "shopping" the subject was required to purchase 5 common grocery items. The number of items correctly selected and the number of latencies/omissions/mis-identifications was recorded. The task is designed with increasing levels of difficulty, characterized by the progressive increase of the number of distractors and of their similarity to the target, i.e. of the characteristics to be considered to recognize the correct item among other products. The subject could move to the next level of difficulty after the proper purchase (1 error at the most) of the articles in two consecutive shopping sessions. From the sixth level, the shopping list is hidden, to stimulate memory.

3.2   Assessment of Cognitive Response

In order to verify the positive effects of the training benefits on cognitive and functional capabilities, before the experimental phase (t0), and at the end of the 6 weeks of training (t1), both the experimental and the control group underwent a full neuropsychological assessment. Mini Mental State Examination (MMSE), Rey Auditory Verbal Learning Test (RAVLT), Frontal Assesment Battery (FAB), Rey-Osterrieth Complex Figure Test (ROCFT), Verbal Fluency (VF), Trail Making Test A and B (TMT-a, TMT-b) and Attentive Matrices (AM) were administered for cognitive evaluation. The Functional Activities Questionnaire (FAQ) was used to assess activities of daily living.

These scales tests return numeric values, which can be considered continuous and allow for the comparison of means. For this first pilot phase, t-tests were conducted to compare the scale scores at t0 and t1 within each group, and the changes in scores between t0 and t1 between experimental and control groups.

3.3   Assessment of Physiological Response

Oxidative stress plays an essential role in the pathogenesis of neurodegenerative diseases as it has been suggested that damage caused by Reactive Oxygen Species (ROS) may result in neuronal cell death. Electron Paramagnetic Resonance (EPR) may evaluate oxidative stress measuring the ROS production. Micro-invasive analytic technique for detection ROS concentration by EPR is now demonstrated suitable to monitor physiological and pathological conditions [6].

The physiological impact of training has been evaluated by the assessment of the heart rate profile, the average work rate and ROS production in both the experimental and control groups at t0 and t1.

4 Results and Discussion

4.1 Assessment of Cognitive Response

Participants had a mild cognitive impairment (MMSE = 23 ± 3.4) and a mild functional impairment (FAQ = 9.7 ± 7.3), of borderline significance. In each group we included three subjects with Mild cognitive impairment (i.e. cognitive impairment in the absence of significant impairment of autonomy) and two patients with mild dementia, (i.e. a mild cognitive impairment and a mild/moderate impairment of instrumental skills of daily living). During the trial, two male participants (one belonging to the experimental group and one to the controls) dropped, both due to hospitalization for reasons unrelated to their cognitive impairment.

In Fig. 4, the mean changes in the corrected test scores between t1 and t0 of experimental and control group are shown. The experimental subjects showed a slight improvement in the MMSE, in visual-constructive test and visuospatial tests of attention, while the controls worsened. The experimental group had a greater improvement than controls in the executive test, memory functions and verbal fluency, while showed a greater worsening of Activities of Daily Living (ADL). None of the comparisons within and between groups reached statistical significance at t-tests, reasonably due to small sample, which amplifies the effect of the slight heterogeneity in scores between subjects.

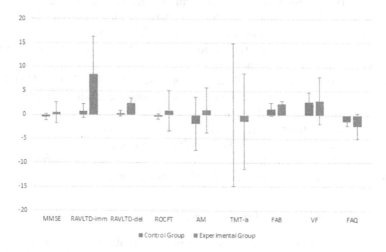

Fig. 4. Mean change scores between the baseline and the end of experimental phase (calculated as t1–t0 scores, except for TMT tests and FAQ implying decreasing scores in relation to better performance, and for which the changes were calculated as t0–t1).

4.2 Assessment of Physiological Response

The compliance to the training regimen was evaluated as "high" (96% of all training sessions were completed as scheduled). Comparing the average work rate performed during the first and the last training sessions a slightly increase was observed whereas heart rate was kept constant.

Compared to the control subjects, in the experimental group after training intervention ROS production rate resulted statistically ($p < 0.05$) lower (2.58 ± 0.32 vs 2.03 ± 0.23 $\mu mol \cdot min^{-1}$ respectively) (Fig. 5).

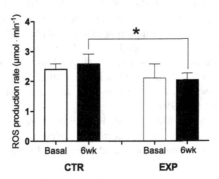

Fig. 5. Histogram plot (mean ± SD) of the absolute ROS production rate ($\mu mol \cdot min^{-1}$) obtained from capillary blood in the control (CTR) and experimental (EXP) groups before and after 6 weeks.

After 6 weeks, ROS productions tend to increase with respect to basal value in the control group (2.39 ± 0.18 vs 2.58 ± 0.32 $\mu mol \cdot min^{-1}$) and tend to decrease in the experimental group (2.10 ± 0.48 vs 2.03 ± 0.23 $\mu mol \cdot min^{-1}$).

This evidence supports the hypothesis that the use of the training protocol may help to delay neurodegenerative damage caused by oxidative stress.

5 Conclusions

The preliminary results of this pilot suggest that the proposed preventive program should be a feasible and effective tool for physical and cognitive stimulation. Further studies, involving more participants, are needed in order to confirm these findings in a larger population.

Acknowledgments. The project was supported by grants "Progetto di interesse Invecchiamento CNR: Goji and WP3.7".

References

1. Gregory, S.M., Parker, B., Thompson, P.D.: Physical activity, cognitive function, and brain health: what is the role of exercise training in the prevention of dementia? Brain Sci. **2**, 684–708 (2012)
2. Che, M.R., Gramegna, S.M., Biamonti, A.: Virtual reality in assessing the supportive environment that promotes navigability of persons with Alzheimer's disease. Stud. Health. Technol. Inform. **6**, 217–951 (2015)
3. Hort, J., Laczo, J., Vyhnalek, M., Bojar, M., Bures, J., Vicek, K.: Spatial navigation deficit in amnestic mild cognitive impairment. Proc. Natl. Acad. Sci. **104**, 4042–4047 (2007)
4. Sacco, M., Redaelli, C., Zangiacomi, A., Greci, L., Di Santo, S., Leone, A., Vezzoli A.: GOJI an Advanced Virtual Environment Supporting Training of Physical and Cognitive Activities to Prevent Dementia Occurrence in Elderly with Minor Cognitive Disorders. In: Ambient Assisted Living. Biosystems & Biorobotics, vol. 11, pp. 429–437. Springer, Cham (2015)
5. Kawada, T., Sunagawa, G., Takaki, H., Shishido, T., Miyano, H., Miyashita, H., Sato, T., Sugimachi, M., Sunagawa, K.: Development of a servo-controller of heart rate using a treadmill. Jpn. Circ. J. **63**, 945–950 (1999)
6. Mrakic-Sposta, S., Gussoni, M., Montorsi, M., Porcelli, S., Vezzoli, A.: A quantitative method to monitor reactive oxygen species production by electron paramagnetic resonance in physiological and pathological conditions. Oxid. Med. Cell. Longev. **2014**, 306179 (2014)

A New Personalized Health System: The SMARTA Project

Massimo W. Rivolta[1(✉)], Paolo Perego[2], Giuseppe Andreoni[2],
Maurizio Ferrarin[3], Giuseppe Baroni[4], Corrado Galzio[4], Giovanna Rizzo[5],
Marco Tarabini[6], Marco Bocciolone[6], and Roberto Sassi[1]

[1] Dipartimento di Informatica, Università degli Studi di Milano, Crema, Italy
massimo.rivolta@unimi.it
[2] Design Department, Politecnico di Milano, Milan, Italy
[3] IRCCS Fondazione Don Carlo Gnocchi Onlus, Milan, Italy
[4] Flextronics Design Srl, Milan, Italy
[5] Istituto di Bioimmagini e Fisiologia Molecolare, CNR, Segrate, Italy
[6] Dipartimento di Meccanica, Politecnico di Milano, Milan, Italy

Abstract. The growing number of elderly people with health issues is
the consequence of the increase in life expectancy. Tele-homecare applications have already reported promising results on reducing health care
costs and improving quality of life. In this study, we present the SMARTA
platform (www.smarta-project.it): a fully integrated system capable to
monitor its user's health condition. The latest telemedicine and wearable
technologies have been used to make cooperating users and caregivers.
The system integrates wearable (ECG and accelerometry), non-wearable
(temperature, weight, blood pressure etc.) and environmental (light,
refrigerator etc.) sensors.

Keywords: Telemedicine · Tele-homecare · Wearable · Accelerometry ·
ECG · Heart rate · Integrated system

1 Introduction

As reported in the fourth World Population Aging 2013 report [11], United
Nations, NY, 2013, *"Population ageing is taking place in nearly all the countries
of the world. Ageing results from decreasing mortality, and, most importantly,
declining fertility. ... Globally, the number of older persons (aged 60 years or
over) is expected to more than double, from 841 million people in 2013 to more
than 2 billion in 2050."* (p. xii). Moreover, *"The older population is itself ageing.
Globally, the share of older persons aged 80 years or over (the "oldest old") within
the older population was 14% in 2013 and is projected to reach 19% in 2050."*
(p. xiii).

Along with the increase in life expectancy, a growing number of elderly people
with health issues and their related chronic co-morbidities is present as well [5].
To worsen the scenario, more than 50% of elderly patients receiving polypharmacy fail in adhering to the therapy when discharged from hospital [6], causing

© ICST Institute for Computer Sciences, Social Informatics and Telecommunications Engineering 2017
P. Perego et al. (Eds.): MobiHealth 2016, LNICST 192, pp. 375–380, 2017.
DOI: 10.1007/978-3-319-58877-3_47

drug reaction and possible need of permanent hospitalization [1]. Such scenario represents an important issue for the public health systems and the economic development.

Even though telemonitoring is still being debated [4], especially for its unpredictable economical advantage, there are evidences of reduced costs for tele-homecare applications [8]. In particular, they are found to reduce the use of hospitals, improving patient compliance, satisfaction and quality of life. Also, the use of current technology, *i.e.*, the Internet of Things paradigm, for health care applications at home, could help to restructure the old healthcare system, still based on a relationship between patient and physician in an ambulatory setting [9].

In this study, we present a fully integrated system, *i.e.*, the SMARTA platform[1], for monitoring the health of elderly people at their home with the aim of improving the quality of life and the subject compliance to therapies, as well as promoting their active aging. Such platform have been developed accordingly to the SMARTA project[2].

2   Methods

2.1   Main Scope

The SMARTA platform is designed to monitor the health status of the user by means of an integrated system. Moreover, the platform is meant to be used in cooperation with the physician or the caregiver. In particular, the physician defines the variables to be collected (*e.g.*, temperature, heart rate *etc.*) and the frequency of the measurements, and can visualize the time evolution of the measured quantities using a web-app application. On the user-side, an automatic notification system reminds the measurements to be performed and provides audio guidelines. The user can constantly see the scheduled tests without any interaction with the system.

Along with the monitoring of the health status, environmental variables are tracked as well. Tap water leakage, lights on, refrigerator door opening are several examples of environmental variables observed.

In the following sections, the hardware and software architecture of the SMARTA platform will be described. Figure 1 shows the scheme of the platform developed.

2.2   Hardware Architecture

The hardware architecture of the SMARTA platform is composed by: (i) wearable, non-wearable and environmental sensors; (ii) gateway and middleware; and (iii) user interface.

---

[1] Sistema di Monitoraggio Ambientale con Rete di sensori e Telemonitoraggio indossabile a supporto di servizi di salute, prevenzione e sicurezza per l'Active Aging.

[2] The work was supported by the project "SMARTA" (code: 40628684, www.smarta-project.it), funded by Regione Lombardia, Italy, through the call "Smart cities 2013".

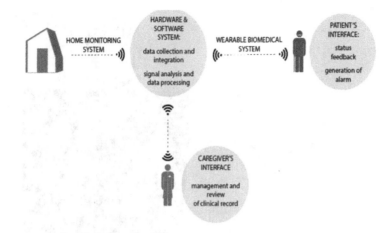

Fig. 1. SMARTA platform architecture.

First, sensors includes

1. a Bluetooth (ver 2.1) weight scale (UC-351PBT-Ci model, A&D Medical Inc., USA) for body weight measurement;
2. a multipurpose device (PC-304 Spot-Check Monitor, CMI Health Inc., USA) for measuring the heart rate, ear temperature, blood pressure, blood oxygen saturation and glycaemia;
3. a wearable fall detection device (SmartWalk, H&S Quality in Software Srl, Italy);
4. a wearable device named "SMARTA patch" for recording a single lead ECG (LSB=$4.8081e-05$ mV, 24 bit and sampling rate of 250 Hz) and 3D accelerometry (±8 g, 16 bit and sampling rate of 52 Hz);
5. the Konnex (KNX) home automation system to monitor tap water, refrigerator and dishwasher.

The SMARTA patch is specifically designed for the SMARTA project (Flextronics Design Srl, Italy; Fig. 2). Its dimensions and weight are $78\times35\times11.5$ mm and 30 g, respectively. ECG signals are collected by using self-adhesive electrodes made of biocompatible material placed directly on the skin, or by plugging the SMARTA patch to a T-shirt (PoliMI Design, Italy), or a chest band for women.

Second, the gateway (Datamed Srl, Italy) collects the raw data coming from all the sensors using a Bluetooth Low Energy protocol, and communicates with the middleware, *i.e.*, a desktop PC configured with common web service settings, that is responsible of the storage and processing of the recorded data.

Third, the user interface is simply a personal computer with internet connection for the physician or caregiver and a touch-screen monitor, plugged to an audio system for interacting with the user.

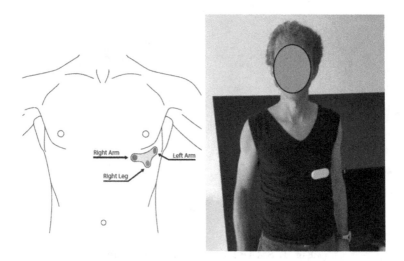

Fig. 2. The SMARTA patch. Left panel shows the approximate position of the SMARTA patch, while on the right panel, the real setting is shown (SMARTA patch + T-shirt).

2.3   Software Architecture

The software can be separated into four parts accordingly to the objective; specifically: (i) data transmission; (ii) data storage; (iii) data processing/data mining; and (iv) user interface.

First, data transmission is performed by integrating the Bluetooth proprietary protocols of the off-the-shelves sensors and by creating an *ad-hoc* Bluetooth Low Energy protocol for the SMARTA patch.

Second, data storage uses the SQL technology to keep track of the clinical information such as age, weight, height *etc*, at time of enrollment of the user, to store raw data from sensors and to schedule the tests to perform by the user.

Third, the data processing software library is meant to process the raw signals, *i.e.*, ECG and accelerometry, and to extract useful information for the physician or caregiver. In particular, the raw ECG signal is used to obtain the time evolution of the heart rate, while the accelerometry is employed to estimate the risk of falling accordingly to the Tinetti test [10], using an automatic intelligent algorithm [7]. Raw data are processed using a software library that integrates Matlab, C and Delphi routines.

Data storage and processing are performed on the middleware.

Finally, the user interface is based on a web-app application. The caregiver can manage the clinical information of the user, the scheduled tests and check the time evolution of the measured variables (such as ECG from wearable, blood pressure from non-wearable and light-on duration from environmental data). On the other hand, the user can visualize the tests to perform. The notifications of the tests for the user are audio messages.

3   Conclusion

In this paper, we described the hardware and software architecture of a new integrated system for tele-homecare monitoring and promoting active ageing: the SMARTA platform.

The prototype was tested at the Smart Home in the DAT department of Fondazione don Gnocchi (Milan, Italy) by enrolling 32 volunteers. The system obtained a good perception among the participants (results are out of the scope of this article). Also, its reliability was on average good, though some technical issues need to be fixed in future releases (*e.g.*, sensor disconnection). Overall, the system was highly appreciated by both physicians and users.

4   Future Works

Four main future activities might be performed to improve the SMARTA platform.

First, we tested whether actigraphy measured at the chest (accordingly with the position of the SMARTA patch) was capable to determine the sleep quality [2] (typically accelerometers are located on the wrist for this purpose). The research provided promising results but needed further investigation.

Second, we implemented a new system capable to detect falls using sensorized garments and accelerometers fixed on the ground [3]. In particular, the accelerometers located on the floor, after a calibration session meant to describe its material, were capable to detect vibrations propagated radially from the fall position.

Third, a cloud-based architecture for the data storage and data processing software would help data privacy and security.

Finally, a physical activity log system (such as number of steps, activity counts *etc.*) was also developed but still not integrated.

Acknowledgment. This work was financially supported by a grant from Regione Lombardia (Bando "Avviso pubblico per la realizzazione di progetti di ricerca industriale e sviluppo sperimentale nel settore delle smart cities and communities (d.d.u.o. n. 2760/2013 - POR-FESR 2007-2013 asse 1 - Linea di intervento 1.1.1.1. azione E)".

Authors thank all partners of the project (www.smarta-project.it): Datamed S.r.l., Flextronics Design S.r.l., Argonet S.r.l., Software Team S.r.l., Electron, Fondazione Don Carlo Gnocchi Onlus, Dipartimento di Informatica of Università degli Studi di Milano, Dipartimento di Meccanica e Design of Politecnico di Milano, Consiglio Nazionale delle Ricerche and CoDeBri.

References

1. Ahmad, A., Mast, M.R., Nijpels, G., Elders, P.J., Dekker, J.M., Hugtenburg, J.G.: Identification of drug-related problems of elderly patients discharged from hospital. Patient Prefer Adherence **8**, 155–165 (2014)
2. Aktaruzzaman, M., Rivolta, M.W., Karmacharya, R., Pugnetti, L., Garegnani, M., Bovi, G., Ferrarin, M., Sassi, R.: Use of detrended fluctuation analysis for sleep vs wake classification from heart rate variability. In: Conference Proceedings of ESGCO, Lancaster, UK (2016)

3. Andreoni, G., Tarabini, M., Gocanin, F., Perego, P., Bocciolone, M.: Smart ambient& wearable integrated monitoring at home for elderly. In: Conference Proceedings of IEEE Engineering in Medicine and Biology Society, Milan, Italy. IEEE (2015)
4. Ekeland, A.G., Bowes, A., Flottorp, S.: Effectiveness of telemedicine: a systematic review of reviews. Int. J. Med. Inform. **79**(11), 736–771 (2010)
5. Gavrilov, L.A., Heuveline, P.: Aging of Population, pp. 32–37. Macmillan Reference USA, New York (2003)
6. Pasina, L., Brucato, A.L., Falcone, C., Cucchi, E., Bresciani, A., Sottocorno, M., Taddei, G.C., Casati, M., Franchi, C., Djade, C.D., Nobili, A.: Medication non-adherence among elderly patients newly discharged and receiving polypharmacy. Drugs Aging **31**(4), 283–289 (2014)
7. Rivolta, M.W., Aktaruzzaman, M., Rizzo, G., Lafortuna, C., Ferrarin, M., Bovi, G., Bonardi, D.R., Sassi, R.: Automatic vs. clinical assessment of fall risk in older individuals: a proof of concept. In: Conference Proceedings of IEEE Engineering in Medicine and Biology Society, Milan, Italy, pp. 6935–6938 (2015)
8. Rojas, S.V., Gagnon, M.P.: A systematic review of the key indicators for assessing telehomecare cost-effectiveness. Telemed. J. E-Health **14**, 896–904 (2008)
9. Silva, B.M., Rodrigues, J.J., de la Díez, I.T., López-Coronado, M., Saleem, K.: Mobile-health: a review of current state in 2015. J. Biomed. Inform. **56**, 265–272 (2015)
10. Tinetti, M.E.: Performance-oriented assessment of mobility problems in elderly patients. J. Am. Geriatr. Soc. **34**(2), 119–126 (1986)
11. United Nations: World Population Ageing. Technical report, Department of Economic and Social Affairs, Population Division, ST/ESA/SER.A/348 (2013)

Advances in Personalized Healthcare Services, Wearable Mobile Monitoring, and Social Media Pervasive Technologies

Identification of Elders' Fall Using the Floor Vibration

Marco Bocciolone, Filip Gocanin, Diego Scaccabarozzi,
Bortolino Saggin, and Marco Tarabini[✉]

Department of Mechanical Engineering,
Politecnico di Milano, Via La Masa 1, Milan, Italy
marco.tarabini@polimi.it

Abstract. This works investigates the possibility of identifying the elders' fall using accelerometers located on the ground. The work is divided in three parts: in the first we have designed a force platform to measure the forces generated during the fall and we have estimated the force generated by the impact of a subject with the floor using a crash test dummy. The effect of the dummy initial posture, of the presence of obstacles on the fall trajectory and of other parameters has been analysed as well. In the second part of the study we have analysed the vibration transmissibility in different dwellings. The final part of the research was focused on the estimation of the force starting from the vibration and from the impedance of the floor. Results have shown the possibility of identifying the elders' falls in the majority of dwellings.

Keywords: Fall detection · Vibration · Impedance

1 Introduction

The continuous improvement of living standard creates a new set of challenges for humanity. Lifespan incline of industrial nation's inhabitants becomes one of the major burdens of a today's society health care. Estimations show that by 2050 we could expect the number of elderly persons, living in their own home but requiring assistance, to triple [1]. The challenge of providing health care to elders even increases in such a case. Many examples demonstrated that in certain situations senior citizens are not capable of autonomously seeking a help.

One of the most hazardous scenarios is fall [1, 2]. Approximately 33% (range: 15 to 44.9%) of community-dwelling USA's elders older than 65 years and up to 60% of nursing home residents fall each year [3]. Falls are the leading cause of death injuries and are one of the major causes for injury-related hospitalization among senior citizens [4]. Different researches were performed all over the globe about elders' falls. For instance, in Swedish elderly people residential care facilities, most common fall locations were found to be bedrooms and bathrooms; the most frequently injured body parts were the head and the hips [5].

In order to help the older ones and at the same time to increase efficiency of health care service many devices and monitoring systems were designed. Most of methods were based on wearable sensors that would detect non-casualties among monitored

© ICST Institute for Computer Sciences, Social Informatics and Telecommunications Engineering 2017
P. Perego et al. (Eds.): MobiHealth 2016, LNICST 192, pp. 383–391, 2017.
DOI: 10.1007/978-3-319-58877-3_48

person daily activities. Bourke and Lyons [6] worked on a threshold-based algorithm able to distinguish between activities of a daily living and actual falls using data measured by a mono-axial gyroscope.

Wu and Xue [7] analyzed the possibility of creating a portable pre-impact fall detector, a gadget that would be able to detect impending falls and then activate inflatable hip pad for preventing fall-related hip fracture. The instrumentation was based on commercially available sensors (triaxial accelerometers and triaxial angular rate sensors) attached to the subject.

Nevertheless, elders show a certain hostility to new technologies and there are cases when seniors refuse to wear instrumented clothes rather than the usual ones. In addition, the most common fall locations are bathroom and bedroom, where subjects are most of the time not wearing the detector. These considerations favor the development of falls detection systems relying on the monitoring signals coming from floor-mounted pickups rather than from wearable devices.

This work presents a feasibility study for the detection of elders' falls using the vibration measured by accelerometers fixed on the floor. The work is a part of the SMARTA project focused on the environmental monitoring for the active aging. There are different aspects that deserve investigation:

- the transmissibility of vibration in different kinds of residential floor have never been studied in the literature: given that the impact location will be in general at variable distances from the sensor positions, it is necessary to identify the vibration transmissibility in order to assess buildings dependent modifications of the signal;
- the force generated by people fall has been studied for frontal falls and rear falls of subjects [8–11]; however, results for elder people are expected to be very different, owing to their limited muscular force and to their reduced mental alertness; and
- In order to identify the fall without false alarms it is necessary to identify different classifiers capable of distinguishing between the falls of subjects, of objects and the common daily activities.

The paper is structured as follows: the proposed method is described in Sect. 2; Sect. 3 describes the preliminary tests. Experimental results are discussed in Sect. 4.

2 Materials and Method

The vibration generated by a fall is generally measured in a position different from that of the impact: consequently, different vibration pickups will measure different vibration time histories depending on their position. In addition, the force generated by the impact is unknown and there may be other events leading to vibration signals that might be similar to that deriving from people's fall. In this study, we have tried to address the first two issues, described in Sects. 2.1 and 2.2 respectively.

The proposed approach is summarized in Fig. 1: the vibration transmissibility through the different floors and the force generated from the different impacts are studied separately in order to be able to predict the vibration generated by different falls on the different floors. In other words, with the separate characterization of the force generated by an impact on an infinitely rigid floor and of the vibration transmissibility through the floor it will be possible to simulate a variety of combinations between impact locations, fall type and floor characteristics. These simulated signals will be used as training phase for the algorithms for the event detection, similarly to what was done in ref. [12].

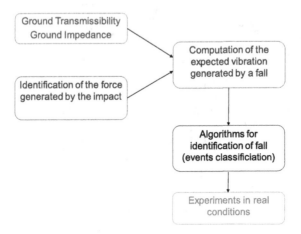

Fig. 1. Scheme of the proposed method.

2.1 Ground Transmissibility

The impact on the ground generates compressive and flexural waves that propagate through the floor from the impact position to the sensor(s) location. The subjects' fall can be identified by observing different features of the signal (in either time or frequency domain) and by using information about the impact location (to discard, for instance, shocks occurring in certain positions). The identification of signals' features requires the knowledge of the frequency response function (FRF) between the impact location and the measurement position while the different methods allowing the identification of the impact location on plates [12–14] require the knowledge of the wave speed in the plate.

The first step for the feasibility study is the identification of the floor vibration transmissibility in residential buildings. Since the vibration transmissibility depends on the mechanical and geometrical characteristics of the base and of the floor, experiments were performed to measure the vibration transmissibility in different conditions. For current purposes, four mono-axial accelerometers Bruel & Kjaer 4508 with nominal sensitivity of 10 mV/(m/s^2) measured the vibration at the positions indicated in Fig. 2; three accelerometers (indicated with the asterisk in the figure) were fixed, while one was moved close to the impact location. The vibration signals were sampled using a National Instruments NI 9234 data acquisition board. The sampling frequency was 2048 Hz in order to be able to evaluate the bandwidth of the stimuli, that were small jumps of a subject landing on the talons with straight knees. Preliminary tests showed that the stimulus' bandwidth was larger than the bandwidth of a subject falling forward on the hands or backwards on the buttocks. Under the hypothesis of linear behavior of the floor, any stimulus with a sufficient bandwidth can be successfully used to identify the vibration transmissibility, given that the transfer function of a linear system is independent from the stimulus.

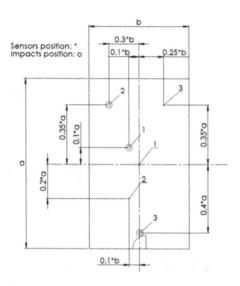

Fig. 2. Position of the accelerometers and of the impact in the transmissibility tests.

To date, the transmissibility has been measured in 30 different rooms, with surfaces between 2 and 50 m², with different pavement materials (wood, stones, tiles) and with different buildings (small residential buildings, condominiums). Tests are still ongoing, with the aim of having a comprehensive statistical description of the floor transmissibility. Experimental results have been summarized by averaging the vibration transmissibility of different buildings; the coherence function and the RMS of the vibration in "quiet" conditions have been evaluated as well.

2.2   Force Generated by Different Falls

There are two separate problems in the identification of the force of elder subjects' falls: the first is the creation of a force platform with a surface of at least 2 m² with a sufficient bandwidth and the second is the creation of a test protocol allowing the simulation of different kinds of falls.

The force platform has been realized using a sandwich honeycomb panel (2.5 × 1.25 m) supported by four piezoelectric load cells PCB 211B. The overall sandwich thickness is 100 mm, with sheets thickness of 1 mm and honeycomb thickness of 50 μm. The theoretical computations pointed out a first resonance frequency of approximately 85 Hz. The dynamic behavior of the force platform has been experimentally verified with an impact hammer and outlined that the frequency pass-band (±3 dB) is 40 Hz. The test protocol includes two groups of tests:

- fall simulations performed by 21 healthy subjects (18 males, 3 females, ages 23–32) falling forward with different arrest strategies: tests are performed on the force platform by healthy subjects starting from standing and sitting posture; the subjects' average weight was 73 kg (standard deviation 12 kg) and the average height was 182 cm (standard deviation of the sample 9 cm);
- fall simulation performed by a dummy: a Humanetics pedestrian dummy (Hybrid III 50th Percentile) is used to identify the force of forward, backwards and lateral falls, upon varying the upper limbs posture.

After the plate metrological calibration, preliminary tests were performed to verify the time histories and the spectral features of the vibration and force signals generated during the impact. A picture of the experimental setup is shown in the figure below.

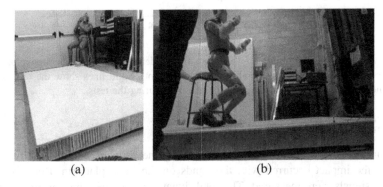

(a)   (b)

Fig. 3. Pictures of the force plate and of the Humanietics dummy.

3 Results

3.1 Ground Transmissibility

The average transmissibility measured in the first 30 tests is shown in Fig. 3a and the average coherence between the input and output positons (asterisks and circles in Fig. 2) is shown in Fig. 3b. Plots include the effect of the different rooms' sizes, of the floor mechanical characteristics and of the different positions of the impact/sensor.

Results show that FRF modulus is averagely lower than 1 in the band between 0 and 150 Hz. The average transmissibility is low below 15 Hz, but the minimum value (0.3) is not critical [15] and does not prevent the measurements in that region. The coherence is larger than 0.8 between 20 and 80 Hz.

The vibration transmissibility and the coherence function depend on the floor type and on the room size: the transmissibility measured on the wooden floors are averagely lower than that on the tiles and stones, especially at high frequencies. As expected, the first resonance frequency depends on the room size, while the effect of the furniture is small in comparison with the effects of floor type and room size (Fig. 4).

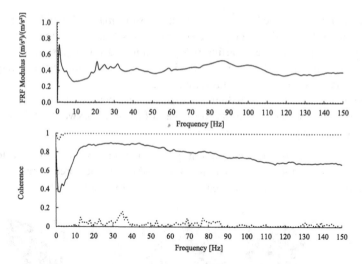

Fig. 4. Averaged transmissibility of the room that underwent to our tests (upper plot) and average coherence of the transmissibility tests (lower plot). Solid lines show the test average, dotted line indicate the maxima and minima measured during the tests.

3.2   Impact Force

Preliminary tests were performed by simulating the forward fall of healthy trained subjects; the impact occurred with the hands on the force platform. Both force and vibration signals were measured. The total dynamic force measured by the four load cells of the force platform (in the range between 1 and 40 Hz) is shown in Fig. 5. The plots show the dynamic forces due to the impact of a subject falling forward from standing position in two tests; although many other tests were performed, results cannot be reported here for sake of brevity.

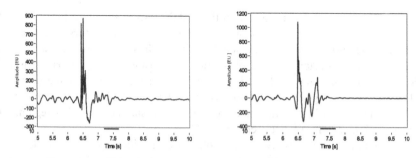

Fig. 5. Time histories of two front falls (Force [N] versus time, frequency range between 2 and 40 Hz)

The frequency content of the signals was at first analyzed using the short-time Fourier transform, but the technique did not allow separating the closely spaced impulses with a sufficient frequency resolution. The problem was overcome by using

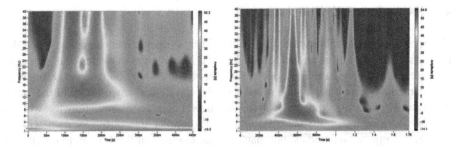

Fig. 6. Wavelet transform of the front fall (left) and back falls (right). Logarithmic scale.

the wavelet transform (4096 scales, time increment of 1 ms); results (Time histories of the left plots in Fig. 5.) are shown in Fig. 6.

In the forward fall, the two impulsive events deriving from the contact of the two hands have a similar frequency content, mostly concentrated at frequencies larger than 8 Hz. In the rear fall, the impulsive events deriving from the impact of the hands have noticeable energetic content above 20 Hz, while the buttocks absorb energy also at lower frequencies. In both front and rear falls, the force spectra include frequency components up to 40 Hz, thus allowing the choice of wide frequency ranges for the identification of falls starting from the floor vibration signals.

The forces generated by the fall of objects were different from those measured during the fall of subjects in terms of both force peak amplitude and event duration, as shown in Fig. 7, evidencing the possibility of discriminating the different events on the basis of the event magnitude and spectral characteristics [16].

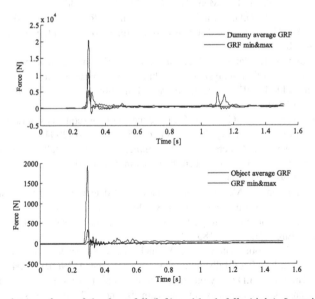

Fig. 7. Wavelet transform of the front fall (left) and back falls (right). Logarithmic scale.

4   Discussion and Conclusions

The results of the feasibility study presented in this paper are encouraging, since the frequency of the fall-generated excitation and the region in which the vibration transmissibility is high are overlapped. The vibration transmissibility is suggesting that in rectangular rooms it is possible to measure the vibration at any position of the room, independently on the impact location, so theoretically one accelerometer will be enough for measuring flexural vibrations. The optimal transducer location will be studied in forthcoming studies, but thanks to the low cost of the MEMS transducers it seems reasonable to put more than one sensor in different room locations. Preliminary analyses showed that the simultaneous use of more transducers allows identifying the impact location, thus allowing a more robust event identification.

The results of the fall-generated excitations presented in this paper were based on falls simulated by young and healthy people; the next steps of the research will be the characterization of the forces generated by falls performed with the instrumented pedestrian dummy and the comparison of different signal processing techniques for the identification and possibly classification of the different types of fall. The research will focus on the identification of the possible features for the signals' classification and on the numerical simulations meant to identify how the ground impedance modifies the force signal at different locations.

References

1. Tinetti, M.E., Speechley, M., Ginter, S.F.: Risk factors for falls among elderly persons living in the community. N. Engl. J. Med. **319**(26), 1701–1707 (1988)
2. Siracuse, J.J., Odell, D.D., Gondek, S.P., Odom, S.R., Kasper, E.M., Hauser, C.J., Moorman, D.W.: Health care and socioeconomic impact of falls in the elderly. Am. J. Surg. **203**(3), 335–338 (2012)
3. Najafi, B., Aminian, K., Paraschiv-Ionescu, A., Loew, F., Bula, C.J., Robert, P.: Ambulatory system for human motion analysis using a kinematic sensor: monitoring of daily physical activity in the elderly. IEEE Trans. Biomed. Eng. **50**(6), 711–723 (2003). doi:10.1109/TBME.2003.812189
4. Salvà, A., Bolíbar, I., Pera, G., Arias, C.: Incidence and consequences of falls among elderly people living in the community. Med. Clin. **122**(5), 172–176 (2004)
5. Sadigh, S., Reimers, A., Andersson, R., Laflamme, L.: Falls and fall-related injuries among the elderly: a survey of residential-care facilities in a Swedish municipality. J. Community Health **29**(2), 129–140 (2004)
6. Bourke, A.K., Lyons, G.M.: A threshold-based fall-detection algorithm using a bi-axial gyroscope sensor. Med. Eng. Phys. **30**(1), 84–90 (2008)
7. Wu, G.E., Xue, S.: Portable preimpact fall detector with inertial sensors. IEEE Trans. Neural Syst. Rehabil. Eng. **16**(2), 178–183 (2008)
8. Tan, J.S., Eng, J.J., Robinovitch, S.N., Warnick, B.: Wrist impact velocities are smaller in forward falls than backward falls from standing. J. Biomech. **39**(10), 1804–1811 (2006)
9. Troy, K.L., Grabiner, M.D.: Asymmetrical ground impact of the hands after a trip-induced fall: experimental kinematics and kinetics. Clin. Biomech. **22**(10), 1088–1095 (2007)

10. DeGoede, K.M., Ashton-Miller, J.A.: Biomechanical simulations of forward fall arrests: effects of upper extremity arrest strategy, gender and aging-related declines in muscle strength. J. Biomech. **36**(3), 413–420 (2003)
11. Kim, K.J., Ashton-Miller, J.A.: Biomechanics of fall arrest using the upper extremity: age differences. Clin. Biomech. **18**(4), 311–318 (2003)
12. Gaul, L., Hurlebaus, S.: Identification of the impact location on a plate using wavelets. Mech. Syst. Signal Process. **12**(6), 783–795 (1998)
13. Meo, M., Zumpano, G., Piggott, M., Marengo, G.: Impact identification on a sandwich plate from wave propagation responses. Compos. Struct. **71**(3–4), pp. 302–306, December 2005. ISSN 0263-8223
14. Choi, K., Chang, F.K.: Identification of impact force and location using distributed sensors. AIAA J. **34**(1), 136–142 (1996)
15. Tarabini, M., Saggin, B., Scaccabarozzi, D., Moschioni, G.: The potential of micro-electro-mechanical accelerometers in human vibration measurements. J. Sound Vib. **331**, 487–499 (2012)
16. Tarabini, M., Moschioni, G., Asensio, C., Bianchi, D., Saggin, B.: Unattended acoustic events classification at the vicinity of airports. Appl. Acoust. **84**, 91–98 (2014)

The Role of Design as Technology Enabler: A Personalized Integrated Predictive Diabetes Management System

Venere Ferraro$^{(\boxtimes)}$ and Venanzio Arquilla

Design Department, Politecnico di Milano, Via Durando 38/A, Milan, Italy
{venere.ferraro,venanzio.arquilla}@polimi.it

Abstract. According to the International Diabetes Federation, in Europe 59.8 million people have diabetes and the number will rise to 71.1 million adults by 2040. Research on new models of care organisation demonstrates that advanced technologies and ICT systems and services may have the potentiality to respond to the increasing burden of diabetes and the complexity of managing it, and, in doing so, to contribute to the sustainability of health and care systems. In this paper we propose the development of a new Personalized Integrated Predictive Diabetes Management System, based on a *design-driven approach* in contrast with the *technology–driven* one generally used in medical field. The Novel System here presented is called Dia_Friend, an integrated care models, oriented to the needs of the user and focused on the way *technology* is used and shaped for him, instead of on the mere instrumental use of it.

Keywords: Design-driven approach · Technology · User experience · Diabetes

1 Introduction

Diabetes mellitus represents a significant burden on individuals and healthcare systems in the European Union and beyond. In the world 415 million adults have diabetes and by 2040 this will rise to 642 million. Type 2 diabetes accounts for approximately 95% of diabetes cases in adult patients and about 20% of them are under insulin treatment.

The management of insulin therapy is indeed often problematic due to the several variables that affect glucose homeostasis and hence exogenous insulin requirement; the most important are food, physical activity, stress, and illness.

Therefore, patients under insulin treatment often suffer for severe glucose oscillations and hyperglycaemic or hypoglycaemic episodes. Hypoglycaemia, in particular, can disrupt many everyday activities and cause well-recognized neurological events such as coma and seizures.

Despite several emerging technologies have been developed, the management of diabetes is still anchored to traditional pathways. ICT services, for example, are not decision-supporting and not empowering the patients to the self-management of the disease. Indeed we want to develop a Novel System, *DIA_Friend,* thanks to which we are willing to re-design a smart health and care systems to develop integrated care models that are more closely oriented to the needs of patients and elderly:

© ICST Institute for Computer Sciences, Social Informatics and Telecommunications Engineering 2017
P. Perego et al. (Eds.): MobiHealth 2016, LNICST 192, pp. 392–397, 2017.
DOI: 10.1007/978-3-319-58877-3_49

multidisciplinary, well-coordinated, anchored in community and home care settings, and shifting from a reactive approach to a proactive and patient-centred care.

The main objective is to go beyond the instrumental aspects of product use and usability and focus on the *user experience* by shaping the technology in a desirable and meaningful way for the user reasoning on the metaphorical and cultural level of the smart system. Briefly our focus is to make the technologies really *enabling and meaningful* for the final user.

2 User Experience and User Oriented Approach

We live in a world pervaded by new advanced technologies that have been changing the way we live and experience the surrounded. New technologies also enable product innovation at different levels. Nevertheless, innovation doesn't lie just in the technological development and in its hard aspects but also in the meaningful use of it for the final user. In order to generate innovative "interconnected" systems a new perspective is needed: the shift from an instrument-oriented view of the technology towards a broader view that includes aspects like aesthetics, acceptance and comfort.

As Pine and Gilmore [1] argue, recently we have moved from a *service* economy to an *experience* economy. A user is more interested in living experiences than in performing actions and in the best way possible the most advanced technologies.

At this point a highlight on technology and experience meaning is needed.

Donald Schön (et al.) defined "extension of human capabilities" as a main goal of technology. Schön [2] Philosopher Peter-Paul Verbeek added the principle that technology is not something that humans work with, but something that is part of being human. Verbeek [3] Indeed, technology is not just a pole of the interaction but a mediator between human beings and the World [4].

Technologies change the way the *people behave* (interact). Different Technologies defines the behaviour of artefacts, environment and system [5].

New Technologies are uncovering new ways to interact with users so as to engage, entertain and inform them, coding new languages of communication and interaction.

Technology, has become deeply embedded in our ordinary everyday experiences that are improving the way our environment helps and entertains us.

The advancement in technology may not be enough for a product to succeed on the market [6] and perceived as useful for the final user. In the history of design, a first phase of products' digitalisation has seen the arising of "smart" concepts, which were technically feasible but not successful on the market. The field of smart home is full of these examples.

For example, although the rapidly emerging "smart homes" movement worldwide, a literature evaluating the validity, efficacy, practicality of smart homes technologies is comparatively sparse [7].

Moreover, the diffusion of home automation technologies is taking place at a slow pace. Such a slow diffusion could be reasonable due to technical reasons (communication standards, for example) or high cost, but to a lack of addressing users real needs. Indeed as different people have varying needs, the system must be tailored to each individual [8].

But while those concepts were not successful, today we are witnessing the development of industrial products with digital interfaces that enable plenty of new functions that users love to have [9].

One good example is in the ICT world: the way mobile phones evolved (compare to refrigerators) into products that offer way more functions than the just the primary one (that is to make phone calls). The success of such development is certainly based both on the technology, that enables the development of the new functions, and on the new experiences of interaction that smart phones elicit (for example the very simple way you can take and share pictures with other people).

This is the reason why it is worth exploring and understanding the relevant role of user experience in smart system.

The user experience of the product is considered the key battlefield to generate a real meaningful level of innovation (Holland 2011). The use of new technologies is indeed useless without paying attention to the user experience.

Designing an experience means to design not only its functional elements, but also the features that should be able to involve the user at a more emotional level.

And, speaking in particular of smart systems, we should focus on the user experience given by the man-product interaction. Indeed, a good experience will make the user have a *good feeling* about a system. In consequence, when a user has a good experience of interacting with a device he/she perceives it as a value of the product. In this perspective, the good experience is a value to seek.

Given these preliminary remarks, we – being design researchers - are interested to design a "meaningful experience".

User experience is at the core of the interaction design discipline that is about making connections *between people through a system*, not connecting to the system itself [10].

There are four approaches to Interaction Design: (i) User-centred design (UCD); (ii) Activity-centred design; (iii) Systems design; (iv) Genius design.

The user category to which Dia_Friend is referred, patient with Diabetes II, has specific needs and requires ad-hoc design solutions. Besides, user experience is dynamic as it is constantly modified over time due to changing usage circumstances and changes to individual systems as well as the wider usage context in which they can be found.

Consequently, authors, as designer researchers decided to put the emphasis on the *user-centred design* approach, in order to develop an innovative System focused not only on *function* and *performance*.

The philosophy behind user-centred design is that users know best. The people who will be using a system know what their needs, goals, and preferences are, and it is up to the designer to find out those things and design for them. Designers focus on what the user ultimately wants to accomplish. The designer then determines the tasks and means necessary to achieve those goals, but always with the users' needs and preferences in mind.

Since the experience is both a user need and an intangible value, we presume that the designers, rather than the engineers, are called to develop it.

As Buchanan states [11], engineers are used to design for the "necessary", while designers design for the "possible".

What we believe is that a real progress is reached when engineers and designers cooperate from the very beginning to the development of products that are not just technically feasible but also useful and enjoyable [12, 13]. In other words, innovation should be driven by design and technology together, not by technology alone.

3 Dia_Friend System

The DIA_Friend System is not an existing concept yet but it is based on theoretical and user studies. The research project was submitted for receiving founding from Horizon 2020 Call on May 2016 but unfortunately it did not succeed. Authors are trying other ways to get founding fro the project execution.

DIA_Friend (Personalized Integrated Predictive Diabetes Management System) main objective will be the development of a new therapeutic strategy aimed to reduce the acute and chronic clinical complications in patients affected by type 2 diabetes mellitus under insulin treatment.

The management of insulin therapy is often problematic due to the several variables that affect glucose homeostasis and hence exogenous insulin requirement; the most important are food, physical activity, stress, and illness. Therefore, patients under insulin treatment often suffer for severe glucose oscillations and hyperglycaemic or hypoglycaemic episodes. The novel system will be based on a decisional support system (DSS) where an algorithm for insulin management has been already validated at pre-clinical level. Dia_Friend will be framed into three major conceptual elements:

- A decisional algorithm. It elaborates three kinds of data: (i) personal data (food and physical activity), (ii) SMBG (self-monitoring of blood glucose) or continuous glucose monitoring (CGM) (iii) insulin treatment.
- Educational tools for favouring patient acceptance and compliance to the therapy with possible teleconsultation.
- A smart system interface to easily update and let the user understand how to manage the disease and hazardous situation.

It plans to provide: (i) the development of a cloud based network between operators and patients as the base for an integrated diabetes management system; (ii) a novel predictive algorithm integrated in a user friendly and personalized interface to support patient empowerment, self-care, adherence to care plans, decision making support and treatment when necessary (sensors, new glucometers, applications).

3.1 The Designer Perspective

Based on the theoretical consideration previously highlighted on *the use* and *the used technology* the solution will pay attention: to overcome barriers from technological, social and organizational points of view especially for the old people; to be personalized on the basis of patients' profiles; to be accepted by users both at social and organizational level. The key innovative elements of the proposed new therapeutic strategy are: (i) A cloud-based infrastructure designed to support the detection of personal physiological data, to simultaneously send them in a centralized repository for their elaboration. This includes new tele-monitoring solutions integrated with new advanced decisional support ICT based to improve the self-management of the therapy; (ii) A clinical DSS, based on the combination of the above reported data, able to generate, thanks to a decisional algorithm, a set of therapeutic options to be validated by the clinicians. It will elaborate these data in order to support through counselling and ultimately propose the right personalized dosage of insulin required by the metabolic conditions of the patient; (iii) A smart user interface to easily update and let the user understand how to manage the disease and the hazardous situations, in order to motivate the patient to accept the technology and solution provided (Fig. 1).

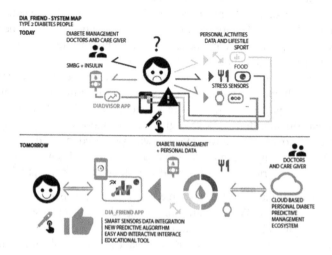

Fig. 1. System framework and novelty

Dia_Friend will mainly consist of a framework that will merge Existing Systems (in term of functions, technological infrastructure, algorithm and interaction) in order to figure out the effective personalized ad-hoc solution for the patient with Diabetes type 2 of the near future.

From Designer Researchers' point of view the lens is on the definition of the Requirements for the System. The requirements from the System Integration will be collected through UCD methods such as Personas and Stakeholders interviews. In our perspective, the Patient (user) is a subject and not an object of the assistance.

ICT based new educational pathways, applications; the system will be designed in order to promote self-management of the therapy. The patient becomes one of the actors involved in the management of diabetes. We focus on the role of psychology of the experience and behaviour modification in addition to education as a cornerstone for self-management.

4   Conclusions

Diabetes mellitus represents one of the major chronic diseases, and it is also a heavy healthcare financial burden. Despite the rapid diffusion of advanced technology the market does not offer solution aimed at support the patient during the management of diabetes disease in a "smart" way. This could be reasonable due to a lack of systems tailored on users real needs. Indeed, the management of diabetes is still anchored to traditional pathways.

In this paper we suggested a new approach and perspective that is to develop solutions focused on the user experience, not only on *function* and *performance*: to go beyond the instrumental aspects of product use and usability and focus on the *user experience* by shaping the technology in a desirable and meaningful way for the user reasoning on the metaphorical and cultural level of the smart system.

With the Novel System *DIA_Friend* we are willing to re-design a smart health and care system closely oriented to the needs of patients. We want to create new scenarios where products, interfaces and services interact smartly by putting the user at the centre, empathizing with him, understanding his needs and behaviours in order to improve his quality of daily life. The user-oriented approach is indeed useful and purposeful to make the technologies really *enabling and meaningful* for the final user.

References

1. Pine, B.J., Gilmore, J.H.: The Experience Economy. Harvard Business Press (2011)
2. Schön, D.: Technology and Change-The New Heraclitus. Delacorte Press, New York (1967)
3. Verbeek, P.-P.: [De daadkracht der dingen. English], What things do: philosophical reflections on technology, agency and design: translated by Robert P. Crease (2005). ISNN 0-271-02539-5
4. Bodker, S.: A human activity approach to user interfaces. Hum. Comput. Interact. **4**, 171–195 (1989)
5. Forlizzi, J., Battarbee, K.: Understanding experience in interactive systems. In: Proceedings of the 2004 Conference on Designing Interactive Systems (DIS 04): Processes, Practices, Methods, and Techniques, pp. 261–268. ACM, New York (2005)
6. Dertouzos, M.L.: The Unfinished Revolution. Human-Centered Computers and What They Can Do For Us. HarperCollins Publishers Inc., USA (2001)
7. Morris, M., Ozanne, E., Miller, K., Santamaria, N., Pearce, A., et al.: Smart technologies for older people: a systematic literature review of smart technologies that promote health and wellbeing of older people living at home. IBES, The University of Melbourne, Australia (2012)
8. Chan, M., Campo, E., Estève, D., Fourniols, J.Y.: Smart homes - current features and future perspectives. Maturitas **64**(2), 90–97 (2009)
9. Stephenson, W.D.: SmartStuff: an introduction to the Internet of Things (2012)
10. Buchanan, R.: Wicked problems in design thinking. Des. Iss. **8**(2), 5–21 (1992)
11. Saffer, D.: Designing for Interaction: Creating Innovative Applications and Devices, 2nd edn. New Riders, USA (2010)
12. Negroponte, N.: Being Digital. Alfred A. Knopf Inc., New York (1995)
13. Nielsen, J., Loranger, H.: Prioritizing Web Usability. New Riders, USA (2006)
14. Kaptelinin, V., Nardi, B.: Acting with Technology: Activity Theory and Interaction Design. The MIT Press, Cambridge (2006)

Detecting Elderly Behavior Shift via Smart Devices and Stigmergic Receptive Fields

Marco Avvenuti, Cinzia Bernardeschi, Mario G.C.A. Cimino$^{(\boxtimes)}$, Guglielmo Cola, Andrea Domenici, and Gigliola Vaglini

Department of Information Engineering, University of Pisa,
Largo L. Lazzarino, 1, 56122 Pisa, Italy
{m.avvenuti,c.bernardeschi,m.cimino,g.cola,
a.domenici,g.vaglini}@iet.unipi.it

Abstract. Smart devices are increasingly used for health monitoring. We present a novel connectionist architecture to detect elderly *behavior shift* from data gathered by wearable or ambient sensing technology. Behavior shift is a pattern used in many applications: it may indicate initial signs of disease or deviations in performance. In the proposed architecture, the input samples are aggregated by functional structures called *trails*. The trailing process is inspired by *stigmergy*, an insects' coordination mechanism, and is managed by computational units called *Stigmergic Receptive Fields* (SRFs), which provide a (dis-)similarity measure between sample streams. This paper presents the architectural view, and summarizes the achievements related to three application case studies, i.e., indoor mobility behavior, sleep behavior, and physical activity behavior.

Keywords: Elderly monitoring · Smart sensing · Stigmergy · Neural receptive field · User's behavior shift

1 Introduction and Motivation

Today there is a great availability of smart devices for health, ranging from general purpose ones (such as phones, watches, clothes, shoes, and socks) for measuring steps, heart rate, body motion, etc., to special medical devices for measuring blood glucose, blood pressure, oximeter, and so on. The term *smart* is commonly due to: miniaturization, physical integration with everyday life, capability of autonomous connection and sharing data through the Web.

However, smart applications should also include mechanisms to prevent cognitive overload. As a matter of fact, most users when equipped with interfaces displaying data or simple activities, like heart rate or pedometer, lose interest after a short period of time. Studies have shown that monitoring and noticing *behavioral events* is more persuasive than displaying sequences of values or labels, because it requires less cognitive work and less user's conscious attention [1].

In the literature, many systems have been developed to detect daily activities, such as feeding, dressing, sleeping, walking, watching TV, etc. as a basis to represent human behavior [2]. The detection of daily activities usually deploys different techniques,

© ICST Institute for Computer Sciences, Social Informatics and Telecommunications Engineering 2017
P. Perego et al. (Eds.): MobiHealth 2016, LNICST 192, pp. 398–405, 2017.
DOI: 10.1007/978-3-319-58877-3_50

including machine learning and probabilistic modeling, to deal with the inherent complex, user-dependent, time varying and incomplete nature of human-driven sensory data and behavioral logic. Actually, much work has to be done before such systems can be regularly managed. Another important problem of this approach is that domain modeling raises proprietary and privacy concerns, due to the direct access and processing of personal data sources and to the explicit modeling and tracking of personal behavior. Moreover, when standardized daily activities are used by health professionals to assess the functional status of people, some important requirements exist: the monitoring system should use a limited amount of states, be highly flexible, handle uncertainty, and allow a personalization of what to monitor and how to notice it.

To cope with the above issues, we present a novel approach, consisting in two paradigm shifts: a different monitoring approach and a novel connectionist architecture with efficient setting and configuration.

The monitoring approach is based on a general-purpose wearable device and minimally affecting the subject's everyday life [3]. The widespread adoption of wearable devices offers an unprecedented opportunity of continuous monitoring of users' health [4]. For example, the use of commonly available smartphones to detect abnormal and potentially dangerous behavior – like falls or deviation in gait pattern – has been extensively investigated in the literature [5, 6]. However, exploiting smartphones to monitor health has some limitations: (i) smartphones are not carried by their users for long periods during the day (e.g., the smartphone may be placed on a desk while being at home); (ii) users can carry the smartphones at different body positions or even in a shoulder bag, making data analysis more difficult and less trustworthy. In this context, a great enhancement could be represented by the adoption of wrist-worn devices, like smartwatches or smart bracelets. These devices can be worn continuously to enable deep analysis of mobility and sleep patterns. Moreover, the position and orientation of the device with respect to the user's body is known in advance. We remark that the approach focuses on detecting *user's behavior shift*, a pattern used here to indicate initial signs of disease [7]. Detection of explicit user activities and diagnosis of specific diseases are not within the scope of the approach.

The proposed architecture relies on advanced bio-inspired techniques to simplify the management effort. In the proposed architecture, the input samples are aggregated by functional structures called *trails*. The trailing process is inspired by *stigmergy* [2, 8], an insects' coordination mechanism, and is managed by computational units called *Stigmergic Receptive Fields* (SRFs), which provide a (dis-) similarity measure between sample streams. SRFs are organized into a multilayer system, and adapted to contextual behavior by means of the Differential Evolution (DE) algorithm [9]. Thus, the novelty of the undertaken study relates to the structure of a receptive field and the way in which such receptive fields are formed and adapted.

The concept of receptive field derives from a computational mechanism employed by biological information processing systems [10]. In our approach to digital information processing, it relates to an architectural style consisting of a collection of general purpose local models (archetypes) that detects a micro-behavior of the entire modeling domain. Since micro-behavior is not individual, a receptive field can be reused for a broad class of patients/users: the use of SRF is then proposed as a more general and effective way of designing micro-pattern detection. Moreover, SRF can be used in a multilayered architecture, thus providing further levels of processing so as to realize a macro analysis.

The paper is structured as follows. Section 2 focuses on the system architecture, including the smart devices adopted, the structure and topology of a multilayer architecture. In Sect. 3, three application case studies are presented. Finally, Sect. 4 summarizes conclusions and future work.

2   System Architecture

In our research different smartwatches and localization systems have been used, differing on accuracy, type of input data, battery duration, and so on. The research regarding sleep analysis was carried out using an *LG Watch R* smartwatch, which ensures battery duration higher than 8 h. The study on physical activity was based on a *Moto 360 Sport* smartwatch (Fig. 1), which provides better accuracy. Both models include an accelerometer, gyroscope, barometric altimeter, and optical hearth rate monitor (PPG), and can be combined with ambient sensors to achieve accurate indoor positioning of the user. An indoor positioning system used in the study of the mobility behavior is the *n-Core* localization system, which exploits a mobile unit worn by the user and a static ZigBee wireless network [2]. This system combines measures such as Receive Signal Strength and Link Quality Indicator with a set of locating techniques to track users' position in real time.

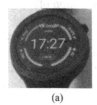   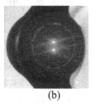

(a)   (b)

Fig. 1.   (a) Front side and (b) back side of the Moto 360 Sport smartwatch.

The processing system periodically takes samples of the user activity parameters as an input and releases a *mark* in a computer-simulated spatial environment, thus allowing the accumulation of marks as a *trail*. A mark is a trapezoid with three attributes: intensity (height), width, and position. The position corresponds to the value of the sample where the mark is left. Mark intensity proportionally decreases with the distance from the position. Mark intensity in the trail has a temporal decay (the percentage of intensity decreased after a step of time). Hence, an isolated mark after a certain time tends to disappear. The time that a mark takes to disappear is longer than the period taken by the system to release a new mark; thus, consecutive samples close to a specific value (clump) will superimpose, so increasing the trail intensity. The trail can then be considered as a short-term and a short-size action memory. Thanks to the width, the trail captures a coarse spatiotemporal structure in the domain space, which hides the micro-complexity and the micro-variability in data. Trails of different sample streams can be compared to provide a degree of similarity between a current micro-behavior, represented by a segment of the time series, and a reference (or archetype) micro-behavior, referring to a pure form time series which embodies a behavioral class. An example of class is *raising heartbeat*, which means that the heartbeat shows a sudden increase of level over time.

The similarity processing is managed by the SRF. Furthermore, an SRF is adaptive: its structural parameters, such as the mark attributes, are tuned by means of the DE algorithm. The use of SRFs is proposed as a more general and effective way of designing micro-pattern detection. Moreover, SRF can be used in a multilayered architecture, thus providing further levels of processing so as to realize a macro analysis. Figure 2 shows the structure of a single SRF. Here, the input is made of the data sample of the reference signal $\bar{d}(k)$, represented in gray color, together with the data samples of the current signal $d(k)$, which periodically feed the SRF. The first three processing modules of the SRF are exactly the same for the reference and the input segment. The modules of the reference signal are represented as gray shadow of the corresponding modules of the input segment.

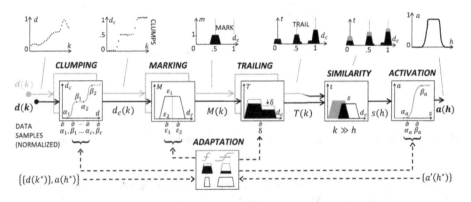

Fig. 2. Structure of a stigmergic receptive field.

A normalization of the continuous-valued samples is assumed. First, normalized data samples undergo the *clumping process*, which is a kind of soft discretization of the samples to a set of levels. Second, the *marking* process produces a *mark* corresponding to each data sample and represented as a trapezoidal form in figure. Third, the *trailing* process creates the *trail* structure exploiting the accumulation and the evaporation over time of the marks. Fourth, *similarity* compares the current and reference (or archetype) trails. Fifth, *activation* increases/decreases the rate of similarity. Here, the term "activation" is taken from neural sciences and it is related to the requirement that a signal must reach a certain level before a processing layer can fire to the next layer [11].

Each SRF should be properly parameterized to enable an effective samples aggregation and output activation. For example, short-life marks evaporate too fast, preventing aggregation and pattern reinforcement, whereas long-life marks cause early activation. The *adaptation* module uses the DE algorithm to adapt the parameters of the SRF with respect to the fitness, which is computed over a tuning set. In Fig. 2 the tuning set is denoted by asterisks: it is a sequence of *(input, desired output)* pairs, represented on the left. In a fitting solution, the desired and *actual output* values (represented on the right) are very close.

Figure 3(a) shows the topology of a *stigmergic perceptron*. In neurocomputing, a perceptron computes a single output value from multiple input values, by forming a linear combination of them, parameterized for achieving some desired mapping. Similarly, the stigmergic perceptron detects the similarity between many reference signals (or archetypes) and the current input samples by forming a linear combination of the most similar SRFs, parameterized for achieving some desired mapping [10].

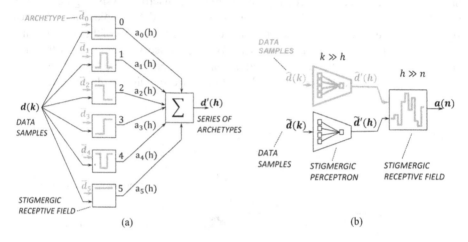

Fig. 3. (a) Topology of a stigmergic perceptron. (b) Topology of a multilayer architecture of SRF.

More specifically, Fig. 3(a) shows six SRFs, whose archetypes are mapped to the natural-valued interval [0, 5]. In the output layer, the average of such natural numbers weighted by the SRF activations is calculated, to provide a linear combination of neighboring archetypes in the real-valued interval [0,5]. Figure 3(b) shows the topology of a multilayer architecture of SRFs. In the first layer, each SRF is fed with the input data series, to provide the degree of similarity to each archetypal pattern. The activation of each SRF is then used to generate a higher level time series through the stigmergic perceptron. In the next layer, another SRF is used to provide the degree of similarity between two time series of archetypes, i.e., current and reference time series. Here, the adaptation is based on similarity samples provided by a human expert. This layer carries out a macro-level similarity between two time series.

An interesting property of the proposed approach is that the provided mapping is not explicitly modeled at design-time and then it is not directly interpretable. This offers a kind of information blurring of the human data, and can be enhanced to solve privacy issues. Indeed, stigmergy preserves privacy since it controls the level of perturbation of information, which means that information is scrambled to be partially hidden but up to preserve its utility. Stigmergy allows masking plain information by replacing it with a mark, as a surrogate keeping some piece of the original information. Furthermore, analog data provided by marker-based stigmergy allows measurements with continuously changing qualities, suitable for multi-valued classification.

3 Application Case Studies

This Section summarizes three application case studies: indoor mobility behavior, sleep behavior, and physical activity behavior.

The research on *indoor mobility behavior* aims to monitor elderly people living alone in their houses, by using a localization system [2]. The purpose is to face in a more proactive and preventive way age-related chronic diseases such as depression, cardiac insufficiency, arthritis, and so on. Indeed, disease situations initially lack noticeable symptoms and then do not cause emotional involvement that could activate decision-making, but gradual deviations of generic behavioral patterns such as mobility or vital parameters. The indoor position of the elderly is periodically estimated by a localization system, and taken as an input to the monitoring system. The similarity between the current and a reference track senses the variation of the current behavior situation with respect to what was judged a normal behavior. The normal behavior of the elderly is established in a long-term period of stable health conditions by a relative and a healthcare professional. The system has analyzed the data collected by a woman aged 90, affected by depression, who has been monitored for 24 days. The system was able to detect behavioral shift caused by depression symptoms, such as decreased appetite and withdrawal from socializing, increased total sleep time and nocturnal awakenings.

The research on *sleep behavior* aims to detect sleep deprivation [12, 13]. Chronic sleep deficit has been linked to long-term health issues such as diabetes, high blood pressure and heart disease, and recent studies suggest that it is the real cause of burnout. Recently developed smart-watches have been used for monitoring sleep patterns variation, because they can also feature sensors. Sensed data, i.e. heartbeat rate and wrist acceleration, are processed to produce a sleep stigmergic trail of the watch wearer. By comparing the current stigmergic trail to a trail produced in normal sleeping, it can be derived a sort of digital sleep diary, enabling the doctor to accurately diagnose any disorder. The system has analyzed the data collected by a woman aged 88, affected by arterial hypertension, who has worn a smartwatch during 20 nights. As a result, the system was able to detect behavioral shift caused by awakenings and an overall sleep quality.

The research on *physical activity behavior* is a part of a larger project whose purpose is to detect frailty in older adults [14]. Physical activity is important for healthy ageing. Better insight into objectively measured activity levels in older adults is needed, since most previous studies employed self-report. This is particularly important for the elderly population, as a healthier lifestyle would enable independent living to occur for a longer period of time. The effect of leading an increasing sedentary lifestyle is also not evident straightaway. Thus, an alert on a behavioral shift event is significant to the user. Data have been collected among 60 + , 70 + and 80 + years old subjects, measuring heartbeat rate, acceleration and pedometer in a variety of physical activity levels. The system generates an activity trail of the elderly, which can be compared with a reference trail to provide physical activity levels. As a result, it is able to detect behavioral shift caused by physical weakness and loss of strength.

The first experimentation of the proposed system was carried out in the indoor mobility behavior study. Subsequently, the system was improved with additional modules/features, and then experimented in the sleep behavior study. Recently, modules/features have been included for the study on physical activity behavior. The modules/features experimented in each application case study are shown in Table 1.

Table 1. Case studies and related modules/features experimented.

Module/Feature type	Application case study and related module/feature		
	Indoor mobility behavior	Sleep behavior	Physical activity behavior
Smart device	Localization system	Smartwatch	Smartwatch
Sampling rate	1 sample/5 min.	10 samples/s	10 samples/s
Input	- Indoor position	- Wrist acceleration - Heartbeat rate	- Wrist acceleration - Heartbeat rate - Pedometer
1D/2D Input	2D	1D	1D
Processing modules	- Marking - Trailing - Similarity - Activation	- Normalization - Clumping - Marking - Trailing - Similarity - Activation - Adaptation - Perceptron - Multilayer	- Normalization - Clumping - Marking - Trailing - Similarity - Activation - Adaptation - Perceptron - Multilayer - Multichannel
Output	Behavioral shift caused by depression	Behavioral shift caused by awakenings and sleep quality	Behavioral shift caused by physical weakness and loss of strength
Subject	Woman aged 90	Woman aged 88 Man aged 72	Men aged 60+, 70+, 80+
Observation period	24 days	20 nights	30 days

4 Conclusions and Future Work

This paper summarizes our research activity on monitoring *elderly behavior shift*. A novel approach based on stigmergic computing paradigm and smart devices is proposed. The challenges in the field are outlined, the novel architectural approach is illustrated and applied to three different application case studies. The proposed architecture has been developed and experimented, making possible the initial roll-out of the approach into real environments. Other pilot case studies are currently undertaken, to demonstrate that the system is effective in achieving the expected performance on a number of cases.

Acknowledgments. This research was supported in part by the PRA 2016 project entitled "Analysis of Sensory Data: from Traditional Sensors to Social Sensors", funded by the University of Pisa.

References

1. Hänsel, K., Wilde, N., Haddadi, H., et al.: Challenges with current wearable technology in monitoring health data and providing positive behavioural support. In: 5th EAI International Conference on Wireless Mobile Communication and Healthcare (MOBIHEALTH 2015), Brussels, Belgium, pp. 158–161 (2015)
2. Barsocchi, P., Cimino, M.G.C.A., Ferro, E., Lazzeri, A., Palumbo, F., Vaglini, G.: Monitoring elderly behavior via indoor position-based stigmergy. Pervasive Mobile Comput. **23**, 26–42 (2015). Elsevier Science
3. Boletsis, C., McCallum, S., Landmark, B.F.: The use of smartwatches for health monitoring in home-based dementia care. In: Zhou, J., Salvendy, G. (eds.) DUXU 2015. LNCS, vol. 9194, pp. 15–26. Springer, Cham (2015). doi:10.1007/978-3-319-20913-5_2
4. Abbate, S., Avvenuti, M., Light, J.: MIMS: a minimally invasive monitoring sensor platform. IEEE Sens. J. **12**(3), 677–684 (2012)
5. Abbate, S., Avvenuti, M., Bonatesta, F., Cola, G., Corsini, P., Vecchio, A.: A smartphone-based fall detection system. Pervasive Mobile Comput. **8**(6), 883–899 (2012)
6. Cola, G., Avvenuti, M., Vecchio, A., Yang, G.Z., Lo, B.: An on-node processing approach for anomaly detection in gait. IEEE Sens. J. **15**(11), 6640–6649 (2015)
7. Aztiria, A., Farhadi, G., Aghajan, H.: User behavior shift detection in ambient assisted living environments. JMIR Mhealth Uhealth **1**(1), e6 (2013)
8. Avvenuti, M., Cesarini, D., Cimino, M.G.C.A.: MARS, a multi-agent system for assessing rowers' coordination via motion-based stigmergy. Sensors **13**(9), 12218–12243 (2013). MDPI
9. Cimino, M.G.C.A., Lazzeri, A., Vaglini, G.: Improving the analysis of context-aware information via marker-based stigmergy and differential evolution. In: Rutkowski, L., Korytkowski, M., Scherer, R., Tadeusiewicz, R., Zadeh, L.A., Zurada, J.M. (eds.) ICAISC 2015. LNCS, vol. 9120, pp. 341–352. Springer, Cham (2015). doi: 10.1007/978-3-319-19369-4_31
10. Cimino, M.G.C.A., Pedrycz, W., Lazzerini, B., Marcelloni, F.: Using multilayer perceptrons as receptive fields in the design of neural networks. Neurocomputing **72**(10–12), 2536–2548 (2009). Elsevier Science
11. Cimino, M.G.C.A., Lazzeri, A., Vaglini, G.: Enabling swarm aggregation of position data via adaptive stigmergy: a case study in urban traffic flows. In: Proceedings of IEEE The Sixth International Conference on Information, Intelligence, Systems and Applications (IISA 2015), Greece, pp. 1–6 (2015)
12. Shinar, Z., Akselrod, S., Daga, Y., et al.: Autonomic changes during wakesleep transition: a heart rate variability based approach. Auton. Neurosci. **130**(12), 17–27 (2006)
13. Mendez, M.O., Matteucci, M., Castronovo, V., et al.: Sleep staging from heart rate variability: time- varying spectral features and hidden markov models. Int. J. Biomed. Eng. Technol. **3**(3/4), 246–263 (2010)
14. Jansen, F.M., Prins, R.G., Etman, A., et al.: Physical activity in non-frail and frail older adults. PLoS ONE **10**(4), e0123168 (2015)

A Pilot Study of a Wearable Navigation Device with Tactile Display for Elderly with Cognitive Impairment

Rosalam Che Me, Venere Ferraro[✉], and Alessandro Biamonti

Design Department, Politecnico di Milano, Via Durando 38/A, Milan, Italy
{rosalam.che,venere.ferraro,alessandro.biamonti}@polimi.it

Abstract. It is typical for the older adults with or without cognitive impairment to manifest sensory declines. This indirectly affects their sense of direction and wayfinding ability as oriented search is linked with sensory, mainly the visual. The deterioration of spatial navigation skill due to aging and cognitive decline is well recognized. We present the conceptual design of a wearable navigation device with tactile display and its prototype development, aimed to assist the navigation of individuals with cognitive impairment. The results of a pilot test conducted on individuals with dementia using the working prototype are also presented and discussed. The experiment intended to verify the positive outcomes of using the haptic modality for navigation and its wearability. Results suggest that the haptic stimulus is a helpful signal for wayfinding. From the user assessment however, some limitations are traceable due to the wearable design of the device. This is needed to be improved and emphasized in our future works.

Keywords: Wearability · Haptic-feedback · Navigation · Cognitive impairment · Pilot study

1   Introduction

With the increasing aging population, the number of elderly with cognitive impairment due to dementia is simultaneously increased [1]. In parallel, although age is not the main factor of dementia, yet, most of the reported cases reside among the elderly [2]. It is very common for the older adults to be linked with the memory loss, cognitive decline and sensory changes, as they grow older [3, 4].

For the elderly with cognitive impairments, one of the ways to maintain the normal social functioning is the mobility skill [5]. In fact, mobility keeps the performance of activity of daily living and at the same time reduces the dependency. Nevertheless, individuals with cognitive impairment, mainly dementia are typically diagnosed with the decline of spatial navigation skill, the process of determining and maintaining trajectory from one point to another [6].

The declines of mobility, wayfinding and spatial ability according to age and severity of cognitive impairment have been recognized [7, 8]. Moreover, older adults with dementia also manifest sensory declines, similar to senescence (biological aging). These issues worsen their spatial ability in general, because oriented search is relatively connected with sensory acuity, mainly the visual [9] and at times auditory.

© ICST Institute for Computer Sciences, Social Informatics and Telecommunications Engineering 2017
P. Perego et al. (Eds.): MobiHealth 2016, LNICST 192, pp. 406–414, 2017.
DOI: 10.1007/978-3-319-58877-3_51

Unfortunately, the most affected sensory for elderly with or without dementia are vision and hearing [10]. This initiates the idea of using alternative sensory/modality to assist their wayfinding. Thus, the paper aims to investigate how older adults with cognitive impairment mainly due to dementia perceive haptics a modality of navigation. A review on the selected existing studies is presented to highlight the potential of haptic/tactile applications for navigational purposes.

2 Related Works

Current navigational devices take advantage of the emerging technological applications, but the common methods of navigation are predominantly based on visual interactions and auditory support. While navigating in the actual environments, obliging to concentrate on the surrounding and visual display of the navigation device at the same time may be very distracting. In the case of dementia, one of the most important aspects to avoid during wayfinding is confusion [11]. Therefore, a possible alternative sensory that should be further explored for wayfinding purpose is the sense of touch.

Similar to vision and hearing, tactile perception is gradually diminished due to the age-related impairment of sensorimotor and cognitive abilities [12]. However, individuals with dementia maintained intact haptic priming, despite the weakened recognition performances [13]. Besides, although individuals with dementia have the difficulties to learn incipient things, the implicit recollection for haptically-explored objects is preserved in those in early stages [13].

There is a growing body of research at present on the use of haptic modality in a variety of applications, such as the system to sense the virtual objects, in surgical tasks, designing the human-computer interfaces and also for wayfinding/navigation purposes. As the focus of the study, the examples of haptic modality for navigation include: (i) a mobile navigational assistance with Microsoft Kinect and optical marker tracking to help the indoor navigation of individuals with visual impairments [11], (ii) a wearable navigation system using haptic directional display integrated with a vest [14], and (iii) a blind navigation system with a Kinect 3D sensor range camera and a vibrotactile helmet [15].

Nevertheless, like the abovementioned studies, the existing body of works often focuses on individuals with visual impairment or blind people, and not specifically for the persons with cognitive impairment. Closer to our goal, [16] investigate the applicability of tactile signals to assist the wayfinding of persons with dementia. They developed a wearable belt with vibrating motors and participants were asked to navigate in a series of routes with the assistance of the built-in vibrotactile signals. This study is a good example that highlights and proves the potentials of haptic stimuli to assist the wayfinding of individuals with cognitive impairments.

Furthermore, this modality as a form of signal provides a simple, yet a promising form of directional cues that allows users to concentrate on the surrounding with other senses (vision and hearing) during wayfinding [17]. Besides, the vibrotactile signals that created the haptic simulation are less disruptive as compared to the auditory instructions, which is a suitable substitute for continuous feedback.

Equally important, most of the navigational assistances described above are wearable devices. This is most probably because designing devices to be wearable improve the practicality of handling and operating. Also, the reason of the "wearable" choice is indeed, readable in the meaning of the word wearable: fully functional, self-powered, self-contained computer. It is worn on the body and provides access to information, and interaction with information, anywhere and at any time [18].

Wearable device refers to the electrical or mechanical systems, which are worn on the human body by means of incorporation into items of clothing, or as an additional apparatus, which is fixed, by straps or harnesses [19]. The advantage of making a device to be wearable is it blends between the technological applications with human body in a natural harmony. In next section, we present a conceptual design of a navigation device that employs the hybrid approaches between; (i) the advantage of haptic/tactile applications, and (ii) the device wearability. We posited based on the previous studies, that the use of haptic stimulus as a form of signal could be a good substitute to the current wayfinding modality for elderly with cognitive impairment.

3   Method

The apparatus for this pilot test is a prototype that integrates tactile displays, instead of the conventional graphic interface. Users are not required to read a map display and listen to speech instruction because the device uses haptic stimuli as the "input". Part from dynamic aspect, the device is designed to be wearable for our designated users since it may support the capabilities of the wearers while preserving personal privacy and functioning over a wide range of situations and contexts [20]. Other comfort issues to the wearers may occur if it is designed without considering their limitations [21].

Similarly important, simplified interface is crucial to avoid distraction or confusion. For this reason, our device provides the simplest possible information of navigational instructions, which is: go to the left or to the right. The prototype system consists of; (1) the input that made of the sensor, (2) the process, and (3) the output which is the tactile display. The prototype is created as two main parts: the tactile display and the other built-in system's hardware (placed in a hard case), as shown in Fig. 1. This is to allow the tactile display to be adjusted for different (body part) positions.

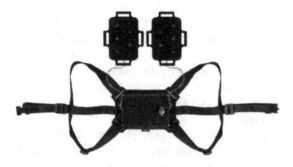

Fig. 1. The two main parts of the wearable navigation device prototype

We previously conducted a preliminary assessment using a survey, mainly for the design concept of the device. Based on the results, two most preferred positions for the tactile display are: (i) waist and (ii) shoulder. Thus, this prototype is adjustable according to body size and the tactile display can be adjusted for these two positions. We adopt the wearable feature of the conventional backpack and body harness for this purpose. As shown in Fig. 1, the hard case that contains the hardware is connected to the adjustable and buckled straps. The tactile display is made of multiple mini vibration motors embedded onto the fabric to create the haptic-feedback. The built-in haptic stimuli from the tactile display are intended as the directional cues/signals in the course of navigation

The assessment of the pilot test is divided into two main sections: (1) navigation test using the device prototype, and (2) a questionnaire for the subjective assessment of the device prototype. Therefore, two substantial decisions were primarily made before starting the experiment: (i) the selections of the participants, and (ii) the methods to test the device prototype.

The experiment was conducted with the cooperation of Fondazione Manuli, a dementia therapy center in Milan, Italy. The experiment started with the orientation or training phase to get the subjects familiarized with the device system and experimental procedures. Since the navigation test could be difficult for the elderly with dementia, we needed to identify the appropriate subjects. First, experimenters put on the wearable device onto the subjects' body and observe their reaction or acceptance. Afterward, only if the subjects reacted well to this wearable device, they will be then asked if they can feel and indicate which side (left/right) of the haptic signals on both waist and shoulder positions. Only the subjects who succeeded this orientation phase were allowed to proceed to the next phase (navigation test). For the test, two routes with same difficulty (same number of turns and distance) level were created, as shown below (Fig. 2).

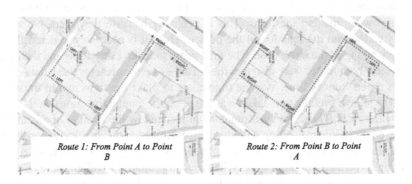

Route 1: From Point A to Point B   Route 2: From Point B to Point A

Fig. 2. The navigation routes with same difficultly level

The severities of cognitive impairment of the subjects are varied and based on their cognitive-based ratings of Mini Mental State Score (MMSE). The MMSE scores ranged from the minimum of 17 and maximum of 27, with average of 21. Those who passed the first phase are able to walk properly with no serious mobility issues. Subjects ranged in age from 74 to 81 years old, with the average age being 78.5. In total, ten subjects partaken in the first phase (three of them are male). From the total of ten, six of them succeeded the first phase (orientation) and recruited for second phase (navigation test). During the test, subjects were required to make the left/right turns at the junctions accordingly, whenever they sense the haptic stimuli from the device. Each subject travelled in both routes, but with the different positions of the tactile display. The test started with the first route (from point A to point B in Fig. 2), but the position of tactile display was randomly decided. If they started on shoulder in the first route, they continued with the waist positions for the second phase, and vice versa.

One important data to be recorded before starting the navigation test was the walking speed of each subject. The recorded walking speeds (m/s) are to be compared with the walking speed while navigating with the device. This justifies the effective walking (based on the walking speed or time taken) when and when not using the device during navigation. In the tests, haptic signals were initiated before subjects reached the junctions, and stopped after they were in the correct turns. We set the constant length of as 6 m for this haptic signal to be stimulated in every junction. For comparison, the subjects' walking speeds, which were recorded beforehand, were calculated as the travelled distance (of 6 m) divided with the time taken. During the navigational test of each subject, experimenters recorded the: (i) Decision making time in making the turns, (ii) Numbers of direction errors made, and (iii) time taken to finish the task. After each navigational test, subjective assessments were carried out.

4   Results

The recorded walking speeds of each subject were compared with the walking speed while navigating with the device. Subjects tended to make mistakes (especially in the first route) when making the turns. This is probably because they were not able to perfectly understand the function of the device. Thus, it is necessary to determine the effective walking of the navigation. The time taken to make every turns and the overall time to finish both routes were also recorded. Table 1 below presents these data of each subject's speed, control time, average time taken to make the turns and to finish both routes. The shown average time taken was based on the cumulative time taken for each turn of both routes. The score was somehow influenced by the number of mistakes (or direction errors) while navigating with the device. However, the justification on average time influences the overall time taken is not necessarily accurate. This is falsified when comparing these data in both routes. What we can primarily highlight here is, even if the subjects took less time to finish the routes as compared to the others, it does not mean they scored the highest effective walking while navigating with the device. This depends on their walking speeds and the hesitation before making the turns.

Table 1. The summary of recorded data for the navigation tests

Subjects	MMSE score	Walking speed (m/s)	Number of errors	Control time (s)	Average time taken to make the turns (s)	Overall time (s)
Route: 1						
6	20	0.79	3	7.56	18.85	776.43
8	17	0.68	3	8.86	23.55	956.43
4	21	0.78	3	7.74	17.62	733.81
9	20	0.51	1	11.08	16.34	682.27
3	27	1.08	–	5.53	6.24	337.82
10	–	0.73	2	8.15	16.56	602.05
Route: 2						
6	20	0.79	2	7.56	11.52	567.01
8	17	0.68	2	8.86	16.23	797.92
4	21	0.78	1	7.74	10.41	526.07
9	20	0.51	1	11.08	14.67	647.72
3	27	1.08	–	5.53	6.19	321.43
10	–	0.73	1	8.15	11.81	512.45

We compared the number of direction errors made by each subject for both routes. The comparison showed that the numbers of direction errors for all the subjects decreased when navigating in the second route. This is indeed an interesting indication, where it is possibly suggests that the participants have started to learn and understand how to navigate with the assistance of the device in the second route.

Subject 9 demonstrated the best navigational performance amongst others. It is mostly related to the fact that he has the highest score of MMSE. For the other participants, the MMSE score are varied from 17 to 21, which is way lower than subject 9's score. According to [22], comparing the MMSE score in terms of description and stage, (i) 26 to 30 could be normal, (ii) 25–20 is mild and in early stage, and (ii) 19–10 is moderate and middle stage. Hence, Subject 4, 6 and 9 have the similar range, which is in the mild condition and only Subject 8 is in the moderate conditions. Nevertheless, we cannot simply justify that subjects in early stage has better navigational performance with or without the device than those in middle stage. This is because Subject 6 who has the MMSE score of 20 did the same number of directional errors with subject 8 with the MMSE score of 17. But then again, the other participants (with mild condition) demonstrated average or moderate navigational performances. A subjective assessment based on user perception was carried out as well. Here after the Table 2 shows the results.

The subjective assessment proved that patients can appropriately sense the vibration and the most preferred position for the tactile display is the waist (4 out 6 subjects). 83.3% agreed that they were comfortable wearing the device as they rated 3 over 3. This is in contrast with subjects' perspective on the device's usefulness, where they mostly gave a lower score to Q3 and moderate to Q4. The average score for Q3 is 1.67 shows that they are not so keen to have and use the device. Meanwhile for Q4, 4 subjects

(66.7%) rated 2 over 3. The data from the last two questions may explain the preceded scores. Indeed, it shows that the user familiarization is a crucial.

Table 2. The Subjective Assessment Questions and the Scales given by subjects

Questions (Scale of 1 to 3)	Subjects and Scale					
	6	8	4	9	3	10
Q1	Do you properly sense the vibration?	3	3	2	2	3	3
Q2	Are you comfortable wearing the device	3	3	2	3	3	3
Q3	Would you like to have the device and use it?	2	2	1	2	1	2
Q4	Do you think the device is useful?	2	2	2	3	3	2
Q5	Do you need more time to learn to use it?	3	3	3	2	1	3
Q6	If you are given more time to use it, will you perform better?	2	3	3	3	3	3

5   Conclusions and Further Development

In this paper, we proposed a new wearable navigation device with tactile display and we developed its prototype systems. We used a working prototype to evaluate the possibilities for practical use by conducting the pilot test on the actual participants (i.e. elderly with dementia). The analysis of the test results proved the potentiality of haptic modality in supporting the target users' wayfinding, despite several noticeable weaknesses of the prototype that leads to the efficacy and practically issues. These positive outcomes from the pilot test lies mainly on the decreasing of (i) overall time taken and (ii) the numbers of errors, when comparing subjects' navigational performance in both routes accordingly. Nonetheless, a new intervention should be appropriately introduced to avoid the misconception and for the familiarization purpose [23]. The wearable form of assistive navigation device is totally new for our participants. Thus, the importance of proper training is proved when subjects demonstrated better navigational performance in the second route. It is supported by the analysis of subjective assessment where the subjects needed ample time to learn to use the device. The responds from the subjects also suggest that the physical appearance of the device needs some improvement since it caused the wearability issues. In our future works, we will develop an improved version of the prototype mainly from wearable point of view. Once the new prototype is developed, we will conduct a following test to the same population but with bigger samples and use the similar experimental procedures in this study. This further development is essential in shaping the wearable form of haptic-feedback technology, making it desirable, acceptable, and pleasurable for the final users.

References

1. Fratiglioni, L., Grut, M., Forsell, Y., Viitanen, M., Grafström, M., Holmén, K., et al.: Prevalence of Alzheimer's disease and other dementias in an elderly urban population: relationship with age, sex, and education. Neurology **41**, 1886–1892 (1991)

2. Lazarczyk, M.J., Hof, P.R., Bouras, C., Giannakopoulos, P.: Preclinical Alzheimer disease: identification of cases at risk among cognitively intact older individuals. BMC Med. **10**, 127 (2012)
3. Lin, F.R., Yaffe, K., Xia, J., Xue, Q.-L., Harris, T.B., Purchase-Helzner, E., et al.: Hearing loss and cognitive decline in older adults. JAMA Int. Med. **173**(4), 293–299 (2013)
4. Collie, A., Maruff, P., Shafiq-Antonacci, R., Smith, M., Hallup, M., Schofield, P.R., et al.: Memory decline in healthy older people: implications for identifying mild cognitive impairment. Neurology **56**(11), 1533–1538 (2001)
5. Whelan, M.: The elderly and mobility: by. Building (255), 118 (2006)
6. Lithfous, S., Dufour, A., Despres, O.: Spatial navigation in normal aging and the prodromal stage of Alzheimer's disease: insights from imaging and behavioral studies. Ageing Res. Rev. **12**(1), 201–213 (2013). http://www.ncbi.nlm.nih.gov/pubmed/22771718. Accessed 2 Jun 2014. Elsevier B.V
7. Monacelli, A.M., Cushman, L.A., Kavcic, V., Duffy, C.J.: Spatial disorientation in Alzheimer's disease: the remembrance of things passed. Neurology **61**(11), 1491–1497 (2003)
8. Cushman, L.A., Stein, K., Duffy, C.J.: Detecting navigational deficits in cognitive aging and Alzheimer disease using virtual reality. Neurology **71**, 888–895 (2008)
9. Golledge, R.G.: Wayfinding behavior: cognitive mapping and other spatial processes. J. Reg. Sci. 428 (1999)
10. Fozard, J.L., Gordon-Salant, S., Birren, J.E., Schaie, K.W.: Changes in vision and hearing with aging. In: Handbook of the Psychology of Aging, 5th edn., pp. 241–266 (2001). http://search.ebscohost.com/login.aspx?direct=true&db=psyh&AN=2001-18327-010&site=ehost-live
11. Zöllner, M., Huber, S., Jetter, H.-C., Reiterer, H.: NAVI – A proof-of-concept of a mobile navigational aid for visually impaired based on the microsoft kinect. In: Campos, P., Graham, N., Jorge, J., Nunes, N., Palanque, P., Winckler, M. (eds.) INTERACT 2011. LNCS, vol. 6949, pp. 584–587. Springer, Heidelberg (2011). doi:10.1007/978-3-642-23768-3_88
12. Dinse, H.R., Kleibel, N., Kalisch, T., Ragert, P., Wilimzig, C., Tegenthoff, M.: Tactile coactivation resets age-related decline of human tactile discrimination. Ann. Neurol. **60**(1), 88–94 (2006)
13. Ballesteros, S., Reales, J.M.: Intact haptic priming in normal aging and Alzheimer's disease: evidence for dissociable memory systems. Neuropsychologia **42**(8), 1063–1070 (2004)
14. Ertan, S., Lee, C., Willets, A., Tan, H., Pentland, A.: A wearable haptic navigation guidance system. In: Digest of Papers Second International Symposium on Wearable Computers (Cat No98EX215) (1998)
15. Mann, S., Huang, J., Janzen, R., Lo, R., Rampersad, V., Chen, A., et al.: Blind navigation with a wearable range camera and vibrotactile helmet. In: Proceedings of the 19th ACM International Conference on Multimedia - MM 2011, p. 1325 (2011)
16. Grierson, L.E.M., Zelek, J., Lam, I., Black, S.E., Carnahan, H.: Application of a tactile wayfinding device to facilitate navigation in persons with dementia. Assist. Technol. **23**, 108–115 (2011)
17. Heuten, W., Henze, N., Boll, S., Pielot, M.: Tactile wayfinder: a non-visual support system for wayfinding. In: Proceedings of the 5th Nordic Conference on Human-Computer Interaction: Building Bridges, pp. 172–181 (2008)
18. Mann, S.: Wearable computing: a first step toward personal imaging. Computer (Long Beach Calif) **30**(2), 25–32 (1997)
19. Farringdon, J., Moore, A.J., Tilbury, N., Church, J., Biemond, P.D.: Wearable sensor badge and sensor jacket for context awareness. In: Digest of Papers Third International Symposium on Wearable Computer, pp. 107–113 (1999)

20. Buttussi, F., Chittaro, L.: MOPET: a context-aware and user-adaptive wearable system for fitness training. Artif. Intell. Med. **42**(2), 153–163 (2008)
21. Mahoney, E.L., Mahoney, D.F.: Acceptance of wearable technology by people with Alzheimers disease: issues and accommodations. Am. J. Alzheimers Dis. Other Demen. **25**(6), 527–531 (2010)
22. Galea, M., Woodward, M.: Mini-mental state examination (MMSE). Aust. J. Physiother. **51**(3), 198 (2005)
23. Charuvastra, A., Marder, S.R.: Unconscious emotional reasoning and the therapeutic misconception. J. Med. Ethics **34**(3), 193–197 (2008)

Author Index

Abbondanza, Paolo   289
Abdullah, A.H.   65
Adorni, Fulvio   45
Ahmed, Mobyen Uddin   144
Alsalamah, Mashail   260, 269
Amici, Cinzia   310
Amin, Saad   260, 269
Andreeva, Elena   85
Andreoni, Giuseppe   53, 100, 187, 200, 375
Angelini, Lucia   138
Antonietti, Alberto   359
Argyros, Antonis A.   328
Arquilla, Venanzio   392
Ascolese, Antonio   53
Atkinson, Sarah   45
Avvenuti, Marco   217, 398

Bagot, Mathieu   79
Balaji, Advait   177
Barbieri, Massimo   200
Baroni, Giuseppe   375
Barrett-Baxendale, Mark   321
Barshan, Billur   225
Barua, Shaibal   144
Basteris, Angelo   297
Baths, Veeky   177
Battaglia, Edoardo   328
Begum, Shahina   144
Beigl, Michael   164
Bernardeschi, Cinzia   251, 398
Biamonti, Alessandro   406
Bianchi, Matteo   328
Bicchi, Antonio   328
Bocciolone, Marco   375, 383
Borboni, Alberto   310
Borodin, Alexander   85
Brazzoli, Elena   138
Buraschi, Riccardo   310
Burgess-Gallop, Ebony   297

Calabrò, Emanuele Maria   345
Calatroni, Alberto   207
Caon, Maurizio   38, 53

Carbonaro, Nicola   337
Carbone, Marina   345
Caroppo, Andrea   367
Carrara, Sandro   71
Carrino, Stefano   38, 53
Castelnuovo, Gianluca   195
Caulfield, Brian   151
Chan Kylar, Yuk Kai   29
Che Me, Rosalam   406
Chen, Hsinchun   233
Cimino, Mario G.C.A.   251, 398
Ciotti, Simone   328
Cola, Guglielmo   217, 398
Condon, Laura   45, 53
Conxa, Castell Abat   45
Correal, Darío   160
Corti, Andrea   302
Crespi, Chiara   45
Crovato, Diego   310
Curran, Kevin   151
Cutolo, Fabrizio   345

De Micheli, Giovanni   71
De Pietro, Giuseppe   278
Demarchi, Danilo   71
Dhingra, Piyush   177
Di Santo, Simona Gabriella   367
Domenici, Andrea   251, 398
Du, Wenjing   11

Eapen, Bell Raj   160
Esposito, Massimo   278
Exler, Anja   164

Facchinetti, Sara   53
Fedeli, Cristina   138
Ferrara, Marinella   187
Ferrari, Vincenzo   345
Ferrarin, Maurizio   375
Ferraro, Venere   392, 406
Ferrero, Renato   241
Fusca, Marcello   100

Galzio, Corrado   375
Gandolla, Marta   359
Giancola, Silvio   289, 302
Gobbo, Massimiliano   310
Gocanin, Filip   383
Gomez, Santiago Felipe   45
Götzinger, Maximilian   91
Guarneri, Maria Renata   187
Guckenberger, Matthias   207
Guidec, Frédéric   79

Hardegger, Michael   207
Hemmatpour, Masoud   241
Hickey, Luke   297

Ivanov, Kamen   11

Jantsch, Axel   91
Jesuthasan, Nithiya   367

Kadyrov, Samat   132
Karageorgos, Grigorios Marios   3
Kelly, Daniel   151
Khaled, Omar Abou   38
Klaas, Vanessa C.   207
Kropf, Johannes   132
Kuznetsova, Tatyana   85
Kwan, Kin Chung   29

Lang, Alexandra   45
Launay, Pascale   79
Lavalle, Eleonora   71
Leone, Alessandro   367
Li, Huihui   11
Liljeberg, Pasi   19, 91
Lim, T.H.   65
Lopomo, Nicola Francesco   310

Maereg, Andualem Tadesse   321
Makris, Alexandros   328
Malamateniou, Flora   125
Manopoulos, Christos   3
Martin, Anne   45
Marzorati, Mauro   367
Mauri, Giancarlo   195
Mazzola, Marco   53
McCloughan, Lucy   45
McKinstry, Brian   45
Megalooikonomou, Vasileios   225

Mei, Zhanyong   11
Meriggi, Paolo   138
Minutolo, Aniello   278
Mireia, Espallargues Carreras   45
Molteni, Franco   302, 359
Montagnani, Giovanni Ludovico   138
Montrucchio, Bartolomeo   241
Moretti, Sarah   367
Motto Ros, Paolo   71
Moutschen, Cedric   321
Mrakic-Sposta, Simona   367
Mugellini, Elena   38, 53

Nagar, Atulya Kumar   321
Nefti-Meziani, Samia   337
Negrini, Stefano   310
Nguyen Gia, Tuan   19
Nikita, Konstantina   3
Novoa, Mónica Paola   160
Ntanasis, Periklis   225

Oikonomidis, Iason   328
Olivieri, Ivana   138
Özdemir, Ahmet Turan   225

Pang, Wai-Man   29
Papakonstantinou, Despina   125
Pathinarupothi, Rahul Krishnan   168
Pedler, Ashley   297
Pedrocchi, Alessandra   359
Perego, Paolo   53, 375
Piazza, Pierpaolo   217
Pietrabissa, Giada   195
Pippa, Evangelia   225
Pollreisz, David   107
Porta, Mauro   100
Prentza, Andriana   125
Prinelli, Federica   45
Puigdomènech, Elisa   45

Rahmani, Amir M.   19, 91
Rangan, Ekanath   168
Rashid, Rajeeb   45
Rebaudengo, Maurizio   241
Reid, David   321
Rivolta, Massimo W.   375
Rizzo, Giovanna   375
Rodocanachi, Marina   138
Roedl, Lukas   132

Rossini, Mauro   359
Russo, Stefania   337

Sacco, Marco   367
Sáenz, Juan Pablo   160
Saggin, Bortolino   383
Sala, Remo   289, 302
Santoro, Eugenio   195
Sassi, Roberto   375
Scaccabarozzi, Diego   383
Scataglini, Sofia   100
Schankin, Andrea   164
Scurati, Diana   138
Secco, Emanuele Lindo   321
Serpelloni, Mauro   310
Sicurello, Ferancesco   195
Silvestro, Clara   310
Standoli, Carlo Emilio   187
Sterling, Michele   297
Stradolini, Francesca   71

TaheriNejad, Nima   107
Taherinejad, Nima   91
Tarabini, Marco   289, 375, 383
Taylor, Isobel   115
Tcarenko, Igor   19
Tenhunen, Hannu   19, 91

Thandayam, Sai Ruthvik   177
Theile, Gudrun   207
Themistocleous, Marinos   125
Tognetti, Alessandro   337
Tröster, Gerhard   207
Tsangaris, Sokrates   3
Tsoli, Aggeliki   328

Urschel, Matthias   164

Vaglini, Gigliola   251, 398
Valliappan, C.A.   177
Vassilacopoulos, George   125
Vecchio, Alessio   217
Velickovski, Filip   53
Vezzoli, Alessandra   367

Wang, Lei   11
Westerlund, Tomi   19
Wong, Man Wai   29

Ye, Qing   29
Yu, Shuo   233

Zangiacomi, Andrea   367
Zoppis, Italo   195